Get Through
Final FRCA: MCQs

Nawal Bahal BSc(Hons) MBBS FRCA
Specialty Registrar, Oxford Deanery

Mubeen Khan MBBS DA FCPS DNB FRCA
Specialty Registrar, London Deanery

Aliki Manoras BSc(Hons) MBBS FRCA
Specialty Registrar, Oxford Deanery

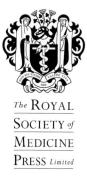

The ROYAL
SOCIETY *of*
MEDICINE
PRESS *Limited*

© 2010 Royal Society of Medicine Press Ltd

Published by the Royal Society of Medicine Press Ltd
1 Wimpole Street, London W1G 0AE, UK
Tel: +44 (0)20 7290 2921
Fax: +44 (0)20 7290 2929
Email: publishing@rsm.ac.uk
Website: www.rsmpress.co.uk

British Library Cataloguing in Publication Data
A catalogue record for this book is available from the British Library

ISBN: 978-1-85315-995-4

Distribution in Europe and Rest of the World:
Marston Book Services Ltd
PO Box 269
Abingdon
Oxon OX14 4YN, UK
Tel: +44 (0)1235 465500
Fax: +44 (0)1235 465555
Email: direct.order@marston.co.uk

Distribution in the USA and Canada:
Royal Society of Medicine Press Ltd
c/o BookMasters Inc
30 Amberwood Parkway
Ashland, OH 44805, USA
Tel: +1 800 247 6553/+1 800 266 5564
Fax: +1 419 281 6883
Email: order@bookmasters.com

Distribution in Australia and New Zealand:
Elsevier Australia
30–52 Smidmore Street
Marrickville, NSW 2204, Australia
Tel: +61 2 9517 8999
Fax: +61 2 9517 2249
Email: service@elsevier.com.au

Typeset by Techset Composition Limited, Salisbury, UK
Printed and bound in India by Replika Press Pvt. Ltd.

Contents

Preface   v
Introduction   vii
Guidelines and recommendations for the Final FRCA examination   ix

1. Practice Paper 1: Questions   1
   Answers   17
2. Practice Paper 2: Questions   62
   Answers   78
3. Practice Paper 3: Questions   121
   Answers   137
4. Practice Paper 4: Questions   180
   Answers   196
5. Practice Paper 5: Questions   240
   Answers   256

Relevant studies for the Final FRCA: Trials   304

Contents

Dedicated to Victoria Bahal, Dr Razina Khan and Carlton Morris. For all of our families, Marina and Bambos Manoras, Sabiha Khan and the late Dr Hamid Khan. In addition, the following doctors have had a profound impact on our careers thus far, and we remain indebted to them: Iram Ahmed, Wynne Davies, Beena Kamdar, Paul Kitchen, Satish Kulkarni, Sarah Leonard, Andrew Levison, Morton Lim, Don Miller, Maria Okoisor, Andrew Papanikitas, Chet Patel, Jairaj Rangasami, Stuart Robertson, Clare Stapleton, Peter Walker, Jonathan Watkiss, Julian Webb, Thusith Wickrama and David Wilkinson.

Finally, we are indebted to Hannah Wessely and Sarah Ogden at RSM Press for their hard work, co-operation, and above all, patience.

Preface

This book is a culmination of years of study and hard work, multiplied three times over. Each of the authors has passed all components of the Fellowship of the Royal College of Anaesthetists (FRCA) examination at their first sitting. It is this dedication and perseverance that we hope will be passed on to you through this publication. We believe that our questions are challenging, of the appropriate standard and, with our answers and references which act as a source of further reading, will serve to plug any gaps in your knowledge.

The Final FRCA exam is notoriously difficult, but, along with practice and commitment, we hope this book will help you on your way to successful completion of a major hurdle in your professional life.

NB, MK, AM

Introduction

Get Through Final FRCA: MCQs has been designed to encompass the syllabus of the final examination of the Fellowship of the Royal College of Anaesthetists (FRCA). This book contains five complete examinations, each comprising 90 multiple choice questions (MCQs). The subject breakdown has been carefully designed to match that of the actual examination, as set by the College, and is as follows:

- 40 Anaesthesia, Pain and Basic Sciences
- 20 Medicine and Surgery
- 20 Intensive Care Medicine
- 10 Clinical Measurement

We have included answers – concise or detailed as necessary, but often with up-to-date, relevant references for those who wish to explore the subject matter further. Each candidate will adapt their own techniques in answering MCQs, and although you might be able to argue the point, in the end it comes down to a 'True' or 'False' answer. To some, this is unjust, but is nevertheless the way of the College. In 2008, the College changed the structure of the examination to remove negative marking. As such, the tips we can provide for the day itself are:

- Read each stem very carefully (including units)
- Read each possible True/False stem against the original question before answering
- Be careful not to miss a question if transcribing answers onto the optical mark reader sheets
- 'Practice makes perfect'

At the time of writing, the Final FRCA examination is due to undergo change again with the introduction of 30 single best answer (SBA) questions. We felt that until the format of these questions is better understood, it would not be beneficial to the candidate for us to include these in this publication.

In addition to five complete papers, we have included two extra sections on landmark studies and guidelines relevant to the FRCA. While it was beyond the scope of this book to give detailed explanations or critical appraisal of the contents of these publications, we have included Internet links or complete references for those who wish to explore them further. We believe that these chapters will be useful not only for the written component of the examination but also, in time, for the Structured Oral Examinations (SOEs) or 'vivas'.

There are many ways up the mountain, but the view from the top is exactly the same. Good luck!

Guidelines and recommendations for the Final FRCA examination

Increasingly, care in anaesthesia and intensive care is guided by consensus or expert opinion. The FRCA examination expects the candidate to have current knowledge of important guidelines and recommendations. What follows is a brief synopsis of important guidelines from recent years (many of which have been the topic of conversation in the vivas). Bear in mind that these publications are updated regularly and the subject matter may be challenged by many anaesthetists. We recommend that this section be used as a guide for further reading.

Association of Anaesthetists of Great Britain and Ireland (AAGBI)
Website: www.aagbi.org

The AAGBI represents the interests of anaesthetists in the UK and Republic of Ireland. In addition to the promotion of research, the AAGBI publishes the following guidelines on a range of issues of concern to the anaesthetist:

Do Not Attempt Resuscitation (DNAR) Decisions in the Perioperative Period. 2009. Available at: www.aagbi.org/publications/guidelines/docs/dnar_09.pdf
Describes perioperative management of patients with 'do not resuscitate' decisions

Interhospital Transfer. 2009. Available at: www.aagbi.org/publications/guidelines/docs/interhospital09.pdf
Guidelines regarding preparation, equipment and documentation for transferring patients between hospitals

Pre-Hospital Anaesthesia. 2009. Available at: www.aagbi.org/publications/guidelines/docs/prehospital_glossy09.pdf
Guidelines for pre-hospital practitioners performing anaesthetic procedures outside the hospital setting

Suspected Anaphylactic Reactions Associated with Anaesthesia. 2009. Available at: www.aagbi.org/publications/guidelines/docs/anaphylaxis_2009.pdf
Updated since 2003; management plan, confirming significance of early diagnosis of anaphylaxis with early intravenous injection of adrenaline

Blood Transfusion and the Anaesthetist – Red Cell Transfusion. 2008. Available at: www.aagbi.org/publications/guidelines/docs/red_cell_08.pdf
Recommendations for transfusion of blood products and importance of documentation

Independent Practice. 2008. Available at: www.aagbi.org/publications/guidelines/docs/independent_practice_08.pdf
Guidelines regarding private practice for fully trained and qualified anaesthetists

Infection Control in Anaesthesia 2. 2008. Available at: www.aagbi.org/ publications/guidelines/docs/infection_control_08.pdf
Measures recommended for anaesthetists to reduce infection rates in the perioperative setting

Assistance for the Anaesthetist. 2007. Available at: www.aagbi.org/ publications/guidelines/docs/assistanceforanaesthetist07.pdf
Recommends changes involving training of anaesthetic assistants and ready availability of trained help when need arises

Management of a Malignant Hyperthermia Crisis. 2007. Available at: www.aagbi.org/publications/guidelines/docs/malignanthyp07amended.pdf
Anaesthetic management of this emergency

Management of Severe Local Anaesthetic Toxicity. 2007. Available at: www.aagbi.org/publications/guidelines/docs/latoxicity07.pdf
Anaesthetic management plan, including the use of Intralipid

Perioperative Management of the Morbidly Obese Patient. 2007. Available at: www.aagbi.org/publications/guidelines/docs/Obesity07.pdf
Guidelines for anaesthetic management; includes organizational and clinical problems associated with morbidly obese patients

Standards of Monitoring During Anaesthesia and Recovery, 4th edn. 2007. Available at: www.aagbi.org/publications/guidelines/docs/ standardsofmonitoring07.pdf
Specifications of monitoring required in theatre and recovery areas

Consent for Anaesthesia. 2006. Available at: www.aagbi.org/ publications/guidelines/docs/consent06.pdf
Ethical, professional and legal responsibilities of the anaesthetist regarding consent

Controlled Drugs in Perioperative Care. 2006. Available at: www. aagbi.org/publications/guidelines/docs/controlleddrugs06.pdf
Guidelines on storage and use of controlled drugs, in compliance with the various governing Acts

Transfer of Patients with Brain Injury. 2006. Available at: www.aagbi. org/publications/guidelines/docs/braininjury.pdf
Recommendations for improving the quality of transfer and outcome of head-injured patients

Anaesthesia Team. 2005. Available at: www.aagbi.org/publications/ guidelines/docs/anaesthesiateam05.pdf
Considers the functions and training of individual members of the anaesthetic theatre team, with special reference to 'Anaesthetic Theatre Practitioners'

Day Surgery 2. 2005. Available at: www.aagbi.org/publications/ guidelines/docs/daysurgery05.pdf
Recommendations for perioperative care in day surgery anaesthesia

Jehovah's Witnesses, 2nd edn. 2005. Available at: www.aagbi.org/ publications/guidelines/docs/jehovah.pdf

Recommendations for perioperative management of this subgroup of patients

Obstetric Anaesthesia Services. 2005. Available at: www.aagbi.org/publications/guidelines/docs/obstetric05.pdf
Administrative recommendations for anaesthetic set-up in a delivery suite

Checking Anaesthetic Equipment 3. 2004. Available at: www.aagbi.org/publications/guidelines/docs/checking04.pdf
Guidelines for performing preoperative checks on anaesthetic machines and equipment and importance of documentation

Fatigue and Anaesthetist. 2004. Available at: www.aagbi.org/publications/guidelines/docs/fatigue04.pdf
Highlights the dangers of tiredness and recommends changes in work environment and schedules to prevent work-related fatigue

Good Practice in the Management of Continuous Epidural Analgesia in the Hospital Setting. 2004. Available at: www.aagbi.org/publications/guidelines/docs/epidanalg04.pdf
Recommendations for patient selection when performing continuous epidural blocks; also covers management and staffing requirements for setting up this service in hospitals

Syringe Labelling in Critical Care Area (Update). 2004. Available at: www.aagbi.org/publications/guidelines/docs/syringelabels(june)04.pdf
Safety measures for naming individual syringes and strengths of drugs in critical areas

Theatre Efficiency. 2003. Available at: www.aagbi.org/publications/guidelines/docs/theatreefficiency03.pdf
Guidelines regarding organization and administration within operating theatre suites

Immediate Post-anaesthetic Recovery. 2002. Available at: www.aagbi.org/publications/guidelines/docs/postanaes02.pdf
Recommendations for patients transferred to recovery areas following an anaesthetic procedure with or without surgery

MRI – Provision of Anaesthetic Services in Magnetic Resonance Units. 2002. Available at: www.aagbi.org/publications/guidelines/docs/mri02.pdf
Administrative recommendations for anaesthetic set-up in an MRI suite

Care of the Elderly. 2001. Available at: www.aagbi.org/publications/guidelines/docs/careelderly01.pdf
Guidelines on preoperative assessment and perioperative management of patients over the age of 80 years

Pre-operative Assessment – The Role of the Anaesthetist. 2001. Available at: www.aagbi.org/publications/guidelines/docs/preoperativeass01.pdf
Recommendations for examination and various investigations performed during the pre-anaesthetic assessment

Royal College of Anaesthetists (RCoA)
Website: www.rcoa.ac.uk

The RCoA runs an annual National Clinical Audit Project (NAP):

NAP 4: 4th National Audit Project (in progress). Available at: www.rcoa.ac.uk/index.asp?PageID=1089
Major complications of airway management

NAP 3: 3rd National Audit Project. 2009. Available at: www.rcoa.ac.uk/index.asp?PageID=717
Major complications of central neuraxial blocks

NAP 2: 2nd National Audit Project. 2003. Available at: www.rcoa.ac.uk/docs/AuditReportv16.pdf
Place of mortality and morbidity review meetings

NAP 1: 1st National Audit Project. 2003. Available at: www.rcoa.ac.uk/docs/AuditReportv16.pdf
Supervisory role of consultant anaesthetists

National Patient Safety Agency (NPSA)
Website: www.nrls.npsa.nhs.uk

The NPSA has a remit to lead and contribute to improved, safe patient care by informing, supporting and influencing organizations and people working in the health sector. It commissions CEMACH and NCEPOD (see below). Relevant NPSA Alerts include:

Throat Packs during Surgery. 2009. Available at: www.nrls.npsa.nhs.uk/resources/type/alerts/?entryid45=59853

WHO Surgical Safety Checklist. 2009. Available at: www.nrls.npsa.nhs.uk/resources/type/alerts/?entryid45=59860

Reducing Risk of Overdose with Midazolam Injection in Adults. 2008. Available at: www.nrls.npsa.nhs.uk/resources/type/alerts/?entryid45=59896&p=2

Clean Hands Save Lives. 2008. Available at: www.nrls.npsa.nhs.uk/resources/type/alerts/?entryid45=59848&p=2

Technical Patient Safety Solutions for Ventilator-Associated Pneumonia in Adults. 2008. Available at: www.nrls.npsa.nhs.uk/resources/type/alerts/?entryid45=59879&p=2

Infusions and Sampling from Arterial Lines. 2008. Available at: www.nrls.npsa.nhs.uk/resources/type/alerts/?entryid45=59891&p=2

Reducing Dosing Errors with Opioid Medicines. 2008. Available at: www.nrls.npsa.nhs.uk/resources/type/alerts/?entryid45=59888&p=2

Chest Drains: Risks Associated with the Insertion of Chest Drains. 2008. Available at: www.nrls.npsa.nhs.uk/resources/type/alerts/?entryid45=59887&p=2

Epidural Injections and Infusions. 2007. Available at: www.nrls.npsa.nhs.uk/resources/type/alerts/?entryid45=59807&p=3

Reducing the Risk of Hyponatraemia when Administering Intravenous Infusions to Children. 2007. Available at: www.nrls.npsa.nhs.uk/resources/type/alerts/?entryid45=59809&p=4

Right Patient, Right Blood: Advice for Safer Blood Transfusions. 2006. Available at: www.nrls.npsa.nhs.uk/resources/type/alerts/?entryid45=59805&p=4

High Dose Morphine and Diamorphine Injections. 2006. Available at: www.nrls.npsa.nhs.uk/resources/type/alerts/?entryid45=59803&p=5

Safer Patient Identification. 2005. Available at: www.nrls.npsa.nhs.uk/resources/type/alerts/?entryid45=59799&p=5

Reducing Harm caused by the Misplacement of Nasogastric Feeding Tubes. 2005. Available at: www.nrls.npsa.nhs.uk/resources/type/alerts/?entryid45=59794&p=5

Protecting People with Allergy Associated with Latex. 2005. Available at: www.nrls.npsa.nhs.uk/resources/type/alerts/?entryid45=59791&p=5

Improving Infusion Device Safety. 2004. Available at: www.nrls.npsa.nhs.uk/resources/type/alerts/?entryid45=59788&p=5

Potassium Solutions: Risks to Patients from Errors Occurring During Intravenous Administration. 2002. Available at: www.nrls.npsa.nhs.uk/resources/type/alerts/?entryid45=59882&p=6

The Confidential Enquiry into Maternal and Child Health (CEMACH)

Website: www.cmace.org.uk/getattachment/05f68346-816b-4560-b1b9-af24fb633170/Saving-Mothers'-Lives-2003-2005_ExecSumm.aspx

This is a triennial independent report formed in 2003 from the Confidential Enquiry into Stillbirths and Deaths in Infancy and the Confidential Enquiry into Maternal Deaths. The remit is to 'improve the health of mothers, babies and children by carrying out confidential enquiries on a nationwide basis and then widely disseminating their findings and recommendations.'

The National Confidential Enquiry into Patient Outcome and Death (NCEPOD)

Website: www.ncepod.org.uk

Formed in 1999, the remit of NCEPOD is to assist in maintaining and improving standards of medical and surgical care for the benefit of the public by reviewing the management of patients, by undertaking confidential surveys and research, and by maintaining and improving the quality of patient care and by publishing and generally making available results of such activities:

Acute Kidney Injury: Adding Insult to Injury. 2009. Available at: www.ncepod.org.uk/2009aki.htm
To assess if acute kidney injury in hospital was caused by clinical or organisational deficiencies

Systemic Anti-Cancer Therapy: for Better, for Worse? 2008. Available at: www.ncepod.org.uk/2008sact.htm
To assess if cancer-related mortality in hospital was due to toxicity of drugs, disease progression or an unrelated cause

Coronary Artery Bypass Grafts: The Heart of the Matter. 2008. Available at: www.ncepod.org.uk/2008cabg.htm
To assess if there was identifiable change in care processes that affect the outcome following a first-time bypass

Sickle: A Sickle Crisis? 2008. Available at: www.ncepod.org.uk/2008sc.htm
To review data regarding mortality from haemoglobinopathy in order to obtain baseline data and recommend changes in practice if appropriate

Trauma: Who Cares? 2007. Available at: www.ncepod.org.uk/2007t.htm
To assess the management of a trauma patient from site of incident to hospital admission

Emergency Admissions: A Journey in the Right Direction? 2007. Available at: www.ncepod.org.uk/2007ea.htm
To assess organizational and clinical aspects of emergency patient care and recommend changes

The Coroner's Autopsy: Do We Deserve Better? 2006. Available at: www.ncepod.org.uk/2006.htm
To examine the use of the coroner's report as a tool for educational purposes, answering questions regarding mortality and addressing queries from relatives of the deceased

Abdominal Aortic Aneurysm: A Service in Need of Surgery? 2005. Available at: www.ncepod.org.uk/2005aaa.htm
To assess perioperative diagnosis and management of abdominal aortic aneurysms particularly as emergency admissions

An Acute Problem? 2005. Available at: www.ncepod.org.uk/2005aap.htm
To assess critical services provided to severely ill patients admitted to hospital

Scoping our Practice. 2004. Available at: www.ncepod.org.uk/2004sop.htm
To assess and recommend changes for improving the practice of gastrointestinal endoscopies performed by medical, surgical and radiological teams

Who Operates When? II. 2003. Available at: www.ncepod.org.uk/2003wow.htm
The follow-up report of which operations should be performed as emergencies and which staff should be performing them

Functioning as a Team? 2002. Available at: www.ncepod.org.uk/2002fat.htm
To assess how individual members in a hospital function as a team and to improve weaknesses within the system; including documentation in detail

Changing the Way we Operate. 2001. Available at: www.ncepod.org.uk/2001cwo.htm
To keep up with changing trends and patient clinical presentations by members in a hospital performing multidisciplinary audits and updates of information systems

Then & Now. 2000. Available at: www.ncepod.org.uk/2000tan.htm
A randomized comparison of mortality in hospital of two selected periods, 10 years apart

Percutaneous Transluminal Coronary Angioplasty. 2000. Available at: www.ncepod.org.uk/2000ptca.htm
To assess the mortality associated with coronary angioplasty and recommend changes

Interventional Vascular Radiology and Interventional Neurovascular Radiology. 2000. Available at: www.ncepod.org.uk/2000ir.htm
To assess relevance and safety of various invasive radiological procedures performed

Extremes of Age. 1999. Available at: www.ncepod.org.uk/1999ea.htm
To assess and recommend changes in the clinical and organizational services provided to children and elderly patients

Perioperative Deaths: The 1996/7 Report of NCEPOD. Available at: www.ncepod.org.uk/1996_7.htm
To assess and recommend changes in mortality occurring for surgical related procedures in hospital

Perioperative Deaths: The 1995/6 Report of NCEPOD. Available at: www.ncepod.org.uk/1995_6.htm

National Institute for Health and Clinical Excellence (NICE)
Website: www.nice.org.uk

NICE is an independent organization that provides national guidance for promotion of good health and prevention and treatment of ill health. NICE produces guidance in three key areas:

- *Public health*
- *Health technologies*
- *Clinical practice*

Child Maltreatment: Guidance on When to Suspect Child Maltreatment. 2009. Available at: guidance.nice.org.uk/CG89

Ultrasound-guided Regional Nerve Block. 2009. Available at: guidance. nice.org.uk/IPG285

Ultrasound-Guided Catheterisation of the Epidural Space. 2008. Available at: guidance.nice.org.uk/IPG249

Sleep Apnoea: Continuous Positive Airway Pressure for the Treatment of Obstructive Sleep Apnoea/Hypopnoea Syndrome. 2008. Available at: guidance.nice.org.uk/TA139

Perioperative Hypothermia (Inadvertent): Management of Inadvertent Perioperative Hypothermia in Adults. 2008. Available at: guidance. nice.org.uk/CG65

Technical Patient Safety Solutions for Ventilator-associated Pneumonia in Adults. 2008. Available at: www.nice.org.uk/guidance/index.jsp? action=byID&o=12053

Pain (Chronic Neuropathic or Ischaemic): Spinal Cord Stimulation. 2008. Available at: guidance.nice.org.uk/TA159

Venous Thromboembolism: Reducing the Risk of Venous Thromboembolism (Deep Vein Thrombosis and Pulmonary Embolism) in Inpatients Undergoing Surgery. 2007. Available at: guidance.nice.org.uk/CG46

Acutely Ill Patients in Hospital. 2007. Available at: guidance.nice. org.uk/CG50

Head Injury: Triage, Assessment, Investigation and Early Management of Head Injury in Infants, Children and Adults. 2007. Available at: guidance.nice.org.uk/CG56

Obesity: The Prevention, Identification, Assessment and Management of Overweight and Obese Adults and Children. 2006. Available at: guidance.nice.org.uk/CG43

Endovascular Closure of Patent Ductus Arteriosus. 2004. Available at: guidance.nice.org.uk/IPG097

Intra-operative Blood Cell Salvage in Obstetrics. 2005. Available at: guidance.nice.org.uk/IPG144

Extracorporeal Membrane Oxygenation in Adults. 2004. Available at: guidance.nice.org.uk/IPG39

Off-pump Coronary Artery Bypass (OPCAB). 2004. Available at: guidance.nice.org.uk/IPG35

The Clinical Effectiveness and Cost Effectiveness of Electroconvulsive Therapy (ECT) for Depressive Illness, Schizophrenia, Catatonia and Mania. 2003. Available at: guidance.nice.org.uk/TA59

Infection Control, Prevention of Healthcare-associated Infection in Primary and Community Care. 2003. Available at: guidance.nice.org. uk/CG2

The Use of Routine Preoperative Tests for Elective Surgery. 2003. Available at: guidance.nice.org.uk/CG3

The Clinical Effectiveness and Cost Effectiveness of Ultrasonic Locating Devices for the Placement of Central Venous Lines. 2002. Available at: guidance.nice.org.uk/TA49

Rheumatoid Arthritis: The Management of Rheumatoid Arthritis in Adults. 2009. Available at: guidance.nice.org.uk/CG79

Prophylosis Against Infective Endocarditis. 2008. Available at: guidance. nice.org.uk/CG64

Cardiac Resynchronisation Therapy for the Treatment of Heart Failure. 2007. Available at: guidance.nice.org.uk/TA120

Diagnosis and Management of Type 1 Diabetes in Children, Young People and Adults. 2004. Available at: guidance.nice.org.uk/CG15

Surviving Sepsis Campaign
Website: www.survivingsepsis.org

This is an international collaboration between the European Society of Intensive Care Medicine, the International Sepsis Forum and the Society of Critical Care Medicine. Their remit is to improve the management, diagnosis and treatment of sepsis. They make detailed recommendations and grade their evidence base. The most recent update was in 2008.

The Intensive Care Society (ICS)
Website: www.ics.ac.uk

The ICS is the representative body in the UK for intensive care professionals. It is responsible for the production of guidelines and standards:

Standards and Recommendations for the Provision of Renal Replacement Therapy on Intensive Care Units in the United Kingdom. 2009. Available at: www.ics.ac.uk
Current options and best evidence available for the provision of renal replacement therapy in critically ill patients

Standards for the Management of Patients after Cardiac Arrest. 2008. Available at: www.ics.ac.uk
Comprehensive guide to the management of patients after cardiac arrest

British Consensus Guidelines on Intravenous Fluid Therapy for Adult Surgical Patients (GIFTASUP). 2008. Available at: www.ics.ac.uk

Venous Thromboprophylaxis in Critical Care. 2008. Available at: www.ics.ac.uk

Care of the Adult Patient with a Temporary Tracheostomy. 2008. Available at: www.ics.ac.uk

Organ and Tissue Donation. 2005. Available at: www.ics.ac.uk

Evaluation of Spinal Injuries in Unconscious Victims of Blunt Polytrauma; Guidance for Critical Care. 2005. Available at: www.ics.ac.uk
Provides recommendations for investigation and management of patients with potential spinal injuries whose consciousness is impaired either as a result of the primary injury or because of the requirement for sedation to facilitate other critical care interventions

Limitation of Treatment. 2003. Available at: www.ics.ac.uk
Guidelines for withdrawal of treatment from critically ill patients

The Process of Consent within the Intensive Care Unit. 2003. Available at: www.ics.ac.uk

Transport of the Critically Ill. 2002. Available at: www.ics.ac.uk

Sedation Guidelines. 2007. Available at: www.ics.ac.uk

Weaning Guidelines. 2007. Available at: www.ics.ac.uk

Association of Paediatric Anaesthetists of Great Britain and Ireland (APAGBI)
Website: www.apagbi.org.uk

Guidelines on the Prevention of Post-Operative Vomiting in Children. 2009. Available at: www.apagbi.org.uk/docs/Final%20APA%20POV %20Guidelines%20ASC%2002%2009%20compressed.pdf

Consensus Guidelines on Perioperative Fluid Management in Children. 2007. Available at: www.apagbi.org.uk/docs/Perioperative_Fluid_ Management_2007.pdf

Royal College of Surgeons of England (Faculty of Dental Surgery) (RCSENG)
Website: www.rcseng.ac.uk

General Anaesthesia in Paediatric Dentistry. 2008. Available at: www. rcseng.ac.uk/fds/clinical_guidelines/documents/Guideline%20for%20 the%20use%20of%20GA%20in%20Paediatric%20Dentistry%20May %202008%20Final.pdf

Scottish Intercollegiate Guidelines Network (SIGN)
Website: www.sign.ac.uk

Management of Chronic Heart Failure. 2007. Available at: www.sign.ac. uk/pdf/sign95.pdf

Safe Sedation of Children undergoing Diagnostic and Therapeutic Procedures. 2004. Available at: www.sign.ac.uk/pdf/qrg58.pdf

British Thoracic Society (BTS)
Website: www.brit-thoracic.org.uk

Guideline for Emergency Oxygen use in Adult Patients. 2008. Available at: www.brit-thoracic.org.uk/Portals/0/Clinical%20Information/ Emergency%20Oxygen/Emergency%20oxygen%20guideline/THX-63-Suppl_6.pdf

Management of Asthma. 2008. Available at: www.brit-thoracic.org.uk/ Portals/0/Clinical%20Information/Asthma/Guidelines/Asthma_ fullguideline_2009.pdf

Management of Community Acquired Pneumonia in Adults. 2004. Available at: www.brit-thoracic.org.uk/Portals/0/Clinical%20Information/ Pneumonia/Guidelines/MACAPrevisedApr04.pdf

Management of Suspected Acute Pulmonary Embolus. 2003. Available at: www.brit-thoracic.org.uk/Portals/0/Clinical%20Information/ Pulmonary%20Embolism/Guidelines/PulmonaryEmbolismJUN03.pdf

American College of Cardiology (ACC)
Website: www.acc.org

American Heart Association (AHA)
Website: www.americanheart.org

ACCF/AHA Guidelines for the Diagnosis and Management of Heart Failure in Adults. *J Am Coll Cardiol* 2009; **53**: 1343–82 and *Circulation* 2009; **119**: 1977–2016. Available at: content.onlinejacc.org/cgi/reprint/53/15/1343.pdf and at: circ.ahajournals.org/cgi/reprint/CIRCULATIONAHA.109.192064

ACC/AHA 2007 Guidelines on Perioperative Cardiovascular Evaluation and Care for Noncardiac Surgery. *J Am Coll Cardiol* 2007: **50**: 159–202 and *Circulation* 2007; **116**: 1971–96. Available at: content.onlinejacc.org/cgi/content/full/j.jacc.2007.09.003 and at: circ.ahajournals.org/cgi/reprint/CIRCULATIONAHA.107.185699

ACC/AHA/ASE 2003 Guideline Update for the Clinical Application of Echocardiography. Available at: www.acc.org/qualityandscience/clinical/guidelines/echo/index_clean.pdf

Other relevant guidelines

British Committee for Standards in Haematology. Insertion and management of central venous access devices in adults. *Int J Lab Hem* 2007; **29**: 261–78. Available at: www.bcshguidelines.com/pdf/cv_management_guidelines.pdf

European Respiratory Society. Weaning from mechanical ventilation. *Eur Resp J* 2007; **29**: 1033–56. Available at: www.ers-education.org/media/2007/pdf/44001.pdf

Royal College of Obstetricians and Gynaecologists. *Management of Severe Pre-Eclampsia and Eclampsia*. London: RCOG, 2006. Available at: www.rcog.org.uk/womens-health/clinical-guidance/management-severe-pre-eclampsiaeclampsia-green-top-10a

UK Working Party on Acute Pancreatitis. UK guidelines for the management of acute pancreatitis. *Gut* 2005; **54**: 1–9

Royal College of Physicians. *Latex Allergy: Occupational Aspects of Management*. London: RCP, 2008. Available at: www.rcplondon.ac.uk/pubs/contents/f0ba0178-f790-48e8-a764-b319357f974a.pdf

1. Practice Paper 1: Questions

1. 48 hours following a blast injury, a patient becomes anuric; acute tubular necrosis (ATN) is likely if:
   a. Urinary sodium is <20 mmol/day
   b. Urine osmolality is <300 mOsm/kg
   c. Fractional excretion of sodium is <1%
   d. Urine : plasma creatinine ratio is <10
   e. Hyaline casts are present in the urine

2. A reduction in cardiac output is expected after administration of the following:
   a. Histamine
   b. Adenosine
   c. Inhaled nitric oxide
   d. Amiodarone
   e. Dantrolene

3. Drugs with a large apparent volume of distribution V_D include:
   a. Amiodarone
   b. Aspirin
   c. Digoxin
   d. Remifentanil
   e. Warfarin

4. Following intra-arterial injection of thiopentone, the following is appropriate:
   a. Stellate ganglion blockade
   b. Intra-arterial injection of procaine
   c. Intra-arterial administration of papaverine
   d. Interscalene blockade
   e. Intra-arterial heparin

5. Features of hypocalcaemia include:
   a. Prolonged QT interval on ECG
   b. J-waves on ECG
   c. Stridor
   d. Convulsions
   e. Cullen's sign

6. Risk factors for the development of uterine atony include:
   a. Oxytocin-augmented labour
   b. Precipitous labour
   c. Magnesium sulphate administration
   d. Chorioamnionitis
   e. Dantrolene administration

7. A patient presents for free flap surgery to undergo resection of a head and neck malignancy; intraoperative management priorities include:
   a. Maintenance of haematocrit $>40-50\%$
   b. Maintenance of a hyperdynamic circulation
   c. Hypothermia to reduce vasodilatation and blood loss
   d. CVP values $3-5$ cmH$_2$O above baseline unless contraindicated
   e. Avoidance of systemic vasodilators

8. When treating patients of Jehovah's Witness faith:
   a. Advanced directives must be respected
   b. They will not accept blood products
   c. Children can be given blood products in an emergency
   d. In an emergency, one is obliged to care for patients in accordance with their wishes
   e. Anaesthetists can refuse to work with the patient

9. Double-lumen endobronchial tubes incorporating a carinal hook include:
   a. Robertshaw
   b. Carlens
   c. Bryce-Smith
   d. Bryce-Smith–Salt
   e. White

10. The following diseases are notifiable in the UK:
    a. *Haemophilus influenzae* type B
    b. Viral meningitis
    c. Leptospirosis
    d. Tetanus
    e. Chickenpox

11. Cardioplegia:
    a. Crystalloid solutions should be calcium-free
    b. Is administered retrograde via the aortic root
    c. Should be administered antegrade in patients with significant aortic valve incompetence
    d. Is always administered following aortic cross-clamping
    e. Is avoided in aortic cross-clamp fibrillation techniques for coronary artery bypass grafting

12. The Bohr equation:
    a. Is used to derive physiological dead space
    b. Describes a shift to the right of the oxyhaemoglobin dissociation curve
    c. Often ignores F_ICO_2
    d. Is expressed as $V_T = V_A - V_D$
    e. Calculates results as a fraction

13. Concerning the decontamination of medical equipment:
    a. Semi-critical items are those in contact with mucous membranes
    b. Glutaraldehyde is a high-level disinfectant
    c. Re-usable laryngeal mask airways can be sterilized using ethylene oxide
    d. Glutaraldehyde cannot be used to disinfect laryngeal mask airways
    e. High-level disinfection is required for critical items

14. Regarding the use of arterial tourniquets:
    a. The pneumatic cuff should have a width >20% of the diameter of the upper arm
    b. Expressive exsanguination is contraindicated in patients with a deep vein thrombosis
    c. Application is absolutely contraindicated in sickle cell trait
    d. Larger-diameter nerve fibres are most susceptible to pressure injury
    e. Application of bilateral thigh tourniquets adds 15% to circulating volume

15. Pneumoperitoneum results in decreased:
    a. Functional residual capacity (FRC)
    b. Pa_{CO_2}
    c. Systemic vascular resistance (SVR)
    d. Cerebral blood flow
    e. Cardiac output

16. Breathing 100% oxygen for 24 hours leads to:
    a. Peripheral vasodilatation
    b. Convulsions
    c. Tunnel vision
    d. A reduction in lung compliance
    e. A reduction in vital capacity

17. A patient due for an hour-long inter-hospital transfer is ventilated with 100% oxygen, using an Oxylog 3000 portable ventilator, and has a minute ventilation (MV) of 6 L/min; the following statements are correct:
    a. A size D oxygen cylinder will meet the patient's absolute minimum oxygen requirement for the journey
    b. A size E cylinder will provide exactly double the patient's absolute minimum oxygen requirement for the journey
    c. This ventilator contains a Venturi device
    d. Cycling in this ventilator is powered electrically
    e. Inspiratory flow in this ventilator is powered electrically

18. **Benefits of central neuraxial blockade (CNB) include:**
    a. Reduction in deep vein thrombosis (DVT) following hip fracture surgery
    b. Reduced mortality following thoracoabdominal surgery
    c. Less blood loss during caesarean section
    d. Decreased rates of operative delivery in parturients
    e. Improved neonatal condition after caesarean section

19. **Concerning benzodiazepines:**
    a. Conductance of chloride ions at $GABA_B$ receptors is increased
    b. Midazolam has active metabolites
    c. Lorazepam exhibits tautomerism
    d. They provide retrograde amnesia
    e. Diazepam has a low hepatic extraction ratio

20. **A man undergoing transurethral resection of the prostate (TURP) under spinal anaesthesia becomes confused and agitated; immediate management includes the following:**
    a. Intravenous administration of 40 mg furosemide
    b. Intravenous administration of 100 mL 20% mannitol
    c. Conversion to general anaesthesia
    d. Administration of 100% oxygen and check arterial blood gases
    e. Stop surgery and give intravenous fluid therapy

21. **The Eastern Association for the Surgery of Trauma (EAST) clinical criteria for clearing cervical injuries include:**
    a. Full range of active neck movements
    b. Lateral neck X-ray to include all cervical vertebrae
    c. No history of significant distracting injuries
    d. GCS of 15
    e. CT scan of head and neck using 1 mm slice thickness

22. **Carboprost:**
    a. Is prostaglandin E_1
    b. Is first-line drug treatment for postpartum haemorrhage
    c. Total dose should not exceed 2 mg
    d. Commonly causes diarrhoea and vomiting
    e. Is contraindicated in asthma

23. **A primigravida is undergoing elective caesarean section under spinal anaesthesia; indications of a high spinal block include the following:**
    a. Bronchospasm
    b. Difficulty breathing with maintained cough reflex
    c. Nasal congestion
    d. Fetal bradycardia
    e. Horner's syndrome

24. **Recovery discharge criteria following day-case surgery include:**
    a. Use of the Modified Aldrete Score
    b. Core temperature $\geq 35°C$
    c. Oral fluid intake
    d. Ambulation
    e. Blood pressure within 20 mmHg of preoperative levels

25. **Breakdown products of codeine include:**
    a. Codeine-6-glucuronide
    b. Morphine
    c. Codeine-3,6-glucuronide
    d. Norcodeine
    e. Acetic acid

26. **Concerning intra-abdominal pressure (IAP):**
    a. Normal values are up to 5 mmHg
    b. Intra-abdominal hypertension is defined as abdominal perfusion pressure ≤ 60 mmHg
    c. Fluid administration can cause secondary abdominal compartment syndrome
    d. The reference standard for intermittent measurement is via the bladder with an instillation volume of 25 mL of sterile saline
    e. The femoral vein can be used to provide accurate measurements

27. **The vacuum-insulated evaporator (VIE):**
    a. Utilizes liquid nitrogen to store oxygen below its critical temperature
    b. Stores liquid oxygen below its boiling point
    c. Stores oxygen at a pressure of 5–10 bar
    d. Contains a safety valve that actuates at 17 bar
    e. Contains a Bourdon pressure gauge that indicates the oxygen content of the vessel in kPa

28. **Magnesium:**
    a. Is the second most abundant intracellular cation
    b. Can be described as the physiological antagonist of sodium
    c. Causes coronary artery constriction
    d. Enhances coagulation, making it safe in eclampsia
    e. Has normal plasma concentrations of 0.5–0.7 mmol/L

29. *Legionella pneumophila:*
    a. Should be tested for in all patients admitted for community-acquired pneumonia
    b. Is not associated with a history of travel
    c. Is most commonly seen in elderly patients
    d. Is a Gram-positive bacillus
    e. Is sensitive to macrolides

30. **In rhabdomyolysis:**
    a. Plasma creatine kinase levels are the most sensitive diagnostic test
    b. Statin therapy is a cause
    c. Intravenous infusion of bicarbonate is indicated
    d. Mannitol is contraindicated
    e. Myoglobin-induced renal failure has a poor prognosis

31. **Damping in a measurement system:**
    a. Is the progressive diminution of frequency of oscillations in a resonant system
    b. Causes a phase shift if excessive
    c. Causes overshoot when over-damped
    d. Is 'optimal' when damping factor = 1.0
    e. Produces no overshoot when 'optimal'

32. **Causes of hyperkalaemia include:**
    a. Spironolactone
    b. Alkalosis
    c. Digitalis toxicity
    d. Thrombocytosis
    e. β-agonists

33. **Absolute indications for one-lung anaesthesia include:**
    a. Bronchopleural fistula
    b. Pneumonectomy
    c. Giant unilateral cyst in right lung
    d. Unilateral bronchopulmonary lavage
    e. Right upper lobectomy

34. **Gabapentin:**
    a. Can be administered intravenously in an emergency
    b. Acts at GABA receptors
    c. Is used both as an anticonvulsant and in the treatment of chronic pain
    d. Can induce ataxia and tremor
    e. Potentiates the analgesic effect of morphine

35. **A 75 kg patient develops pain while undergoing a hand procedure under regional anaesthesia following interscalene blockade with 40 mL 0.25% bupivacaine; the following management is appropriate:**
    a. Intravenous sedation with midazolam
    b. Top-up injection of local anaesthetic to the brachial plexus
    c. Conversion to general anaesthesia
    d. Intravenous fentanyl and consult with surgical team regarding duration
    e. Request the surgeon infiltrate 10 mL 0.5% bupivacaine to the surgical site

36. **Concerning the jugular venous pressure (JVP) waveform:**
    a. Kussmaul's sign is an increase in JVP with inspiration
    b. The *a* wave is reduced in atrial fibrillation
    c. Cannon waves are large *c* waves occurring in complete heart block
    d. When raised it is predictive of increased mortality in heart failure
    e. Friedreich's sign is characteristic of constrictive pericarditis

37. **Regarding the myocardial blood supply:**
    a. The right and left coronary arteries arise from the posterior and anterior sinuses of the ascending aorta respectively
    b. The right coronary artery supplies the sinoatrial and the atrio-ventricular node in the majority of people
    c. The right marginal branch anastomoses with the circumflex artery
    d. The endocardium has no direct blood supply
    e. 5% of the cardiac output is supplied to the heart at rest

38. **The Humphrey ADE system:**
    a. Is efficient for both spontaneous and controlled ventilation
    b. Consists of a lever, the position of which determines the nature of the breathing circuit
    c. Behaves as a Mapleson D system in the ventilator mode
    d. Exists as both parallel and co-axial systems
    e. Is appropriate for paediatric use

39. **Levosimendan:**
    a. Increases intracellular calcium concentration
    b. Has no active metabolites
    c. Stabilizes the complex between calcium and troponin C
    d. Is an inodilator
    e. Can be used during active myocardial ischaemia

40. **The diaphragmatic foramina transmit the following structures:**
    a. Inferior vena cava at T8
    b. Aorta at T10
    c. Right phrenic nerve at T10
    d. Azygos vein at T12
    e. Vagus nerve at T8

41. **Causes of a lack of train-of-four (TOF) response when using nerve stimulators to monitor depth of non-depolarizing neuromuscular blockade include:**
    a. Cholinesterase genotype Ea:Ea
    b. Diabetes
    c. Myasthenia gravis
    d. Dry electrodes
    e. Aminoglycoside therapy

42. **The British Thoracic Society guidelines for severe asthma (2008) recommend:**
    a. Supply of high-flow oxygen as essential
    b. Intravenous aminophylline as a bolus of 5 mg/kg as essential
    c. Intravenous magnesium sulphate at a dose of 1.2–2 g
    d. Heliox based on level 1 evidence
    e. Intravenous co-amoxiclav as a single bolus

43. **Apnoea in the premature infant:**
    a. Is preceded by hyperventilation
    b. Occurs in >80% when severely premature
    c. Is pathological when lasting 15 s in the absence of other features
    d. Is most commonly central in origin
    e. Occurs frequently in the postoperative period

44. **When measuring cardiac output using pulse contour analysis (PiCCO):**
    a. Subjects treated for mania with lithium chloride are excluded
    b. The arterial waveform is obtained from the femoral, axillary or brachial arteries
    c. A central venous catheter is required for calibration
    d. Beat-to-beat cycles are averaged over a 60 s cycle to display a numerical value
    e. Arrhythmias affect readings

45. **A young man is extracted from a house fire and brought to A&E; the following features suggest carbon monoxide poisoning:**
    a. Bullous skin lesions
    b. Ataxia
    c. Arterial oxygen saturation of 85%
    d. Papilloedema
    e. Bright red retinal veins on fundoscopy

46. **Regarding anticholinergics:**
    a. Atropine is active as the D-isomer only
    b. Atropine has greater cardiac action than hyoscine
    c. Atropine has greater antisialagogue action than hyoscine
    d. Atropine and hyoscine are structural isomers
    e. Glycopyrrolate and hyoscine are quaternary amines

47. **Extravascular lung water (EVLW):**
    a. Is normally 4–7 mL/kg
    b. Utilizes a fibreoptic catheter for detection of indicators
    c. Has a linear thermodilution curve
    d. May be calculated by subtracting pulmonary blood volume from pulmonary thermal volume
    e. Is reduced effectively in capillary leak with the use of diuretics

48. The volatile anaesthetics listed have the correct colour-coding for key filling mechanisms:
    a. Halothane: red
    b. Isoflurane: green
    c. Desflurane: blue
    d. Sevoflurane: yellow
    e. Enflurane: orange

49. Concerning thromboelastography (TEG) of whole blood without additives; the following values are normal:
    a. r-time: 15–30 minutes
    b. K-time: 6–12 minutes
    c. α-angle: 60–70°
    d. Maximum amplitude: 30–40 mm
    e. LY30: >7.5%

50. Average normal daily requirements in adults are:
    a. Water   30–40 mL/kg
    b. Energy   30–40 kcal/kg
    c. Calcium   0.1–0.2 mmol/kg
    d. Magnesium   0.1–0.2 mmol/kg
    e. Phosphate   2–5 mmol/kg

51. The ideal gas law:
    a. Can be stated as $PV = nRT$
    b. R is the Boltzmann constant
    c. n is the number of moles of gas
    d. Is a combination of Boyle's law, Charles' law, Gay-Lussac's law and Avogadro's hypothesis
    e. Is true only for perfect gases

52. The following organisms are positive on Gram-staining:
    a. *Streptococcus pneumoniae*
    b. *Staphylococcus aureus*
    c. *Clostridium difficile*
    d. *Legionella pneumophila*
    e. *Neisseria meningitidis*

53. A 52-year-old man had been extricated from a road traffic accident suffering bilateral femoral fractures 2 days ago; findings consistent with fat embolism syndrome include:
    a. Pao_2: 80 mmHg (Fio_2 0.4)
    b. Raised haematocrit
    c. Axillary petechiae
    d. Pulmonary oedema
    e. Hypocalcaemia

54. **Digoxin:**
    a. Contains a steroid nucleus
    b. Causes tunnel vision as a side-effect
    c. Reduces vagal tone
    d. Decreases atrioventricular nodal conduction
    e. Is indicated in Wolff–Parkinson–White syndrome

55. **The following criteria should mandate patient referral to a specialist burns centre:**
    a. $\geq 10\%$ total body surface area burns in adults
    b. Burns of the perineum
    c. Any burn with associated trauma
    d. Full-thickness area burns $>5\%$ total body surface area
    e. Burns with concomitant shock

56. **A drug that stimulates H_2-receptors will:**
    a. Activate guanylyl cyclase
    b. Increase gastric acid production
    c. Increase pacemaker rate
    d. Act postsynaptically
    e. Stimulate histamine release

57. **Remifentanil:**
    a. Has an octanol : water partition coefficient of 2
    b. Is metabolized by butyrylcholinesterase
    c. Is 68% ionized at pH 7.4
    d. Has a pK_a of 8.0
    e. Contains four ester linkages

58. **Systemic inflammatory response syndrome (SIRS) is defined as the combination of two or more of the following:**
    a. Temperature $>38°C$ or $<36°C$
    b. Heart rate >100/min
    c. Respiratory rate >20/min
    d. White cell count $>12\,000$ or <4000/mm^3
    e. Presence of infection

59. **The Armitage regimen for caudal block recommends:**
    a. 0.25% bupivacaine
    b. 0.25 mL/kg for lumbosacral blockade
    c. 0.75 mL/kg for upper abdominal blockade
    d. 1.5 mL/kg for midthoracic blockade
    e. 0.9% saline : local anaesthetic in a ratio of 1 : 3 for larger volumes

60. **Osmolality:**
    a. Is defined as the number of osmoles per litre of solvent
    b. Is measured using the principles of Henry's law
    c. Is independent of the size and weight of particles in solution
    d. Is a property of solution independent of a membrane
    e. A 5% glucose solution is iso-osmolar compared with plasma

61. **In porphyria:**
    a. Inheritance is X-linked
    b. Suxamethonium is contraindicated
    c. Phenytoin is contraindicated
    d. Females are more commonly affected
    e. Psychosis is a presenting feature

62. **Obesity is associated with:**
    a. Increased growth hormone release
    b. Increased plasma leptin concentrations
    c. Body mass index (BMI) $>30 \text{ kg/m}^2$
    d. An increased alveolar–arterial gradient
    e. An increased relative blood volume

63. **Regarding local anaesthetic drugs:**
    a. Esters are comparatively unstable in solution
    b. All have a pK_a value above 7.4
    c. They are weak bases
    d. At neutral pH they exist predominantly in the un-ionized form
    e. Potency is related to pK_a

64. **A venous air embolus causes a reduction in end-tidal carbon dioxide (ETCO$_2$) measurement due to:**
    a. Arrhythmias
    b. Fall in cardiac output
    c. Increased airway pressure
    d. Increased dead space
    e. Reduced diffusion of gas

65. **A large right-to-left cardiac shunt:**
    a. Results in pulmonary hypertension
    b. Leads to a prolonged inhalational induction of anaesthesia
    c. Leads to a prolonged intravenous induction of anaesthesia
    d. Is a feature of tetralogy of Fallot
    e. Classically features a mill-wheel murmur

66. According to the National Prospective Post-Tonsillectomy Audit (2005), risk factors for postoperative bleeding include:
    a. Children
    b. Adults
    c. Tonsillectomy performed for quinsy
    d. Use of diathermy
    e. Use of blunt dissection

67. Naloxone:
    a. Precipitates acute withdrawal symptoms in opiate addicts
    b. Is a competitive antagonist at μ-opioid receptors only
    c. Is presented as a clear solution containing 0.4 mg/mL
    d. Alleviates the pruritus associated with spinal opioid use
    e. Undergoes extrahepatic conjugation

68. Features of sarcoidosis include:
    a. Caseating granulomas
    b. Bilateral hilar lymphadenopathy
    c. Lymphocytosis
    d. Hyperprolactinaemia
    e. Erythema marginatum

69. The Modified Day-Surgery Discharge Criteria include the following parameters for assessment:
    a. Nausea and vomiting
    b. Blood pressure
    c. Site of incision
    d. Surgical bleeding
    e. Cognitive dysfunction

70. Features of phaeochromocytoma include:
    a. 10% are benign tumours
    b. An association with neurofibromatosis
    c. Raised urinary 5-HIAA levels
    d. Dilated cardiomyopathy as a recognized complication
    e. Persistent hypertension as the most common presenting feature

71. Amide local anaesthetics include:
    a. Cocaine
    b. Tetracaine
    c. Prilocaine
    d. Etidocaine
    e. Bupivacaine

72. Appropriate anaesthetic management for a patient with known malignant hyperthermia undergoing appendicectomy includes:
    a. A rapid sequence induction using thiopentone and suxamethonium with maintenance on propofol and remifentanil
    b. A spinal anaesthetic
    c. A modified rapid sequence induction with thiopentone and rocuronium with maintenance on ether and remifentanil
    d. A modified rapid sequence induction with thiopentone and rocuronium with maintenance on sevoflurane
    e. An induction with ketamine and rocuronium and maintenance on propofol and remifentanil

73. The following statements are correct for WHO Clinical Staging of HIV/AIDS (2007):
    a. Persistent generalized lymphadenopathy occurs in Stage 1
    b. >10% loss in measured body weight occurs in Stage 2
    c. Applies to individuals aged 15 and over
    d. A CD4 count is required
    e. There are four stages

74. Application of positive end-expiratory pressure (PEEP):
    a. Improves left ventricular function in patients with congestive heart failure
    b. Increases right ventricular afterload
    c. Is termed 'best' when producing maximal oxygen delivery
    d. Increases venous return to the right heart
    e. May compromise portal venous drainage

75. The Braden scale for predicting pressure ulcer risk includes the following parameters:
    a. Comorbidity
    b. Skin moisture
    c. Mobility
    d. Patient sensory perception
    e. Reason for admission

76. A patient who has been declared brainstem-dead is undergoing a beating-heart organ retrieval; intravenous administration of the following is appropriate:
    a. Growth hormone
    b. T_3
    c. T_4
    d. Insulin
    e. Desmopressin

77. **Features associated with Down's syndrome include:**
    a. Leukaemia
    b. Atrial septal defect
    c. Atlantoaxial subluxation
    d. Hypertonicity
    e. Trisomy 18

78. **Regarding acute pancreatitis:**
    a. Diagnosis is preferably made by amylase estimation
    b. A Glasgow score of 3 indicates severe acute pancreatitis
    c. Enteral route is preferred for nutritional support
    d. The Balthazar severity index is used for biopsy staging
    e. Renal failure is a cause of increased amylase and lipase

79. **Causes of thrombocytopenia include:**
    a. Vitamin B_{12} deficiency
    b. Trimethoprim administration
    c. Hypersplenism
    d. Disseminated intravascular coagulation (DIC)
    e. Splenectomy

80. **Intraosseous cannulation in children:**
    a. Is contraindicated if proximal fractures exist
    b. Is contraindicated if osteomyelitis is present
    c. Can be performed in the femur
    d. Requires aspiration of blood for confirmation of placement
    e. Does not allow administration of bretylium

81. **Intra-aortic balloon pump counter-pulsation:**
    a. Describes inflation in early systole and deflation in diastole
    b. Is a Class I indication for cardiogenic shock
    c. Is contraindicated in aortic stenosis
    d. Uses N_2 as the inflation gas
    e. Requires the tip of the balloon catheter to be distal to the origin of the left subclavian artery

82. **Regarding community-acquired pneumonia**
    a. *Haemophilus influenzae* is the most frequent pathogen
    b. Pneumococcal antigen should only be performed in severe cases
    c. Severity is assessed using CURB-65 score
    d. Mortality rate for severe cases admitted to ICU is 33%
    e. Leukocytosis has a stronger association with mortality than leukopenia

83. **Bedside tests for detecting autonomic neuropathy include:**
    a. Valsalva manoeuvre
    b. Sustained hand grip
    c. Romberg's test
    d. Maddox wing test
    e. Postural blood pressure measurement

84. **Features of hypopituitarism include:**
    a. Hypoglycaemia
    b. Hyper-pigmentation
    c. Osteoporosis
    d. Morning cortisol level of 600 nmol/L
    e. Central obesity

85. **Expected blood results for an infant with uncorrected pyloric stenosis would include:**
    a. Hypochloraemia
    b. Hypokalaemia
    c. Hypernatraemia
    d. Metabolic acidosis
    e. Aciduria

86. **The following are correct of adverse drug reactions (ADRs):**
    a. Anaphylaxis is a Type A reaction
    b. Type B reactions are dose-related
    c. Only serious reactions should be reported on the Yellow Card Scheme
    d. Only health-care professionals can report using the Yellow Card Scheme
    e. The Yellow Card Scheme does not apply to herbal remedies

87. **A 42-year-old inpatient has been suffering from intermittent generalized convulsions for 45 minutes without regaining consciousness; management should include:**
    a. Diagnosing the type of epilepsy immediately
    b. Non-depolarizing muscle relaxant after general anaesthetic to terminate seizure
    c. A bolus of glucose if the blood glucose level cannot be ascertained
    d. Administration of a phenytoin bolus 15–17 mg/kg over 1 minute
    e. Fosphenytoin administration as an alternative to phenytoin

88. **Predisposing factors for dissecting aneurysms of the thoracic aorta include:**
    a. Coarctation of the aorta
    b. Oriental race
    c. History of trauma
    d. Unicommisural aortic valve
    e. Syphilis

89. Features of ankylosing spondylitis include:
    a. Association with HLA-B27
    b. Male predominance
    c. Aortic regurgitation
    d. Foramen magnum stenosis
    e. Raynaud's phenomenon

90. In a chronic smoker undergoing routine surgery, the following alterations in respiratory physiology would be expected:
    a. The oxyhaemoglobin dissociation curve is shifted to the right
    b. FEV_1 declines at the rate of 110 mL/year
    c. Closing capacity is increased
    d. Normal pulse oximetry readings
    e. Carbon monoxide levels may be increased up to 5 times

I. Practice Paper I: Answers

1a. **False**
1b. **True**
1c. **False**
1d. **True**
1e. **False**
ATN is heralded by an acute decrease in glomerular filtration rate (GFR), followed by a rise in plasma urea and creatinine concentrations. There follows a maintenance phase usually lasting 1–2 weeks where GFR remains reduced, leading to further rises in urea and creatinine, and a final phase where tubular function recovers and large volumes of urine are often produced. Hyaline casts can occur under normal circumstances, but tubular epithelial casts indicate renal injury. The following indices are found in prerenal failure and acute renal failure caused by ATN:

Measurement	Prerenal failure	ATN
Urine osmolality (mOsm/kg)	>500	<300
Urine sodium concentration (mmol/L)	<20	>40
Fractional excretion sodium (%)	<1	>1
Urine : plasma creatinine ratio	>40	<10
Urine microscopy	Normal	Epithelial casts

Ronco C, Bellomo R, Kellum JA. *Critical Care Nephrology*, 2nd edn. London: Saunders, 2008.

2a. **False**
2b. **True**
2c. **False**
2d. **True**
2e. **False**
Histamine acts on H_2-receptors within the myocardium and has positive chronotropic and inotropic effects. Amiodarone and adenosine are both negatively inotropic and chronotropic. Amiodarone reduces diastolic depolarization and depresses atrioventricular nodal automaticity and conduction. Adenosine reduces sinoatrial and atrioventricular nodal conduction, thus terminating paroxysmal supraventricular tachycardias; it has an extremely short plasma half-life of 10 s. Inhaled nitric oxide is a selective pulmonary vasodilator and therefore does not affect the myocardium. Finally, dantrolene may have antiarrhythmic properties in humans, but it does not affect force of contraction within the myocardium.

Sasada M, Smith S. *Drugs in Anaesthesia and Intensive Care*, 3rd edn. Oxford: OUP, 2003.

3a. True
3b. False
3c. True
3d. False
3e. False
V_D is defined as the volume into which the amount of drug would need to be uniformly distributed to produce the observed blood concentration. It is extremely large for amiodarone, which tends to accumulate in adipose tissue.

Drug	V_D (L/kg)
Amiodarone	50–100
Aspirin	0.2
Digoxin	5–11
Remifentanil	0.3–0.5
Warfarin	0.1–0.16

Burton ME, Shaw LM, Schentag JJ, Evans W, eds. *Applied Pharmacokinetics and Pharmacodynamics: Principles of Therapeutic Drug Monitoring*, 4th edn. Philadelphia: Lippincott Williams & Wilkins, 2005.

4a. True
4b. True
4c. True
4d. True
4e. False
The morbidity associated with intra-arterial injection of thiopentone relates to the change in pH resulting in precipitation of microcrystals from solution and within the artery, causing arterial spasm, endarterial obstruction and release of vasoactive mediators which results in thrombosis and necrosis. Priorities of management are stopping the injection, immediate dilution, followed by methods to establish maximal arterial vasodilatation of the affected limb; this includes sympathetic blockade of the stellate ganglion or brachial plexus blocks. Papaverine is a smooth-muscle relaxant structurally related to atracurium and local anaesthetics, such as lignocaine or procaine, are appropriate options. Intravenous anticoagulation with heparin is also indicated as a priority.

Goldsmith D, Trieger N. Accidental intra-arterial injection: a medical emergency. *Anesth Prog* 1975; **22**: 180–3.

5a. True
5b. False
5c. True
5d. True
5e. False
Calcium is critical for cell homeostasis, involved in many processes including neural transmission, haemostasis and coagulation, muscle contraction,

secretory processes, and skeletal support. 99% of calcium is found in the bony skeleton, the remaining 1% comprises the free diffusible fraction. Plasma calcium (1% of total calcium) is present as free ionized calcium (45%), complexed with anions (10%) and protein-bound, predominantly to albumin (45%). The normal concentration of plasma calcium (ionized and non-ionized) is 2.5 mmol/L; effects of hypocalcaemia are usually present when total calcium is below 2 mmol/L and are due to reduced level of ionized calcium.

Features of hypocalcaemia begin with increased membrane excitability:

- paraesthesia
- spasm
- muscle cramps
- tetany

Tetany leads to the classic Chvostek (facial spasm on tapping VIIth nerve) and Trousseau (carpopedal spasm on inflation of arm tourniquet) signs.

In severe cases, it leads to:

- respiratory insufficiency with bronchospasm and stridor
- reduced myocardial contractility and congestive heart failure
- ECG changes including prolonged QT
- irritability, confusion, extrapyramidal signs and convulsions may all occur
- preterm labour may also occur (due to smooth muscle dysfunction)

J-waves are pathognomonic of hypothermia. Cullen's sign is blue–black bruising around the umbilicus and is classically indicative of pancreatitis, although it was first described for ruptured ectopic pregnancy.

Cullen TS. *Embryology, Anatomy, and Diseases of the Umbilicus Together with Diseases of the Urachus*. Philadelphia: WB Saunders, 1916.
Power I, Kam P. *Principles of Physiology for the Anaesthetist*, 2nd edn. London: Arnold, 2007.

6a. True
6b. True
6c. True
6d. True
6e. True

Uterine atony is the most common cause of postpartum haemorrhage. Risk factors for atony include augmented or prolonged labour, labour lasting less than 3 hours, polyhydramnios, fetal macrosomia associated with diabetes, grand multiparity, chorioamnionitis and tocolytic drugs such as salbutamol, magnesium sulphate and halogenated anaesthetics. Dantrolene as a cause of uterine atony is controversial and disputed but has been reported.

Datta S. *Anesthetic and Obstetric Management of High-Risk Pregnancy*. New York: Springer-Verlag, 2004.
Weingarten AE, Korsh JI, Neuman GG, Stern SB. Postpartum uterine atony after intravenous dantrolene. *Anesth Analg* 1987; **66**: 269–70.

7a. False
7b. True
7c. False
7d. True
7e. True

Principles of anaesthesia and perioperative management for free tissue transfer surgery are aimed at providing optimal physiological conditions for perfusion and flow. Perfusion pressure must be maintained, and excessive vasoconstriction must be avoided since this will compromise blood flow and increase blood viscosity, resulting in flap failure. For these reasons, hypothermia must be avoided. A non-linear relationship exists between blood viscosity and haematocrit and while haemodilution improves flow dynamics, it also reduces the oxygen-carrying capacity of the blood; a haematocrit of 30% is thought to be optimal. Systemic vasodilators should also be avoided because they may cause a steal phenomenon and divert blood away from the flap, since the vessels will already be maximally dilated. A hyperdynamic circulation maintains cardiac output with a low systemic vascular resistance, providing optimal conditions for microcirculatory flap perfusion.

Adams J, Charlton P. Anaesthesia for microvascular free tissue transfer. *Contin Educ Anaesth Crit Care Pain* 2003; 3: 33–7.

8a. True
8b. False
8c. True
8d. True
8e. True

Patients should be individually consulted to ascertain which treatments are acceptable. Advanced directives state the desire of a competent individual and must be respected. In a life-threatening emergency for a child unable to give competent consent, all life-saving treatment should be given, irrespective of the parents' wishes. Departments should keep a regularly updated list of those senior members prepared to care for followers of the Jehovah's Witness faith.

Association of Anaesthetists of Great Britain and Ireland. *Management of Anaesthesia for Jehovah's Witnesses*, 2nd edn. London: AAGBI, 2005.

9a. False
9b. True
9c. False
9d. False
9e. True

Carlens is a left-sided double-lumen tube with one lumen running anterior to the other and a carinal hook to aid correct placement. White is a right-sided version of the Carlens tube. Left-sided tubes are usually preferred, even for right-sided surgery. Right-sided tubes are preferred if the left main bronchus is compressed by an aortic aneurysm, in order to prevent traumatic haemorrhage. The other named tubes are all double-lumen tubes without carinal hooks.

Yentis S, Hirsch N, Smith G. *Anaesthesia and Intensive Care A to Z: An Encyclopaedia of Principles and Practice*, 4th edn. Oxford: Butterworth-Heinemann, 2009.

10a. False
10b. True
10c. True
10d. True
10e. False
Doctors in England and Wales have a statutory duty to notify the local authority of suspected cases of the diseases listed below:

- Public Health (Control of Diseases) Act 1984:
  - cholera, food poisoning, plague, relapsing fever, smallpox, typhus.
- Public Health (Infectious Diseases) Regulations 1988:
  - acute encephalitis, acute poliomyelitis, anthrax, diphtheria, dysentery, leprosy, leptospirosis, malaria, measles, meningitis (all types), meningococcal septicaemia (without meningitis), mumps, ophthalmia neonatorum, paratyphoid fever, rabies, rubella, scarlet fever, tetanus, tuberculosis, typhoid fever, viral haemorrhagic fever, viral hepatitis, whooping cough, yellow fever.

Haemophilus influenzae type B is not notifiable but should be reported to the local authority, as should chickenpox in cases of exposure to immunocompromised patients, pregnant women or neonates.

McCormick A. The notification of infectious diseases in England and Wales. *Commun Dis Rep CDR Rev* 1993; 3: R19–25.

11a. False
11b. False
11c. True
11d. True
11e. True
Cardioplegia is a method of inducing intentional asystole to provide myocardial protection and a motionless field during cardiac surgery with cardiopulmonary bypass. It reduces the metabolic demand of cardiac muscle, often in the context of hypothermia. Cold crystalloid solutions are most commonly employed and do contain calcium. Calcium-free solutions risk causing the *calcium paradox*; this is the phenomenon of massive cell death following restoration of calcium containing perfusate of hearts infused for a brief period with a calcium-free medium. Antegrade cardioplegia is a solution introduced through the aortic sinus and, although practice may vary, administration depends on a competent aortic valve; retrograde cardioplegia is via the coronary sinus. Aortic cross-clamping with induced fibrillation is a technique of brief periods of ischaemia followed by reperfusion and is not a method of myocardial protection, but is an alternative to cardioplegia.

Fawzy EG, Barash PG, Reves JG. *Cardiac Anesthesia: Principles and Clinical Practice*. Philadelphia: Lippincott Williams & Wilkins, 2001.

12a. True
12b. False
12c. True
12d. False
12e. True
The Bohr *effect* is a descreased affinity of haemoglobin for oxygen secondary to a fall in pH and/or a rise in partial pressure of carbon dioxide, with a consequent shift to the right of the oxyhaemoglobin dissociation curve. It favours delivery of O_2 to the tissues. The Bohr *equation* states $V_A = V_T - V_D$, where V_A is the alveolar volume, V_T is the tidal volume and V_D is the dead space. It can also be written as:

$$\frac{V_D}{V_T} = \frac{Pa_{CO_2} - P_{ET}{CO_2}}{Pa_{CO_2}}$$

where Pa_{CO_2} and $P_{ET}{CO_2}$ are the arterial and end-tidal partial pressures of carbon dioxide, respectively.

13a. True
13b. True
13c. False
13d. True
13e. False
The Spaulding classification categorized medical devices according to the risk of infection associated with their use as critical, semi-critical and non-critical; critical items must be sterile because they enter sterile tissue or the vascular system, while semi-critical items describe those in contact with mucous membrane or intact skin. Decontamination processes can be divided into cleaning, low- and high-level disinfection, and sterilization; high-level disinfection kills vegetative bacteria, fungi and viruses (not all endospores) but with sufficient contact time will produce sterilization, provided thorough cleaning has been carried out. Laryngeal mask airways cannot be cleaned with glutaraldehyde, iodine or phenols and should *only* be sterilized using steam autoclaving.

Centers for Disease Control and Prevention. *Guideline for Disinfection and Sterilization in Healthcare Facilities*. Atlanta, GA: CDC, 2008. Available at: www.cdc.gov.

General Cleaning and Sterilization Instructions for Reusable LMA™ Products. Available at: www.lmana.com.

Sabir N, Ramachandra V. Decontamination of anaesthetic equipment. *Contin Educ Anaesth Crit Care Pain* 2004; 4: 103–6.

14a. True
14b. True
14c. False
14d. True
14e. True
Arterial tourniquets are used to provide a bloodless surgical field. American Heart Association guidance states that cuffs should have a width of >20% of the upper arm diameter, or 40% of the circumference of the thigh. Expressive exsanguination is contraindicated in local infection, tumour or

deep vein thrombosis, since fatal pulmonary embolus has resulted. Circulatory overload is also a risk following compression and can lead to left ventricular failure. Pathophysiological effects are local and systemic, leading to depletion of muscle ATP stores and progressive conduction block of motor and sensory nerves, thought to be due to local ischaemia. More permanent tourniquet paralysis has also been described as associated with higher cuff pressures. Recommendations limit tourniquet time to a minimum possible duration; 1.5 to 2 hours is the maximum recommended time for a healthy adult and deflation for 10–15 minutes should precede re-inflation. Complications include nerve injury, muscle injury, local skin necrosis or burns, and vascular injury. In addition, reactive hyperaemia following deflation can present with rising CO_2 partial pressure and acidosis, which can have negative inotropic effects and lead to cardiovascular instability. Use in sickle cell trait is controversial; following complete exsanguination, theoretically risks should be minimized.

Collins C. Orthopaedic surgery. In: Allman KG, Wilson IH, eds: *Oxford Handbook of Anaesthesia*, 2nd edn. Oxford: OUP, 2006.

Deloughry JL, Griffiths RG. Arterial tourniquets. *Contin Educ Anaesth Crit Care Pain* 2009; 9: 56–60.

15a. True
15b. False
15c. False
15d. False
15e. True

Laparoscopy has the following effects:

Respiratory: ↓compliance, ↓FRC (upward shift of diaphragm), ↑$PaCO_2$ (absorption of CO_2, $\dot{V}/\dot{Q}$ mismatch, respiratory depression), ↑end-tidal CO_2 ($ETCO_2$).

Complications: subcutaneous emphysema, endobronchial intubation, pneumothorax.

Cardiovascular: ↓venous return (pooling of blood in limbs, compression of vessels, high venous pressure), ↓cardiac output, ↑SVR (↑intrathoracic pressure, stimulation of peritoneal receptors, ↑vascular resistance of intra-abdominal organs, release of neurohumoral factors, e.g. vasopressin, catecholamines).

Complications: arrhythmias, hypotension, hypertension, gas embolism.

Gastrointestinal: ↑intra-abdominal pressure, ↓lower oesophageal tone.

Complications: Aspiration, vomiting, postoperative nausea and vomiting.

Central nervous system: ↑cerebral blood flow, intracranial pressure.

Renal: ↓GFR, ↓urine output.

Joris JL. Anesthesia for laparoscopic surgery. In: Miller RD, ed. *Miller's Anesthesia*, 7th edn. New York: Churchill Livingstone, 2009.

16a. False
16b. True
16c. True
16d. True
16e. True
Prolonged breathing of high concentrations of oxygen leads to features of pulmonary (Smith effect), central nervous system (Bert effect) and ocular oxygen toxicity; initially retrosternal discomfort occurs with coughing and dyspnoea due to tracheobronchial irritation, and subsequent reductions are seen in vital capacity, lung compliance and diffusing capacity in healthy volunteers after 24 hours. Central nervous system toxicity is manifest by visual defects, tinnitus, nausea and convulsions. The mechanism is thought to be oxidative damage and production of reactive oxygen species leading to oxidative stress at the cellular level; hence oxygen toxicity is worsened by certain drugs, such as disulfiram, which blocks superoxide dismutase.

17a. False
17b. False
17c. True
17d. True
17e. False
A full size D oxygen cylinder contains 340 L, while a size E contains 680 L. An absolute minimum of 360 L (6 × 60 minutes) is required to provide the patient's minimum oxygen requirement for the journey time, with MV of 6 L/min. In practice, modern ventilators consume gas in addition to the patient's actual MV, and oxygen supply must also allow for delays and altered patient demand. The Oxylog 3000 is an electrically powered ventilator but inspiratory flow is *pneumatically* powered; the additional gas consumption in the Oxylog 3000 is a 'bias flow' of 0.5 L/min, which flows through the circuit during expiration and this should be added to the MV when calculating gas requirements for transfers using this ventilator.

Fludger S, Klein A. Portable ventilators. *Contin Educ Anaesth Crit Care Pain* 2008; 8: 199–203.

18a. True
18b. False
18c. True
18d. False
18e. False
A Cochrane review reported a 36% relative reduction in occurrence of DVT with CNB when compared with general anaesthesia (GA) for fractured hip surgery, a 30% fall in mortality for patients undergoing surgery for fractured neck of femur, but no difference in a 3-month or 1-year mortality. A significant reduction in postoperative confusion was noted. Systematic review and analysis have demonstrated improved pain relief and reduced respiratory failure when epidural analgesia was used in conjunction with GA for thoracoabdominal surgery, with no effect on mortality. Epidural analgesia in labour provides effective pain relief but increased rates of instrumental vaginal delivery are reported. A Cochrane review reported a lesser reduction in

haematocrit and lower estimated blood loss during caesarean section with CNB compared with GA, with no impact on neonatal condition.

Afolabi BB, Lesi FEA, Merah NA. Regional versus general anaesthesia for Caesarean section. *Cochrane Database Syst Rev* 2006; (4): CD004350.

Anim-Somuah M, Smyth RMD, Howell CJ. Epidural versus non-epidural or no analgesia in labour. *Cochrane Database Syst Rev* 2005; (4): CD000331.

Parker MJ, Handoll HH, Griffiths R. Anaesthesia for hip fracture surgery in adults. *Cochrane Database Syst Rev* 2001; (4): CD000521.

Seller Losada JM, Sifre Julio C, Ruiz Garcia V. Combined general–epidural anesthesia compared to general anesthesia: a systematic review and meta-analysis of morbidity and mortality and analgesic efficacy in thoracoabdominal surgery. *Rev Esp Anestesiol Reanim* 2008; 55: 360–6.

19a. False
19b. True
19c. False
19d. False
19e. True

Benzodiazepines are a group of drugs with sedative, anxiolytic and anticonvulsant properties and they provide *anterograde* amnesia. They act via GABA-mediated inhibition within the central nervous system and bind allosterically to ionotropic $GABA_A$ receptors, where they increase chloride conductance; $GABA_B$ receptors are G-protein-coupled (metabotropic) receptors. As a group they are highly lipid-soluble and highly protein-bound; diazepam and midazolam have active metabolites, while lorazepam does not. They all have low hepatic extraction ratios, except midazolam. Midazolam exhibits pH-dependent tautomerism – a special form of structural isomerism whereby midazolam interconverts between a closed-ring lipophilic species and its open-ring aqueous form, in which it is stored. Diazepam is on the British National Formulary (BNF) list of drugs unsafe for use in porphyria.

British Medical Association, Royal Pharmaceutical Society of Great Britain. *British National Formulary 58*. Section 9.8.2: Drugs unsafe for use in acute porphyrias. London: Pharmaceutical Press, 2009. Available at: bnf.org/bnf.

20a. False
20b. False
20c. False
20d. True
20e. False

TURP is the surgical treatment of choice for benign prostatic hypertrophy and is usually performed in patients with prostatic weights of <60 g. Intraoperative complications that could account for the confusion include surgical causes such as TURP syndrome and haemorrhage. A high level of suspicion for TURP syndrome should be exercised as it is a clinical diagnosis made more likely with prolonged resection/irrigation time (>1 hour), low venous pressure, preceding blood loss due to open venous sinuses, high irrigation pressures or capsular perforation leading to peritoneal absorption of large volumes of irrigation fluid. Other patient causes include myocardial ischaemia, hypothermia and more rarely pulmonary embolus (air or thrombus). Immediate management prioritizes initial support of breathing and circulation and formulation of a diagnosis; fluid therapy is relatively contraindicated in TURP syndrome (although if serum Na^+ < 120 mmol/L or severe symptoms of hyponatraemia develop, 3% hypertonic saline may be indicated), and if suspected, surgery should be abandoned and fluids stopped. Intravenous diuretic therapy is recommended for treatment of acute pulmonary oedema, and arterial blood gas (ABG) measurement will provide useful information regarding dilutional electrolyte disturbance and assist further diagnosis.

O'Donnell AM, Foo ITH. Anaesthesia for transurethral resection of the prostate. *Contin Educ Anaesth Crit Care Pain* 2009; 9: 92–6.

21a. True
21b. False
21c. True
21d. True
21e. False
The Eastern Association for the Surgery of Trauma (EAST) clinical criteria for clearing cervical spine injury consist of:

- GCS 15; alert and oriented
- no intoxicants or drugs consumed
- no significant distracting injuries
- clinical examination: no midline tenderness or pain; full range of active neck movements; no referable neurological deficit

The EAST criteria for radiological clearance of the cervical spine in the obtunded patient include:

- adequate X-ray: anteroposterior, adequate lateral (defined as showing atlantoaxial joint, all cervical levels and cervicothoracic joint) and PEG views
- CT scans: thin cut axial slices with sagittal reconstruction of C1/C2
- dynamic fluoroscopy

Harrison P, Cairns C. Clearing the cervical spine in the unconscious patient. *Contin Educ Anaesth Crit Care Pain* 2008; 8: 117–20.

22a. False
22b. False
22c. True
22d. True
22e. True
Carboprost (Hemabate) is a prostaglandin $F_{2\alpha}$ and is used as an uterotonic agent for treatment of postpartum haemorrhage caused by uterine atony refractory to conventional treatment of uterine massage and intravenous oxytocin preparations. Side-effects relate to its contractile effect on smooth muscle, commonly leading to vomiting and diarrhoea; bronchospasm, chest

pain and hypertension are also adverse effects and caution should be exercised in individuals with cardiovascular disease.

British Medical Association, Royal Pharmaceutical Society of Great Britain. *British National Formulary 58*. Section 7.1.1: Prostaylandias and oxytocics – Carboprost. London: Pharmaceutical Press, 2009. Available at: bnf.org/bnf.

23a. False
23b. True
23c. True
23d. True
23e. True
Early recognition is the key to effective management of high or total spinal anaesthesia. The constellation of signs and symptoms arise from disruption of the sympathetic autonomics at that level. Initial signs include bradycardia and hypotension, which is accompanied by symptoms of nausea as the earliest sign. Fetal distress can occur if cardiotocography (CTG) monitoring is in place owing to uteroplacental insufficiency, and this can manifest as fetal bradycardia. Difficulty breathing occurs owing to intercostal nerve blockade, but until the phrenic nerve supply (C3, 4, 5) to the diaphragm is interrupted, cough will be relatively maintained. Ensuing paraesthesia in the fingers indicates a high spinal level but in the absence of other signs, can also be caused by hyper-ventilation and hypocapnia. Nasal congestion occurs owing to blockade of the sympathetic vasomotor innervation of the nasal mucosa, and Horner's syndrome is possible and has been described following obstetric spinal and epidural anaesthesia.

Lavi R. Spinal anesthesia for cesarean delivery associated with Horner's syndrome and contralateral trigeminal parasympathetic activation. *Anesth Analg* 2007; 104: 462.

24a. True
24b. False
24c. False
24d. False
24e. True
The Modified Aldrete Score comprises five categories:

Activity: able to move

Four extremities	2
Two extremities	1
No extremities	0

Respiration

Able to breath deeply or cough freely	2
Dyspnoea or limited breathing	1
Apnoea	0

Circulation

BP within 20 mmHg of preoperative value	2
BP within 20–50 mmHg of preoperative value	1
BP $\geq$ 50 mmHg of preoperative value	0

Consciousness

Fully awake	2
Rousable on calling	1
Unresponsive	0

Oxygen saturation

>92%	2
Requires O_2 to maintain >90%	1
<90% with O_2	0

A score of 9 or 10 is required to meet discharge criteria. Other criteria that are also included in local discharge policies include pain control, no nausea or vomiting and wound checks. NICE guidelines concerning inadvertent perioperative hypothermia state that patient core temperature should be checked on arrival and patients should not be discharged to the ward until they are $\geq 36°$C. Oral fluid intake and ambulation are parameters that are usually assessed prior to hospital discharge and increasing evidence suggests that voiding and oral fluid intake are less necessary in the assessment for fitness to street-discharge.

Association of Anaesthetists of Great Britain and Ireland. *Day Surgery 2*. London: AAGBI, 2005. Available at: www.aagbi.org/publications/guidelines/docs/daysurgery05.pdf.

Cahill H, Jackson I, McWhinnie D. *Guidelines about the Discharge Process and the Assessment for Fitness to Discharge*, British Association of Day Surgery Handbook Series. London: British Association of Day Surgery, 2002.

National Institute for Health and Clinical Excellence. *Perioperative Hypothermia (Inadvertent): Management of Inadvertent Perioperative Hypothermia in Adults*. NICE Clinical Guideline. CG65. London: NICE, 2008. Available at: guidance.nice.org.uk/CG65.

25a. True
25b. True
25c. False
25d. True
25e. False
Codeine is metabolized in the liver through three main pathways:

- Glucuronidation to codeine-6-glucuronide (10–20%)
- *N*-demethylation to norcodeine (10–20%)
- *O*-demethylation to morphine (5–15%)

Minor metabolites include normorphine and norcodeine-6-glucuronide. Genetic variability exists within the cytochrome P450 enzyme subset that is responsible for conversion of codeine to morphine; hence some 'fast' metabolizers produce a greater fraction of morphine.

Sasada M, Smith S. *Drugs in Anaesthesia and Intensive Care*, 3rd edn. Oxford: Oxford University Press, 2003.

26a. True
26b. True
26c. True
26d. True
26e. False
The normal range for IAP is 0−5 mmHg and intra-abdominal hypertension is defined as ≥ 12 mmHg or abdominal perfusion pressure (mean arterial pressure − IAP) ≤60 mmHg. The most commonly used and most accurate technique for measurement is intravesical instillation of saline, with zero reference from pubic symphysis or axilla; measurement should be undertaken three times, 4−6 hours apart. Inaccurate techniques include intrafemoral, uterine and rectal pressures. IAP has been classified as below, with suggested management included:

Grade	IAP (mmHg)	Suggested action
I	10−15	Normovolaemic resuscitation
II	16−25	Hypervolaemic resuscitation
III	26−35	Decompression
IV	>35	Decompression and re-exploration

Hopkins D, Gemmel LW. Intra-abdominal hypertension and the abdominal compartment syndrome. *Contin Educ Anaesth Crit Care Pain* 2001; 1: 56−9.
World Society of the Abdominal Compartment Syndrome (WSACS).
    Website: www.wsacs.org.

27a. False
27b. False
27c. True
27d. True
27e. False
A VIE is an efficient method of providing an oxygen supply to a hospital (see Figure 1.1). It consists of a stainless steel vessel that stores up to 1500 L of liquid oxygen, separated from a carbon-steel shell by an insulated gap with a vacuum pressure of 0.16−0.3 kPa. Oxygen has a boiling point of −182°C and it is stored below its *critical* temperature of −119°C at about −160°C to −180°C. The container is pressurized to approximately 10.5 bar and gaseous oxygen passes through a superheater to hospital pipelines via a pressure regulator. At times of high usage, the evaporation of oxygen draws the latent heat of vaporization from the liquid oxygen, maintaining its low temperature; however, at times of excessive demand, a control valve allows oxygen to pass

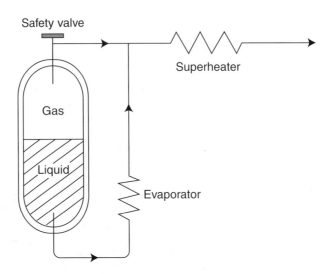

FIGURE 1.1   Vacuum insulated evaporator.

through coils of copper tubing that superheat it to ambient temperature to meet the extra demand. A safety valve that opens at 15–17 bar actuates at times of reduced usage, to prevent a pressure build-up within the container. Finally, the oxygen content of the vessel is estimated using a weighing scale, as it is stored as a liquid; some devices utilize a differential pressure gauge instead.

Al-Shaikh B, Stacey S. *Essentials of Anaesthetic Equipment*, 3rd edn. London: Churchill Livingstone, 2007.

28a. True
28b. False
28c. False
28d. False
28e. False
Magnesium is the fourth most abundant extracellular cation and the second most abundant intracellularly. Normal plasma concentrations are 0.7–1.05 mmol/L. It is an obligatory cofactor in all cells containing adenosine triphosphate (ATP). It helps to maintain the transmembrane sodium and potassium gradient by active involvement in the $Na^+K^+ATPase$ system. High concentrations of magnesium depress myocardial contractility and catecholamine release; its calcium channel blocking effects lead to a decrease in vascular tone resulting in reduced peripheral and pulmonary vascular resistance and coronary vasodilation. It antagonizes calcium at the neuromuscular junction and inhibits release of acetylcholine; it also has a direct action causing decreased excitability of nerves. Magnesium inhibits platelet activity and has been shown to increase bleeding time in pre-eclampsia.

Watson VF, Vaughn RS. Magnesium and the anaesthetist. *Contin Educ Anaesth Crit Care Pain* 2001; **1**: 16–20.

29a. False
29b. False
29c. False
29d. False
29e. True

Legionella pneumophila is a Gram-negative bacillus which is present in water and can survive in ponds, lakes, reservoirs and artificial sources (air-conditioning systems, cooling towers and respiratory therapy equipment). It is aerobic and facultative, replicating within macrophages. It is most commonly seen in younger patients and smokers and a history of travel is often present. Elderly patients tend to present with severe infection. *L. pneumophila* is sensitive to macrolides, fluoroquinolones and rifampicin. The British Thoracic Society recommends investigating for *Legionella* in patients with severe community-acquired pneumonia, for patients with specific risk factors and during outbreaks.

British Thoracic Society. *Guidelines for the Management of Community Acquired Pneumonia in Adults – 2004 Update*. London: BTS, 2004. Available at: www.brit-thoracic.org.uk/Portals/0/Clinical%20Information/Pneumonia/Guidelines/MACAPrevisedApr04.pdf.
Sadashiviah JB, Carr B. Severe community-acquired pneumonia. *Contin Educ Anaesth Crit Care Pain* 2009; **9**: 87–91.

30a. True
30b. True
30c. True
30d. False
30e. False

Rhabdomyolysis describes the disintegration of skeletal muscle, which leads to the release of myocytic enzymes and constituents into the systemic circulation. The most sensitive diagnostic test is plasma creatine kinase levels of which are proportional to the extent of muscle injury. Causes are traumatic (such as crush injury and electrocution) and non-traumatic (including statin therapy, cocaine abuse, sepsis and electrolyte dysfunction). The events leading to myocyte necrosis involve the influx of intracellular calcium, which leads to cytotoxicity and cell death with extrusion of intracellular contents such as myoglobin. Acute renal failure is a common sequel and is thought to be due to myoglobin-induced renal tubular obstruction and renal vasoconstriction resulting in oxidative damage. Management should be directed at prevention of renal failure with aggressive fluid resuscitation and avoidance of life-threatening metabolic disturbances such as hyperkalaemia. In addition, bicarbonate infusion increases urinary pH and reduces precipitation of the acidic myoglobin complex within renal tubules. Diuretics, including mannitol, have been used to maintain urinary flow and reduce complications, but use is controversial. Finally, prognosis is extremely good, with full recovery of renal function expected within 3 months in the majority of patients.

Hunter JD, Gregg K, Damani Z. Rhabdomyolysis. *Contin Educ Anaesth Crit Care Pain* 2006; **6**: 141–3.

31a. False
31b. True
31c. False
31d. False
31e. False

Damping is defined as the progressive diminution of amplitude of oscillation in a resonant system caused by dissipation of stored energy. It is inherent in any system, slowing the rate of change of signal between the patient and trans-ducer. It can be useful by reducing the frequency of the pressure transducing system. The 'damping factor' (*D*) is a measure of damping within a resonant system.

- *Optimally damped* (*D* = 0.7): system responds rapidly with small amount of overshoot
- *Critically damped* (*D* = 1.0): no overshooting, but may be too slow
- *Underdamped* (*D* < 0.7): resonance occurs, signal oscillates and overshoots
- *Overdamped* (*D* > 1.0): signal takes a long time to reach equilibrium, but will not overshoot

Ward MA, Langton SA. Blood pressure measurement. *Contin Educ Anaesth Crit Care Pain* 2007; 7: 122–6.

32a. True
32b. False
32c. True
32d. False
32e. False

Hyperkalaemia is defined as plasma potassium above 5.5 mmol/L. Causes of high potassium include:

Increased intake of potassium

- High input (inappropriate fluids, or supplements)

Reduced loss of potassium

- Decreased excretion ($\downarrow$ GFR, acute kidney injury, $\downarrow$ mineralocorticoids, drugs: K^+-sparing diuretics, ACE-inhibitors, angiotensin II receptor blockers)

Redistribution: An acute shift from intracellular to extracellular compartments

- Acidosis, $\downarrow$ insulin, digitalis toxicity (which inhibits Na^+K^+ATPase), β-blockers, suxamethonium, malignant hyperthermia, rhabdomyolysis and exercise, release of tourniquets

Factitious

- A result of haemolysis, or thrombocytosis and leukocytosis (which secrete K^+ prior to laboratory analysis)

β-agonists such as salbutamol comprise part of the management for acute hyperkalaemia.

33a. True
33b. False
33c. True
33d. True
33e. False
One-lung anaesthesia is indicated in lung, oesophageal, mediastinal and spinal surgery. It is achieved with the use of bronchial blockers or a double-lumen tracheal tube. Indications are absolute and relative.

Absolute

- Massive air leak: bronchopleural fistula, tracheobronchial tree disruption, giant unilateral cyst/bulla, open surgery on main bronchi
- Lung isolation (to avoid contamination): infection, haemorrhage
- Unilateral bronchopulmonary lavage: pulmonary alveolar proteinosis

Relative

- Surgical access: pulmonary, oesophageal, spinal, great vessel surgery
- Severe hypoxaemia due to unilateral lung disease

Eastwood J, Mahajan R. One-lung anaesthesia. *Contin Educ Anaesth Crit Care Pain* 2002; 2: 83–7.

34a. False
34b. False
34c. True
34d. True
34e. True
Gabapentin is an acetic acid derivative and was originally synthesized to mimic the neurotransmitter GABA, hence its name. It is not believed to act at GABA receptors, but at voltage-dependent calcium channels ($\alpha_2\delta$ subunit). Uses include the treatment of neuropathic pain, post-herpetic neuralgia and partial seizures. It is presented as 600/800 mg tablets, 100/300/400 mg capsules and an oral solution of 50 mg/mL. It is given in divided doses up to a total of 1800 mg/day; it is an analgesic and anticonvulsant; side-effects include dizziness, ataxia, tremor, nausea and vomiting. Gabapentin is well absorbed orally, is not metabolized and is excreted generally unchanged in the urine; it can potentiate the analgesic effect of morphine.

Sasada M, Smith S. *Drugs in Anaesthesia and Intensive Care*, 3rd edn. Oxford: OUP, 2003.

35a. False
35b. False
35c. True
35d. True
35e. True
The maximum safe dose of bupivacaine is 2 mg/kg; the 75 kg patient therefore has a maximum safe dose of 150 mg bupivacaine and has already received 100 mg through the interscalene approach to the brachial plexus. Additional local infiltration of up to 50 mg bupivacaine (without adrenaline) may be performed if surgically feasible. Equally, administration of intravenous

analgesia and communication with the surgical team is also appropriate and sensible. Intravenous benzodiazepine sedation does not provide analgesia and a top-up interscalene block is inappropriate and unsafe owing to the risk of intraneural injection, damage to anaesthetized local structures and exceeding the maximum safe dose of bupivacaine.

36a. True
36b. False
36c. False
36d. True
36e. True
The JVP represents an indirect measure of central venous pressure; the following waveforms are present, as illustrated in Figure 1.2:

Waves: upward deflections:
a – right atrial contraction
c – bulging of tricuspid valve into the right atrium during ventricular systole with isovolumetric contraction
v – atrial venous filling occurring in late systole

Descents:
x – atrial relaxation with downward movement of the tricuspid valve and ventricular systole
y – right ventricular filling as tricuspid valve opens

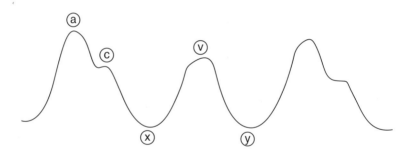

FIGURE 1.2   Venous waveform.

Causes of Kussmaul's sign include constrictive pericarditis, pericardial effusion, and severe right-sided heart failure. The a wave is absent in atrial fibrillation, while cannon waves are large a waves caused by atrial contraction against a closed tricuspid valve. Friedreich's sign is a rapid rise and subsequent fall of the JVP seen in constrictive pericarditis.

Drazner MH, Rame JE, Stevenson LW, et al. Prognostic importance of elevated jugular venous pressure and a third heart sound in patients with heart failure. *N Engl J Med* 2001; 345: 574–81.

37a. False
37b. True
37c. False
37d. True
37e. True
The blood supply to the heart is derived from the right and left coronary arteries, which arise from the right (anterior) and left (posterior) sinuses at the origin of the aorta (see Figure 1.3). The right coronary artery is smaller than the left but supplies the atrioventricular node in 80% and the sinoatrial node in 60% of individuals; thus its compromise may result in arrhythmias. The right coronary artery divides into a marginal branch and continues to give rise to the inferior interventricular artery. The left coronary artery divides into the circumflex and the anterior interventricular artery, which continues to anastomose with the posterior interventricular artery of the right coronary artery.

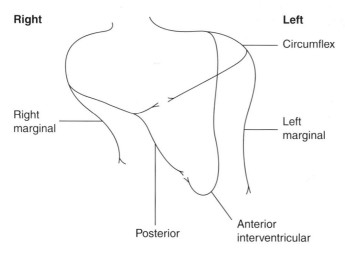

FIGURE 1.3   Coronary arteries.

38a. True
38b. True
38c. False
38d. True
38e. True
The Humphrey ADE is a very versatile system, which can be used in adults and children for spontaneous and controlled ventilation. Parallel and co-axial systems exist. Two smooth-bore 15 mm tubings are connected to the patient, via a Y-piece distally and the Humphrey block proximally. The block has an adjustable pressure-limiting (APL) valve, 2 L reservoir bag, lever to select method of ventilation, ventilator port and safety pressure relief valve. With the lever 'up' (spontaneous mode) the reservoir bag and valve are connected to the breathing system and it performs as a Mapleson A (Magill) system. With the lever 'down' (ventilator mode) the reservoir bag and valve are isolated from the circuit, and thus it performs as a Mapleson E system.

Al-Shaikh B, Stacey S. *Essentials of Anaesthetic Equipment*, 3rd edn. London: Churchill Livingstone, 2007.

39a. False
39b. False
39c. True
39d. True
39e. False
Levosimendan is a calcium-sensitizing agent indicated for the treatment of acutely decompensated chronic heart failure. It is a positive inotrope, vaso-dilator and inodilator (particularly when given concomitantly with β-blockers). It displays calcium-dependent binding of the *N*-terminal domain of cardiac troponin C (TnC), stabilizing the complex between calcium and TnC, which prolongs the actin—myosin association rate. This results in positive inotropy without increasing intracellular calcium concentrations or significantly increasing myocardial oxygen demand. Vasodilatation is achieved through the K^+-ATP-channel opening in cardiac and smooth muscles; right and left ventricular afterload is decreased. Levosimendan has a half-life of $1-3$ hours, undergoes hepatic metabolism to active compounds (which have half-lives of ~75 hours) that are renally excreted and must be used in caution with patients in renal impairment. Use during active ischaemia or obstructive coronary artery disease has resulted in hypotension leading to tachycardia, aggravated ischaemia and myocardial damage.

Cordingley J. Levosimendan. In: Waldmann N, Soni N, Rhodes A, eds. *Oxford Desk Reference: Critical Care*. Oxford: OUP, 2008.

40a. True
40b. False
40c. False
40d. True
40e. False
The diaphragm consists of a central tendon and peripheral muscular part; it has three main openings, which transmit the following structures:

T8 — inferior vena cava and right phrenic nerve (**I R**ead)
T10 — vagus, oesophagus and gastric nerves and vessels (**V**ery **O**ld)
T12 — aorta, thoracic duct and azygos vein (**A**nd **T**orn **A**rticles)

The left phrenic nerve pierces the diaphragm within its central tendon.

41a. False
41b. True
41c. True
41d. True
41e. True
Nerve stimulators can monitor depth of non-depolarizing neuromuscular blockade (NDMB) using the TOF response; causes of lack of response can be divided as follows:

- *Equipment-related*: poor electrode contact, disconnection, misplacement (not overlying a peripheral nerve), faulty equipment, low battery power

- *Patient-related*: any condition leading to disruption of neuromuscular transmission; neuropathy (diabetes, porphyria), myasthenia gravis (increased sensitivity to NDMB), drugs (aminoglycosides), electrolyte imbalance (hypermagnesaemia), nerve transection

Cholinesterase mutations will lead to a varying prolongation of neuromuscular blockade following use of drugs reliant upon cholinesterase for hydrolysis, such as suxamethonium (suxamethonium apnoea).

Hines RL, Marschall KE. *Stoelting's Anesthesia and Co-existing Disease.* Philadelphia: Churchill Livingstone, 2008.

42a. True
42b. False
42c. True
42d. False
42e. False
The British Thoracic Society guidelines on the management of asthma (2008) recommend the following for acute asthma:

- FiO_2 40–60%, high flow
- β_2-agonists (i.e. salbutamol) via a nebulizer or spacer; severe asthma can be managed by continuous nebulization of 5–10 mg/h
- Steroids: prednisolone 40–50 mg per day or hydrocortisone 100 mg four times daily
- Ipratropium bromide 0.5 mg via a nebulizer 4–6 hourly if asthma is acutely severe or life-threatening or there is a poor response to β_2-agonists
- Intravenous $MgSO_4$ 1.2–2 g over 20 minutes with ECG monitoring
- Intravenous aminophylline may be given, although it may not be of much benefit
- Intravenous antibiotics are no longer recommended unless a definite source of infection has been ascertained
- Heliox may be tried, although this is not evidence-based

British Thoracic Society/Scottish Intercollegiate Guidelines Network. British guideline on the management of asthma. *Thorax* 2008; **63**(Suppl 4): iv1–121.

43a. False
43b. True
43c. False
43d. False
43e. True
50 000 premature babies are born in the UK per annum. Mortality remains high at 4.2 per 1000 live births. Prematurity is categorized by gestational age or birth weight as follows:

Category	Birth weight (g)	Gestational age (weeks)
Borderline/near term	<2500	36–37
Moderately premature	<1500	31–36
Severely premature	<1000	24–30

In addition to reduced alveoli, pulmonary capillaries and surfactant production, chemoreceptor responses are blunted in the preterm infant. The normal response to hypoxaemia is biphasic (hyperventilation followed by apnoea or hypoventilation). In the preterm infant this response is monophasic, consisting only of apnoea. Incidence is related to birth weight (25% in borderline babies; 84% in severely premature babies). Apnoeas may be:

- *Central*: diminished hypercapnic response, hypoxic ventilatory depression, active inhibitory reflexes
- *Obstructive*: apposition of soft tissues in the hypopharynx or nose
- *Mixed*: obstruction followed by central pauses; these occur most frequently

Apnoeas are considered pathological if >20 s alone, or <20 s with bradycardia (30 beats/min decline from resting heart rate), cyanosis, pallor or hypotonia. Postoperatively, apnoeas occur frequently within the first 12 hours, but can continue for up to 30 days.

Peiris K, Fell D. The prematurely born infant and anaesthesia. *Contin Educ Anaesth Crit Care Pain* 2009; 9: 73–7.

44a. False
44b. True
44c. True
44d. False
44e. True
PiCCO utilizes pulse contour analysis from the arterial waveform, obtained from femoral, brachial or axillary arterial catheters. Central venous access is required for a transcardiopulmonary thermodilution injectate used for calibration. The area under the waveform is analysed to derive ejection systolic area by identifying ventricular ejection and the dicrotic notch. Beat-to-beat calculations are averaged over 30 s cycles and displayed as a number. Problems may be encountered by abnormal waveforms or arrhythmias. Lithium medication is an exclusion criterion for lithium dilution (LiDCO) measurement.

Allsager M, Swanevelder J. Measuring cardiac output. *Contin Educ Anaesth Crit Care Pain* 2003; 3: 15–19.

45a. True
45b. True
45c. False
45d. True
45e. True
Carbon monoxide (CO) is a colourless, odourless gas produced by incomplete combustion of organic compounds. CO binds to haemoglobin 240 times more avidly than oxygen, causing a left shift in the oxyhaemoglobin dissociation curve, preventing oxygen delivery and utilization at the cellular level. CO toxicity presents with a wide and varying range of symptoms and signs, making misdiagnosis possible. Inhalation injury or burns should always alert the clinician to the possibility of CO exposure. Presentation includes headache,

malaise, fatigue, confusion, nausea and vomiting; the cherry-red appearance is classically reported but occurs uncommonly, while arterial oxygen saturations may be misleadingly high. Eye signs include flame-shaped retinal haemorrhages, papilloedema and bright-red retinal veins (a sensitive early sign).

Gorman D, Drewry A, Huang Y. The clinical toxicology of carbon monoxide. *Toxicology* 2003; 87: 25–38.

46a. False
46b. True
46c. False
46d. False
46e. False
Atropine and hyoscine are naturally occurring esters of tropic acid with tropine and scopine respectively. They are tertiary amines and readily cross the blood–brain barrier, while glycopyrrolate is a quaternary amine with a permanent charge and thus does not. Atropine and hyoscine exhibit optical isomerism and their muscarinic action is due to their L-forms. The order of activity is as follows:

- *Antisialagogue*: glycopyrrolate > hyoscine > atropine
- *Cardiac*: atropine > glycopyrrolate > hyoscine
- *Sedation*: hyoscine > atropine

Hyoscine is contraindicated in porphyria.

British Medical Association, Royal Pharmaceutical Society of Great Britain. *British National Formulary 58*. Section 9.8.2: Drugs unsafe for use in acute porphyrias. London: Pharmaceutical Press, 2009. Available at: bnf.org/bnf.

47a. True
47b. True
47c. False
47d. True
47e. False
EVLW is the volume of water contained within the pulmonary interstitium and alveolar space. Normal EVLW is 4–7 mL/kg, which has been derived postmortem. Increased EVLW is caused by:

- disruption of Starling forces: e.g. left ventricular failure
- damage to integrity of pulmonary and capillary alveolar endothelium: e.g. acute lung injury

The volume of distribution for indicators is derived from dilution curves detected at the femoral artery. Detection is via a fibreoptic catheter with a thermistor tip. The rate of decay of indicators is exponential. EVLW may be calculated by subtracting pulmonary blood volume from pulmonary thermal volume. Treatment of pulmonary oedema by diuresis and ultrafiltration has been shown to be less effective at reducing EVLW in the context of capillary leak compared with congestive heart failure.

Singer M, Webb AR. *Oxford Handbook of Critical Care*, 3rd edn. Oxford: OUP, 2009.

48a. True
48b. False
48c. False
48d. False
48e. True
The key filling systems for modern vaporizers consist of:

- *Filler tube*: It has a base which connects to the bottle and a block which only fits into the correct vaporizer port
- *Collar*: Around the neck of the volatile bottle; has pegs for the corresponding slot in the filler tube base

This closed system prevents filling with incorrect agents, spillage and pollution in theatre. The collar, filler tube base and block are colour-coded for each agent: halothane – red, isoflurane – purple, enflurane – orange, methoxyflurane – green. Sevoflurane and desflurane vaporizers do not utilize the key filling system. They have an agent-specific attachment already on the bottle (desflurane) or fitted to it (sevoflurane).

Yentis S, Hirsch N, Smith G. *Anaesthesia and Intensive Care A to Z: An Encyclopaedia of Principles and Practice*, 4th edn. Oxford: Butterworth-Heinemann, 2009.

49a. True
49b. True
49c. False
49d. False
49e. False
TEG is a method of near-patient coagulation testing that uses whole blood (as opposed to plasma), representing a global test of coagulation. The analyser produces a trace that can quantify the kinetics of clot formation and lysis.

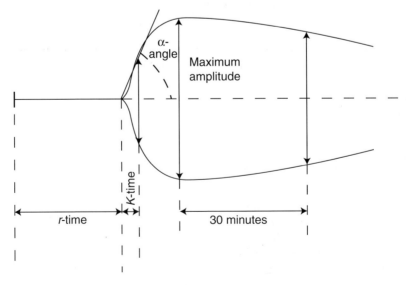

FIGURE I.4 Thromboelastogram.

They have been used successfully in orthotopic liver transplants and cardiac surgery when cardiopulmonary bypass is being used. The five parameters measured are illustrated in Figure 1.4 and are:

r-time (reaction time) (15−30 minutes)

- Time from initiation of test until amplitude reaches 2 mm (initial fibrin formation)
- Functionally related to plasma clotting and inhibitor factor activity
- ↑ anticoagulation/factor deficiencies/hypofibrinogenaemia
- ↓ hypercoagulable states

K-time (6−12 minutes)

- Time from *r*-time until amplitude reaches 20 mm
- 'Clot formation time'
- ↑ anticoagulation/hypofibrinogenaemia/thrombocytopenia
- ↓ hyperfibrinogenaemia/increased platelet function

α-angle (40−50°)

- Tangent of the curve as *K* is reached
- 'Speed at which clot forms'
- ↑ hyperfibrinogenaemia/increased platelet function
- ↓ anticoagulation/hypofibrinogenaemia/thrombocytopenia

MA (maximum amplitude) (50−60 mm)

- Greatest amplitude on curve
- 'Maximal clot strength': quality of fibrin and platelet activation
- ↑ hypercoagulable states/thrombocytosis
- ↓ thrombocytopenia/platelet blocker/fibrinolysis/factor deficiencies

LY30 (<7.5%)

- Based on area under curve 30 minutes after MA
- Measure of fibrinolysis

Curry ANG, Pierce JMT. Conventional and near-patient tests of coagulation. *Contin Educ Anaesth Crit Care Pain* 2007; 7: 45−50.

50a. True
50b. True
50c. True
50d. True
50e. False
Normal requirements in adults includes:

- Water   30−40 mL/kg
- Energy   30−40 kcal/kg
- Sodium   1 mmol/kg
- Potassium   1 mmol/kg
- Calcium   0.1−0.2 mmol/kg
- Magnesium   0.1−0.2 mmol/kg

- Chloride 1.5 mmol/kg
- Phosphate 0.2–0.5 mmol/kg
- Nitrogen 0.2 g/kg

51a. True
51b. False
51c. True
51d. True
51e. True
The ideal gas law is true for a perfect gas, in which intermolecular forces (such as Van der Waals forces) are neglected. In such a gas the ideal gas law can be applied without restriction (unlike in an ideal or a real gas). The nomenclature is as follows (SI units):

- P is the absolute pressure (Pa)
- V is the volume of gas (L)
- n is the number of moles
- R is the universal gas constant ($8.314 \, J \, K^{-1} \, mol^{-1}$)
- T is the absolute temperature (K)

As stated, it is a combination of Boyle's law, Charles' law, Gay-Lussac's law and Avogadro's hypothesis. The Boltzmann constant (k_B) is the universal gas constant (R) divided by the Avogadro constant and describes the relationship between absolute temperature and the kinetic energy contained in each molecule of an ideal gas.

52a. True
52b. True
52c. True
52d. False
52e. False
Gram-staining is a method used to classify bacteria by crystal violet staining following fixation with iodine and alcohol decolorization. Gram-positive organisms have a cell wall that contains peptidoglycans, lipoteichoic acid and polysaccharides. Gram-negative species have an additional outer cell wall layer that contains endotoxin. Examples include:

Gram-positive

- cocci: *Staphylococcus, Enterococcus, Streptococcus*
- bacilli: *Bacillus, Corynebacterium, Mycobacterium, Clostridium*

Gram-negative

- cocci: *Neisseria*
- bacilli: *Enterobacteria, Acinetobacter, Pseudomonas, Camplylobacter, Haemophilus, Legionella, Chylamdia*

53a. False
53b. False
53c. True
53d. True
53e. False

The term fat embolism describes the presence of fat globules in lung parenchyma and the peripheral circulation, usually following long bone injury or major trauma; it is often asymptomatic. *Fat embolism syndrome* can result, producing a distinct pattern of clinical symptoms and signs. Clinical presentation is typically 24–72 hours after injury with a triad of respiratory changes, neurological abnormalities and a petechial rash. Various diagnostic criteria exist, the most commonly used are Gurd's criteria:

Major criteria

- Axillary or subconjuctival petechiae
- Hypoxaemia (PaO_2 <60 mmHg, FiO_2 0.4)
- Central nervous system depression disproportionate to hypoxaemia
- Pulmonary oedema

Minor criteria

- Tachycardia >110/min
- Pyrexia <38.5°C
- Emboli present in the retina on fundoscopy
- Fat present in the urine
- A sudden inexplicable drop in haematocrit or platelet values
- Increasing ESR
- Fat globules present in the sputum

Diagnosis requires at least one major and four minor criteria to be present. Hypocalcaemia is often seen as free fatty acids bind with calcium.

Gupta A, Reilly CS. Fat embolism. *Contin Educ Anaesth Crit Care Pain* 2007; 7: 148–51.

54a. True
54b. False
54c. False
54d. True
54e. False

Digoxin is a widely used cardiac glycoside used to treat supraventricular tachycardias, although it is contraindicated in Wolff–Parkinson–White syndrome. It is derived from the foxglove plant (*Digitalis lanata*) and contains a steroid moiety and carbohydrate moieties, which affect lipophilicity and drug kinetics. Its main effects are decreasing conduction through the atrioventricular node and slowing heart rate by an increase in vagal tone; it also exerts a positive inotropic effect on the myocardium. It binds to the α-subunit of the extracellular membrane Na^+K^+ATPase, blocking its action. This leads to an increase in Na^+ availability intracellularly and, in turn, decreased extrusion of calcium by the Na^+/Ca^+ exchanger. This increases the availability of calcium, thereby increases force of contraction. Digoxin has a narrow therapeutic index; tunnel vision is not a feature, although xanthopsia and colour vision disturbance can occur.

Calvey TN, Williams NE. *Principles and Practice of Pharmacology for Anaesthetists*. Oxford: Wiley-Blackwell, 2001.

55a. True
55b. True
55c. True
55d. True
55e. False
The British Burns Association referral criteria are:

- Burns >10% TBSA for adults and >5% TBSA for children
- Burns >5% TBSA full thickness
- Burns of specialized areas: face, hands, feet, genitalia, perineum, joints
- Burns with associated inhalation injury
- Electrical or chemical burns
- Circumferential burns of limbs or chest
- Burns at extremes of age
- Burns with pre-existing disease that may affect management, recovery or mortality
- Any burn with associated trauma

Hilton PJ, Hepp M. The immediate care of the burned patient. *Contin Educ Anaesth Crit Care Pain* 2001; **1**: 113–16.

56a. False
56b. True
56c. True
56d. True
56e. False
There are four histamine receptors H_1–H_4 and are all G-protein-coupled receptors; H_2-receptor antagonists such as ranitidine and cimetidine are used to reduce gastric acid secretion. H_2-receptors act via cyclic adenosine monophosphate (cAMP) and are found in gastric mucosa, cardiac muscle, mast cells and brain tissue. They are located postsynaptically and stimulation is thought to modulate histamine release via a negative feedback mechanism.

Katzung BG, Masters SB, Trevor AJ. *Basic and Clinical Pharmacology*, 11th edn. New York: McGraw-Hill Professional, 2007.

57a. False
57b. False
57c. False
57d. False
57e. False
Remifentanil is a synthetic pure μ-agonist, which has a pK_a value of 7.1 and is 68% un-ionized at pH 7.4. It is lipophilic with an octanol : water partition coefficient of 17.9. It contains three ester linkages and is rapidly broken down

by non-specific plasma and tissue esterases, which confers its elimination half-life of 3–10 minutes, with a constant context sensitive half-time; it is not a substrate for butyrylcholinesterase (pseudocholinesterase).

Freye E. *Opioids in Medicine: A Comprehensive Review on the Mode of Action and the Use of Analgesics in Different Clinical Pain States.* Dordrecht: Springer, 2008.

58a. True
58b. False
58c. True
58d. True
58e. False

SIRS is a term used to define a clinical state with a myriad of causes, but which all ultimately activate the cytokine cascade. SIRS is defined as the presence of two or more of the following:

- Temperature $>38°C$ or $<36°C$
- Heart rate >90/min
- Respiratory rate >20/min or $PaCO_2$ <4.5 kPa
- White cell count <4000 or $>12\,000$/mm^3 or $>10\%$ immature cells (band forms)

It may result from non-infective disease processes such as trauma or pancreatitis. Sepsis is SIRS plus the presence of an infection.

Brun-Buisson C. The epidemiology of the systemic inflammatory response. *Intensive Care Med* 2000; **26**: 1870.

59a. True
59b. False
59c. False
59d. False
59e. True

Caudal anaesthesia provides sacral and lumbar nerve root blockade, making it useful for perineal surgery. The Armitage regimen for caudal block recommends 0.25% bupivacaine in the following volumes:

- Lumbosacral blockade   0.5 mL/kg
- Upper abdominal blockade   1.0 mL/kg
- Midthoracic blockade   1.25 mL/kg

For volumes above 20 mL the recommendation is to add 0.9% saline in a ratio of 1 : 3 with the bupivacaine.

Vadodaria B, Conn D. Caudal epidural anaesthesia. *Update in Anaesthesia* 1998; Issue 8, Article 3: 1–2.

60a. False
60b. False
60c. True
60d. True
60e. True

Osmolarity is the number of osmoles per *litre* of solution while *osmolality* is defined as the number of osmoles per *kilogram* of solvent and is a measure of the number of particles present within a solution. It is independent of the size or weight of the particles and independent of a cell membrane. It can be determined only by using the colligative properties of solution and is measured using the principles of Raoult's law. Henry's law states that at a constant temperature, the amount of a given gas dissolved in a given type and volume of liquid is directly proportional to the partial pressure of that gas in equilibrium with that liquid.

61a. False
61b. False
61c. True
61d. True
61e. True

Porphyria describes a heterogeneous group of diseases characterized by defects in the enzymes involved in the biosynthesis of haem, resulting in the over-production and excretion of porphyrins. Porphyria is classified as erythropoeitic or hepatic, depending on the site of excess production. Porphyrias are inherited as autosomal dominant disorders and are more common in females, presenting in early adult life. Three hepatic forms affect the conduct of anaesthesia:

- *Acute intermittent porphyria*: most common in Sweden; presentation includes abdominal pain and vomiting (90%), motor/sensory neuropathies (70%), neuropsychiatric dysfunction, convulsions or coma (50%)
- *Variegate porphyria*: most common in South African Afrikaaners; photosensitivity occurs
- *Hereditary coproporphyria*: photosensitivity may occur

Drugs definitely unsafe include barbiturates, etomidate, sulphonamides and phenytoin. A full list of unsafe drugs can be found in the British National Formulary.

British Medical Association, Royal Pharmaceutical Society of Great Britain. *British National Formulary 58*. Section 9.8.2: Drugs unsafe for use in acute porphyrias. London: Pharmaceutical Press, 2009. Available at: bnf.org/bnf.

Kumar P, Clark M. *Kumar and Clark's Clinical Medicine*, 7th edn. London: Saunders, 2009.

62a. False
62b. True
62c. True
62d. True
62e. False
The WHO International Classification states the following BMI ranges:

- Normal: $18.5-24.9$ kg/m^2
- Pre-obese: $25-29.9$ kg/m^2
- Class I obesity (overweight): $30-34.9$ kg/m^2
- Class II obesity (obese): $35-39.9$ kg/m^2
- Class III obesity (morbidly obese): >40 kg/m^2
- Morbidly obese has also been described as Class II with comorbidities

Obesity is associated with numerous hormonal changes influencing fat deposition and distribution. Growth hormone increases utilization of fat and increases availability of free fatty acids, but daily secretion is reduced in obesity. Leptin is a hormone produced by adipocytes and indicates satiety. Obesity is associated with leptin insensitivity but increased plasma levels. Functional residual capacity declines with increasing obesity and the alveolar–arterial gradient increases linearly as the $\dot{V}/\dot{Q}$ mismatch worsens owing to airway collapse and increased shunt. The absolute blood volume is increased, but this value is low relative to actual body weight and this contributes to the increased left ventricular workload, leading to hypertrophy and reduced ventricular compliance.

Bray GA, Bouchard C. *Handbook of Obesity: Etiology and pathophysiology: Volume 1 of Handbook of Obesity.* London: Informa Healthcare, 2004.
Lotia S, Bellamy MC. Anaesthesia and morbid obesity. *Contin Educ Anaesth Crit Care Pain* 2008; 8: 151–6.
World Health Organization. *WHO Expert Consultation on Obesity: Preventing and Managing the Global Epidemic.* Geneva: WHO, 3–5 June 1997.

63a. True
63b. True
63c. True
63d. False
63e. False
Esters are comparatively unstable in solution, unlike amides, which have a shelf-life of up to 2 years. They are weak bases, with pK_a values above 7.4; thus at neutral pH they are predominantly ionized. Onset of action is closely related to pK_a, while potency is related to lipid solubility.

Peck TE, Hill SA, Williams M. *Pharmacology for Anaesthesia and Intensive Care*, 3rd edn. Cambridge: CUP, 2008.

64a. False
64b. True
64c. False
64d. True
64e. False
Prerequisites for venous air embolism (VAE) are a source of gas in communication with the venous system and a driving pressure difference; it is the volume of entrained air and the rate of accumulation that determine the morbidity, in addition to patient positioning. A VAE of approximately 2 mL/kg is associated with tachycardia, hypotension, arrhythmias, increased central venous pressures, a mill-wheel murmur, cyanosis and right heart strain patterns on ECG. Right-sided intracardiac emboli cause 'foaming' of ventricular blood, which results in reduction of effective cardiac output, and dead space ventilation is increased; these changes result in a reduction in $ETCO_2$. Interestingly, if CO_2 is the gas causing the embolization (i.e. during laparoscopic surgery with CO_2 insufflation) a biphasic response is seen on capnography. Initially there will be an increase in $ETCO_2$ due to absorption of CO_2 into the blood and subsequent excretion through the lungs, followed by a drop.

Joris JL. Anesthesia for laparoscopic surgery. In: Miller RD, ed. *Miller's Anesthesia*, 7th edn. New York: Churchill Livingstone, 2009.

65a. False
65b. True
65c. False
65d. False
65e. False
Right-to-left intracardiac shunts result in pulmonary oligaemia as deoxygenated caval blood is diverted from the right to the left systemic circulation. Pulmonary hypertension results from left-to-right shunts, which can progress to Eisenmenger's syndrome in which there is flow reversal across the defect. Prolonged inhalational induction occurs as pulmonary blood flow is diverted systemically without exposure to the anaesthetic agent's alveolar–arterial gradient; conversely, intravenous induction is faster owing to rapid rise in arterial blood levels thence perfusing the brain. A left-to-right shunt occurs in tetralogy of Fallot, which comprises a ventricular septal defect, overriding aorta, pulmonary outflow obstruction and right ventricular hypertrophy. A mill-wheel murmur is classically a feature of air embolism.

66a. False
66b. True
66c. True
66d. True
66e. False
Haemorrhage is one of the most serious complications following tonsillectomy. Primary haemorrhage is that which occurs within the first 24 hours and secondary haemorrhage occurs within 28 days following surgery. The National Prospective Post-Tonsillectomy Bleeding Audit reported:

- Incidence of primary haemorrhage was 0.6%; the majority in the first 6 hours
- Adults were at a higher risk than children

- Operations for quinsy (retropharyngeal abscess) and recurrent tonsillitis had the highest rates
- Blunt dissection techniques had lower rates than diathermy

Ravi R, Howell T. Anaesthesia for paediatric ear, nose and throat surgery. *Contin Educ Anaesth Crit Care Pain* 2007; 7: 33–7.
Royal College of Surgeons of England. *National Prospective Tonsillectomy Audit*. London: RCSENG, 2005.

67a. True
67b. False
67c. True
67d. True
67e. False
Naloxone is a substituted oxymorphone derivative and is used for the reversal of respiratory depression caused by opioid use; it is also used in the treatment of clonidine overdose. It is a competitive antagonist at μ-, δ- and κ-opioid receptor subtypes, and is metabolized in the liver, primarily by conjugation to glucuronide.

Sasada M, Smith S. *Drugs in Anaesthesia and Intensive Care*, 3rd edn. Oxford: OUP, 2003.

68a. False
68b. True
68c. False
68d. True
68e. False
Sarcoidosis is a multisystem disease of unknown aetiology, characterized by *non-caseating* granulomas, its presentation can be identical to berylliosis. It can affect any organ and occur in any age group but most commonly affects young adults, with greater prevalence and severity in populations of African descent. Symptoms are often vague but up to 50% present with respiratory symptoms or CXR findings; other features include fatigue, weight loss, arthralgia, dry eyes, anterior or posterior uveitis, peripheral lymphadenopathy, and erythema *nodosum*. Laboratory investigations can reveal lymphopenia, hypercalcaemia (due to disordered vitamin D metabolism), raised serum ACE levels and hyperprolactinaemia. Lung function classically shows a restrictive defect. Erythema marginatum occurs in rheumatic fever.

69a. True
69b. True
69c. False
69d. True
69e. False

The Modified Day-Surgery Discharge Criteria measure five parameters prior to home discharge:

Vital signs

- 2: Within 20% of preoperative values
- 1: 20–40% of preoperative values
- 0: >40% of preoperative values

Ambulation

- 2: Steady gait
- 1: Requires assistance to walk
- 0: Unable to mobilize

Pain/Surgical bleeding/Nausea and vomiting (for each category)

- 2: Minimal
- 1: Moderate
- 0: Severe

Patients who score a total of 9–10 are considered fit for discharge with an escort.

Association of Anaesthetists of Great Britain and Ireland. *Day Surgery*. London: AAGBI, 2005. Available at: www.aagbi.org/publications/guidelines/docs/daysurgery05.pdf.

Cahill H, Jackson I, McWhinnie D. *Guidelines about the Discharge Process and the Assessment for Fitness to Discharge*. British Association of Day Surgery Handbook Series. London: British Association of Day Surgery, 2002.

70a. False
70b. True
70c. False
70d. True
70e. True

Phaeochromocytoma is a tumour of chromaffin cells and 90% occur within the adrenal medulla; 10% are extraadrenal and 90% are benign. They may secrete adrenaline, noradrenaline or dopamine and the most common presenting feature is sustained hypertension. Phaeochromocytoma can also present with nausea, vomiting, persistent headaches and sweating, and can progress to end-organ damage resulting in acute myocardial infarction, pulmonary oedema and left ventricular failure, dilated cardiomyopathy or cerebrovascular accident. Definitive treatment is surgical, but the patient's blood pressure should be controlled preoperatively using α-blockers, and subsequently β-blockade can be used to control resulting tachycardia. Diagnosis is made biochemically with 24-hour urine collection, by finding raised plasma or urine catecholamine levels or urinary catecholamine metabolites (vanillylmandelic acid (VMA), metadrenaline or normetadrenaline). MRI or CT imaging can localize the tumour, but if it is extraadrenal, an uptake scan (*meta*-iodobenzylguanidine (MIBG) scan) may become necessary. 5-Hydroxyiadoleacetic acid (5-HIAA) is a serotonin metabolite and raised levels are found in carcinoid syndrome.

Marshall P. Endocrine surgery. In: Allman KG, Wilson IH, eds. *Oxford Handbook of Anaesthesia*, 2nd edn. Oxford: OUP, 2006.

71a. False
71b. False
71c. True
71d. True
71e. True
All local anaesthetics consist of a lipophilic aromatic group, an intermediate chain and a hydrophilic tertiary or quaternary amine. The intermediate chain can either be an amide or an ester. The names of amide local anaesthetics have a letter 'i' at some point preceding the '-aine' suffix; esters do not.

Ester local anaesthetics

- Cocaine
- Procaine
- Tetracaine

Amide local anaesthetics

- Lignocaine
- Prilocaine
- Bupivacaine
- Etidocaine

72a. False
72b. False
72c. False
72d. False
72e. True
Malignant hyperthermia is a pharmacogenetic autosomal dominant disorder, characterized by disordered calcium homeostasis within skeletal muscle. The definite triggers for malignant hyperthermia in susceptible patients are suxamethonium and inhalational anaesthetic agents, including ether. Neuraxial anaesthesia would not be appropriate in this instance, owing to pain associated with traction on the mesentery and potential extension of the surgical incision.

73a. True
73b. False
73c. True
73d. False
73e. True
The Clinical Staging System has been designed for use in resource-poor settings. Staging does not require a CD4 count. For the purpose of HIV case definitions for reporting and surveillance, children are defined as being younger than 15 years of age and adults as 15 years or older. The clinical

stages have been shown to correlate with survival, prognosis and progression of clinical disease without antiretroviral therapy in adults and children:

- *Stage 1*: asymptomatic, persistent generalized lymphadenopathy
- *Stage 2*: moderate (<10%) unexplained weight loss
- *Stage 3*: severe (>10%) unexplained weight loss
- *Stage 4*: HIV wasting syndrome

World Health Organization. *WHO Case Definitions of HIV for Surveillance and Revised Clinical Staging and Immunological Classification of HIV-Related Diseases in Adults and Children.* Geneva: WHO, 2007.

74a. True
74b. True
74c. False
74d. False
74e. True

Positive pressure applied at end-expiration during mechanical ventilation is termed positive end-expiratory pressure (PEEP). The same process applied to a spontaneous breathing cycle is named 'continuous positive airway pressure' or CPAP. PEEP is responsible for recruiting functionally closed alveoli, redistributing lung water and therefore reducing ventilation–perfusion (V/Q) mismatch; these factors contribute to an improvement in gas exchange. Successful recruitment results in increased pulmonary compliance; decreased compliance suggests over-distension of alveoli. Increased intrathoracic pressure can decrease venous return to the heart, which can result in a decreased right ventricular (RV) output; thus patients should ideally have an adequate circulating volume before PEEP is applied. Left ventricular (LV) preload is decreased as a function of decreased venous return, decreased ventricular compliance, decreased ventricular contractility and increased RV afterload; these changes result in decreased LV stroke volume. In patients with congestive heart failure, however, diastolic volume is elevated and cardiac output is relatively insensitive to a reduction in venous return. Application of PEEP can result in an increase in LV function as a result of decreased LV transmural pressure leading to decreased LV afterload.

PEEP decreases splanchnic blood flow; hepatic perfusion and portal venous drainage may be compromised. Renal blood flow may also be reduced, depending on the volaemic status and the degree of pressure applied. 'Best' PEEP is that which produces least shunting while minimizing reduction in cardiac output. 'Optimum' PEEP is that which maximizes oxygen delivery with lowest dead space/tidal volume ratio. 'Appropriate' PEEP describes that with the least dead space.

Mascia L, Zanierato M, Ranieri M. Positive end-expiratory pressure. In: Waldmann N, Soni N, Rhodes A. *Oxford Desk Reference: Critical Care.* Oxford: OUP, 2008.

Yentis S, Hirsch N, Smith G. *Anaesthesia and Intensive Care A to Z: An Encyclopaedia of Principles and Practice*, 4th edn. Oxford: Butterworth-Heinemann, 2009.

75a. False
75b. True
75c. True
75d. True
75e. False

The Braden scale for predicting pressure ulcer risk includes the following parameters, each of which are assessed and scored (1–4):

- sensory perception
- skin moisture (influenced by incontinence, sweat)
- activity
- mobility
- nutrition
- friction and shear (worsened by agitation and contractures)

A score ≥ 19 indicates no risk, patients with a score of ≤ 18 are considered to be at risk of developing pressure ulcers, while scores of ≤ 9 indicate very high risk.

Bergstrom N, Braden B, Kemp M, Champagne M, Ruby E. Predicting pressure ulcer risk: a multisite study of the predictive validity of the Braden scale. *Nurs Res* 1998; **47**: 261–9.

76a. False
76b. True
76c. False
76d. True
76e. True

In a brainstem-dead patient undergoing a beating-heart organ donation, endocrine failure dictates a requirement for hormone supplementation. Hypothalamo–pituitary axis dysfunction causes a significant fall in vasopressin (antidiuretic hormone, ADH), resulting in diabetes insipidus and necessitating replacement with desmopressin. Thyroid-stimulating hormone (TSH) levels decrease, leading to a fall in triiodothyronine (T_3). Although debated, the supplementation of T_3 to the donor has been shown to improve donor heart function in the recipient. Thyroxine (T_4) does not appear to undergo peripheral conversion to its active form T_3 in a brain-dead patient. Hyperglycaemia is common and thus insulin is required. The United Network for Organ Sharing recommends a three-drug 'hormone-resuscitation', which has led to a 22% increase in number of organs recovered. It comprises:

- vasopressin: 1 unit bolus, infusion at 0.5–2.5 U/h
- T_3: 4 µg bolus, infusion at 3 µg/h
- Insulin: 1 IU/h minimum titrated to blood glucose

In addition, high-dose methylprednisolone 15 mg/kg is also recommended.

Edgar P, Bullock R, Bonner S. Management of the potential heart-beating organ donor. *Contin Educ Anaesth Crit Care Pain* 2004; **4**: 86–90.

77a. True
77b. True
77c. True
77d. False
77e. False

Described in 1866 by John Langdon Down, the syndrome is the most common chromosomal disorder, affecting 1 in 700 live births. There is an exponential increase in incidence with maternal age (1 in 1400 at 25 years; 1 in 46 by 45 years). Survival is approximately 90% for 1 year and 45% survive until the age of 60 years. 95% of individuals possess trisomy 21, 4% translocation and 1% mosaic trisomy 21. Down's syndrome is a multisystem condition. Features include:

General appearance

- Characteristic appearance: brachycephaly, flat nasal bridge, single palmar crease
- Low birth weight
- Obesity from childhood

Respiratory

- Dysfunctional central respiratory drive
- Subglottic or tracheal stenosis
- Recurrent lower respiratory tract infections
- Obstructive sleep apnoea secondary to craniofacial deformities

Cardiovascular

- Congenital heart disease (16–60%), commonly atrioventricular canal defects, atrial septal defects, ventricular septal defects (most commonly), patent ductus arteriosus and tetralogy of Fallot
- Pulmonary hypertension as a result both of shunts and of obstructive sleep apnoea

Neurological

- Generalized hypotonia
- Laxity of joint ligaments
- Intellectual impairment (IQ 20–80)
- Epilepsy (10%)

Gastrointestinal

- Gastro-oesophageal reflux
- Anomalies (7%): obstruction, atresia, Hirschprung's disease

Others

- Immune system dysfunction making individuals prone to infections
- Polycythaemia (haematocrit values up to 70%)
- Hypothyroidism and type 1 diabetes are more common

- Atlantoaxial instability: excessive movement of spinal vertebrae can lead to compression of spinal cord in the spinal foramen

Trisomy 18 is Edwards' syndrome.

Allt JE, Howell CJ. Down's syndrome. *Contin Educ Anaesth Crit Care Pain* 2003; 3: 83–6.
Carvalho B. Miscellaneous problems. In: Allman KG, Wilson IH, eds. *Oxford Handbook of Anaesthesia*, 2nd edn. Oxford: OUP, 2006.

78a. False
78b. True
78c. True
78d. False
78e. True
Where available, lipase estimation is preferred over amylase for diagnosis of acute pancreatitis. Pancreatic lipase is four times more active than amylase, thus is less likely to be affected by chronic pancreatic insufficiency. Amylase and lipase may both accumulate in renal failure. Amylase may also be elevated in diabetic ketoacidosis, ectopic pregnancy and perforated duodenal ulcer among other pathologies. The Atlanta criteria are recommended for severity scoring, but in the UK the Glasgow system is the most widely used. A score of 3 or more indicates severe acute pancreatitis. Prognostic features that predict complications are clinical impression of severity, obesity, APACHE II >8 within 24 hours of admission and C-reactive protein (CRP) > 150 mg/L, Glasgow score >3 or persisting organ failure after 48 hours. There is no conclusive evidence to support enteral nutrition in all patients, but if support is required it should be used if it can be tolerated. CT grading of severity (Balthazar scale) comprises appearance of pancreas and necrosis to predict complications and death.

UK Working Party on Acute Pancreatitis. UK guidelines for the management of acute pancreatitis. *Gut* 2005; 54: 1–9.
Balthazar EJ. Acute pancreatitis: assessment of severity with clinical and CT evaluation. *Radiology* 2002; 223: 603–13.

79a. True
79b. True
79c. True
79d. True
79e. False
Thrombocytopenia is a platelet count below 100×10^9/L. Bleeding is more likely as the count falls. Thrombocytopenia is due to:

- *Decreased production*: bone marrow failure, B_{12} or folate deficiencies
- *Increased destruction or loss*: haemorrhage, idiopathic thrombocytopenic purpura (ITP), thrombotic thrombocytopenic purpura (TTP), infection, hypersplenism, heparin-induced thrombocytopenia, sulphonamides, quinine
- *Increased consumption*: DIC
- *Dilution*: massive transfusion
- *In vivo aggregation*

Thrombocytosis is uncommon in the ICU patient. Causes include infective or inflammatory processes, splenectomy, myeloproliferative disorders and essential thrombocythaemia.

Singer M, Webb AR. *Oxford Handbook of Critical Care*, 3rd edn. Oxford: OUP, 2009.

80a. True
80b. True
80c. True
80d. False
80e. True

Intraosseous cannulation allows rapid vascular access in an emergency using specially designed needles. The safest and easiest sites are the tibia (2–3 cm below the tibial tuberosity) and the femur (3 cm above the lateral condyle). Proximal fractures and osteomyelitis in the intended site are absolute contraindications. Signs suggesting correct position in the marrow include:

- convincing 'give' on entering the marrow cavity
- cannula staying in an upright position without support
- aspiration of blood

All resuscitation drugs can be given via this route, with the exception of bretylium

Hawkins KC. Transfer of the critically ill child. *Contin Educ Anaesth Crit Care Pain* 2002; **2**: 170–3.

81a. False
81b. True
81c. False
81d. False
81e. True

Counter-pulsation describes balloon inflation at onset of diastole, which cor-responds to the middle of the T-wave on the ECG and deflates immediately before systole (peak of the R-wave). This arrangement results in an increased gradient between aortic diastolic and left ventricular end-diastolic pressures; this optimizes coronary blood flow and systemic perfusion. The balloon is often inflated with helium, which confers rapid gas transfer from console to balloon because of its low density. In the event of balloon rupture, helium is easily absorbed into the bloodstream. Optimal placement for the balloon catheter tip is 2–3 cm distal to the origin of the subclavian artery.

Indications include acute myocardial infarction, acute mitral regurgitation and ventricular septal defects, cardiogenic shock (American College of Cardiology/American Heart Association guidelines consider this as a Class I indication when not reversed by pharmacological therapy) and refractory left ventricular failure. Contraindications include aortic regurgitation (an intra-aortic balloon pump (IABP) would worsen the magnitude), aortic dissection (the balloon may enter the false lumen, leading to further dissection or rupture), abdominal aortic aneurysms and peripheral vascular disease.

Krishna M, Zacharowski K. Principles of intra-aortic balloon pump counterpulsation. *Contin Educ Anaesth Crit Care Pain* 2009; **9**: 24–8.

Ryan TJ, Antman EM, Brooks NH, et al. American College of Cardiology/American Heart Association guidelines for the management of patients with acute myocardial infarction: executive summary and recommendations: a report of the American College of Cardiology/American Heart Association Task Force on Practice Guidelines (Committee on Management of Acute Myocardial Infarction). *Circulation* 1999; **100**: 1016–30.

82a. False
82b. True
82c. True
82d. False
82e. False

Streptococcus pneumoniae is the most frequent pathogen, comprising 36% of community-acquired pneumonia (CAP), 39% of hospital-acquired pneumonia and 21.6% of ICU pneumonia. Measurement of pneumococcal antigen should be reserved for severe cases of CAP. The latest (2004) update to the British Thoracic Society Guidelines has added the CURB-65 system for severity scoring:

- **C**onfusion (Abbreviated Mental Test Score <8)
- **U**rea >7 mmol/L
- **R**espiratory rate ≥30/min
- **B**lood pressure (<90 mmHg systolic or ≤60 mmHg diastolic)
- **A**ge >**65** years

A score of 3 or above is predictive for severe CAP. The mortality rate for severe CAP admitted to ICU is >50% in the UK. Multivariate analyses suggest that leukopenia is more important a variable than leukocytosis.

BTS. British Thoracic Society guidelines for the management of community acquired pneumonia in adults. *Thorax* 2001; 56(Suppl. 4): iv1–64.

83a. True
83b. True
83c. False
83d. False
83e. True

Autonomic neuropathy affects autonomic neurons of parasympathetic or sympathetic nervous systems, or both. It can be classified as:

Central: primary (i.e. Shy–Drager syndrome) or secondary (cerebrovascular accident, infection)
Peripheral: Diabetes mellitus, amyloidosis, Guillain–Barré syndrome, porphyria

Bedside tests of autonomic function include:

- Postural blood pressure: a drop of >30 mmHg in systolic blood pressure when standing indicates dysfunction

- Valsalva manoeuvre
- Sustained hand grip: normal response is tachycardia and an increase
  > 15 mmHg in diastolic blood pressure. Absence indicates presence of
  autonomic neuropathy.

Romberg's test is designed to test the dorsal column of the spinal
cord. Maddox wing tests ocular muscle imbalance.

Yentis S, Hirsch N, Smith G. *Anaesthesia and Intensive Care A to Z: An
Encyclopaedia of Principles and Practice*, 4th edn. Oxford: Butterworth-
Heinemann, 2009.

84a. True
84b. False
84c. True
84d. False
84e. True
Presentation of hypopituitarism depends on hormone deficiency. The
following hormones are secreted from the anterior pituitary, and
deficiencies lead to a wide range of signs and symptoms:

- adrenocorticotropic hormone (ACTH, corticotropin): adrenal
  insufficiency; hypoglycaemia, fatigue, weight loss, hyponatraemia;
  hyperpigmentation is a feature of Addison's disease
- thyroid-stimulating hormone (TSH): hypothyroidism; cold intolerance,
  constipation, weight gain, hair loss, depression
- growth hormone (GH): central obesity, muscle atrophy, growth retardation
  in children
- luteinizing hormone/follicle-stimulating hormone (LH/FSH): oligo/
  amenorrhoea, osteoporosis, infertility, loss of libido

Conversely, hypopituitarism leads to hyperprolactinaemia, due to loss of
inhibitory control by dopamine. Hypopituitarism is excluded by normal
morning cortisol levels (range 80–550 nmol/L).

Steroid and thyroid hormone maintenance therapy is essential for life.

85a. True
85b. True
85c. False
85d. False
85e. True
Presenting in the first 6 months, infantile pyloric stenosis is one of the most
common gastrointestinal abnormalities. It represents a medical emergency,
and correction of acid–base abnormalities and re-hydration are the primary
treatment goals prior to subsequent definitive treatment via a surgical pylor-
otomy. Incidence is 3 per 1000 live births, with a male predominance and
higher incidence in white populations. Typical presentation is in a term infant in
the 3rd to 5th week of life with progressive non-bilious vomiting, which may
become projectile and blood-tinged. Subsequent starvation can lead to glu-
curonyl transferase deficiency and jaundice. The infant may be ravenously
hungry yet fail to gain weight.

Regurgitation and vomiting result in loss of gastric acid, water, sodium, potassium and chloride. In a normal individual, vomiting results in loss of H^+ from the stomach and pancreatic HCO_3^- from the duodenum with a neutral effect on acid/base balance. However, in pyloric stenosis there is loss only of H^+, which results in a net effect of retained HCO_3^- and subsequent metabolic alkalosis. Decreased extracellular fluid (ECF) volume stimulates aldosterone production and the kidney attempts to conserve sodium at the expense of potassium. In an effort to maintain normal pH, H^+ ions in the glomerular filtrate are exchanged for potassium ions; alkalosis also drives an intracellular shift of potassium ions. These factors compound the existing hypokalaemia. When sodium exchange with potassium in the distal renal tubules reaches a maximal level, sodium is forced to exchange with H^+, resulting in the typical 'paradoxical' acidic urine in the context of metabolic alkalaemia.

This results in a *hypochloraemic, hypokalaemic, hyponatraemic metabolic alkalosis* with alkaline urine, which later may become *paradoxically acidic*. Medical management consists of correction of the metabolic abnormalities and restoration of the ECF volume. Surgery cannot commence until this has been achieved.

Fell D, Chelliah S. Infantile pyloric stenosis. *Contin Educ Anaesth Crit Care Pain* 2001; **1**: 85–8.

86a. False
86b. False
86c. False
86d. False
86e. False
ADRs can be divided into the more common Type A (predictable), which are dose-related and an extension of the drug's normal pharmacological response, and Type B (idiosyncratic) which are not dose-related and include anaphylaxis, malignant hyperthermia and halothane hepatitis. Most ADRs are caused by non-steroidal anti-inflammatory drugs (aspirin), diuretics and warfarin and account for approximately 6000 deaths per year in England. The Yellow Card Scheme is run by the Medicines and Healthcare Regulatory Agency (MHRA), advised by the Committee on Safety of Medicines (CSM), and was introduced following the thalidomide disaster in 1964. It allows reporting of suspected ADRs and, more recently, direct reporting by non-health-care professionals; it cover over-the-counter medications and herbal remedies. For long-established drugs, only serious reactions are reported, but for 'black triangle' drugs (newly licensed) all suspected ADRs should be filed as a Yellow Card. The scheme is described as an early warning system for the identification of previously unidentified ADRs.

Pirmohamed M, James S, Meakin S, et al. Adverse drug reactions as a cause of admission to hospital: prospective analysis of 18,820 patients. *BMJ* 2004; **329**: 15–19.

87a. False
87b. False
87c. True
87d. False
87e. True

Generalized convulsive status epilepticus is a medical emergency; it is defined as a generalized convulsion lasting 30 minutes or longer or repeated convulsions over 30 minutes without recovery of consciousness between convulsions. Management consists of:

- Protecting the patient and staff from harm
- Airway, breathing, circulation with 100% oxygen
- Intravenous access and administration of benzodiazepine: lorazepam (0.1 mg/kg) or diazepam (10–20 mg PR)
- Phenytoin infusion (15–17 mg/kg): can cause profound hypotension, thus must be administered slowly (50 mg/min). Fosphenytoin is a safe alternative
- Phenobarbital (10–15 mg/kg; administered 100 mg/min)
- Refractory status epilepticus (60–90 minutes) requires a general anaesthetic

Seizures are central nervous system dysfunctions; while a muscle relaxant may stop physical signs, the seizure may nevertheless continue. Consideration should be given to hypoglycaemia and alcohol withdrawal as causes of seizure activity; accordingly glucose and thiamine may be administered, respectively. Diagnosis is EEG-dependent and must not hinder emergency management.

Walker M. Status epilepticus: an evidence based guide. *BMJ* 2005; **331**: 673–7.

88a. True
88b. False
88c. False
88d. True
88e. False

Aortic dissection describes a tear in the intima that allows a column of blood to enter the aortic wall, separating the intima from adventitia and creating a false lumen. Commonly occurring in men aged 40–70 years, it carries a high mortality: 50% of patients will die within 48 hours, 70% in 1 week and 90% in 3 months. The prime factors for developing a dissecting aneurysm are a combination of high intraluminal pressure and medial damage. Predisposing factors are:

- male sex (M : F ratio of 3 : 1)
- afro-Caribbean race (rare in Oriental people)
- hypertension
- bicuspid or unicommissural aortic valve
- pregnancy
- syndromes (Turner's, Noonan's, Marfan's)

- other connective tissue disorders: Ehlers–Danlos syndrome, systemic lupus erythematosus, relapsing polychondritis, giant cell aortitis
- surgical aortotomy sites

Swanton RH. *Pocket Consultant Cardiology*, 5th edn. Oxford: Blackwell Science, 2003.

89a. True
89b. True
89c. True
89d. False
89e. False
Ankylosing spondylitis is an inflammatory arthritis of the sacroiliac joints and spine; the hallmark is sacroiliitis, leading to ankylosis in later stages of the disease. Prevalence varies between 0.1% and 2%, the male : female ratio is ~5 : 1 and the peak onset is between 15 and 35 years. There exists a strong predisposition associated with human leukocyte antigen (HLA) B27. Diagnosis is difficult owing to the nature of the disease and is usually made at a late stage, although MRI of the sacroiliac joints has proved a useful method. Treatment consists of NSAIDs, physiotherapy and corticosteroid injections into the joint. Extraarticular manifestations include anterior uveitis, aortic incompetence, cardiac conduction defects and pulmonary fibrosis. Foramen magnum stenosis is common in achondroplasia.

McVeigh CM, Cairns AP. Diagnosis and management of ankylosing spondylitis. *BMJ* 2006; 333: 581–5.

90a. False
90b. False
90c. True
90d. True
90e. True
Chronic smoking has a deleterious effect on most of the physiological systems, the most pronounced being the respiratory system.

- Carbon monoxide (CO) levels in smokers can rise to 10% (2% in normal patients). CO has a 240 times greater affinity for haemoglobin than oxygen. It causes a shift of the oxyhaemoglobin curve to the left, since carboxyhaemoglobin (COHb) binds more avidly to the oxygen, thus reducing oxygen delivery at tissue level
- Since the light absorbance of carboxyhaemoglobin is at the same wavelength as that of oxyhaemoglobin, saturation readings may be higher or normal
- FEV_1 declines at the rate of 60 mL/year in smokers compared with a normal decline of 20 mL/year
- Closing capacity and shunt fraction are markedly increased
- Airways of chronic smokers are much more irritable and prone to spasm

Moppett I, Curran J. Smoking and the surgical patient. *Contin Educ Anaesth Crit Care Pain* 2001; 1: 122–4.

2. Practice Paper 2: Questions

1. The Manley MP3 ventilator consists of:
   a. A reservoir bag
   b. Two unidirectional valves
   c. Three sets of bellows
   d. An adjustable pressure-limiting (APL) valve
   e. A cuirass

2. Concerning the premature neonate:
   a. Definition is birth before 37 weeks' gestation
   b. Surfactant production is inadequate before 36 weeks' gestation
   c. Hypoxia stimulates the central chemoreceptors
   d. Apnoea is pathological when >20 s duration
   e. Patent ductus arteriosus presents with central cyanosis

3. A 45-year-old patient admitted to ICU with pneumonia develops an upper gastrointestinal (GI) bleed; the following statements apply:
   a. Mortality is significantly higher for patients who develop bleeds in hospital
   b. The most common cause is varices
   c. The management of patients in specialized units has not shown a statistically significant reduction in mortality
   d. Severity can be determined by using the Rockall score
   e. Heat application is as effective as endoscopic injection of adrenaline

4. Regarding poisoning in children:
   a. Mortality has not declined following the reduction in pack sizes of certain drugs
   b. Carboxyhaemoglobin of 5% is fatal in neonates
   c. Urinary alkalinization increases elimination of drugs with a high pK_a
   d. Ingestion of 100 mg/kg of aspirin is considered toxic
   e. Children do not typically display alkalosis following salicylate overdose

5. Differential diagnoses for a 2-year-old child with inspiratory stridor and a fever include:
   a. Croup
   b. Inhaled foreign body
   c. Bronchiolitis
   d. Bacterial tracheitis
   e. Laryngeal haemangioma

6. **Indications for an emergency laparotomy include:**
   a. A 21-year-old patient with a gunshot wound to the abdomen with a blood pressure of 90/40 mmHg following completion of the primary survey
   b. Fresh rectal bleeding in a 71-year-old man on ICU
   c. Perforated duodenal ulcer with gas under the diaphragm on chest X-ray
   d. Sigmoid volvulus causing obstruction in a 65-year-old woman
   e. Haemoperitoneum following blunt trauma in a 34-year-old man

7. **Features of Paget's disease include:**
   a. Hypercalcaemia
   b. Raised alkaline phosphatase
   c. Loss of hearing
   d. Osteoporosis
   e. Low-output cardiac failure

8. **With regards to tracheal tubes:**
   a. A 15 mm connector at the proximal end is universal
   b. RAE is an acronym for Ring, Adair and Elwyn
   c. Armoured tracheal tubes cannot be cut
   d. A Montadon tube is used for patients with a tracheostomy
   e. The cuff should be filled with saline for laser surgery of the larynx and trachea

9. **During laser surgery for removal of a vocal cord polyp, a supraglottic airway fire occurs in the patient; the following therapeutic measures are appropriate:**
   a. Immediate discontinuation of the laser
   b. Flooding of the supraglottic area with hypertonic saline
   c. Attending to the patient with an ABC approach and ventilating with 100% oxygen
   d. Maintenance of a definitive airway with the existing endotracheal tube
   e. High-dose intravenous steroids

10. **Features of a venous air embolism (VAE) include:**
    a. An increase in Pa_{CO_2}
    b. Retinal gas bubbles
    c. Mill-wheel murmur as a late sign
    d. Rise in central venous pressure
    e. Normal chest X-ray

11. **When performing a sub-Tenon's block:**
    a. It is appropriate for retinal surgery
    b. The conjunctiva is raised in the inferonasal quadrant
    c. Akinesia is superior when compared with a peribulbar block
    d. Tenon's capsule is white
    e. It requires 3–5 mL of local anaesthetic

12. **Expected findings associated with hypothermia include:**
    a. Metabolic acidosis and hyperkalaemia with moderate hypothermia
    b. Dilated pupils with severe hypothermia
    c. U-waves with severe hypothermia
    d. Diuresis with severe hypothermia
    e. Coagulopathy with moderate hypothermia

13. **A man is brought to A&E with suspected organophosphate poisoning; the following is expected:**
    a. Atrioventricular block on ECG monitoring
    b. Paralysis
    c. Mydriasis
    d. Sweating
    e. Symptoms occurring 12–24 hours following exposure

14. **Brain natriuretic peptide (BNP) levels are increased with:**
    a. Acute pulmonary embolus
    b. Sepsis
    c. Renal failure
    d. Old age
    e. Heart failure

15. **A 65-year-old man presents with a suspected massive pulmonary embolus (PE); appropriate investigations and management include:**
    a. D-dimers
    b. CT pulmonary angiography (CTPA) within 1 hour
    c. Alteplase 50 mg intravenously
    d. Leg ultrasound
    e. Intravenous heparin prior to imaging

16. **The following is correct of epilepsy:**
    a. Absence seizures are a form of partial epilepsy
    b. Partial seizures can progress to generalized seizures
    c. Febrile convulsions can lead to an increased risk of developing epilepsy
    d. Consciousness is impaired in simple partial seizures
    e. It is most commonly idiopathic

17. **False low oxygen saturation readings can be expected in the following situations:**
    a. A 65-year-old lady undergoing a parathyroidectomy who is administered methylene blue
    b. An alcoholic patient with severe jaundice
    c. A patient on ICU who is administered indocyanine green for cardiac output measurement
    d. Following a Bier's block with prilocaine
    e. A young man extracted from a house fire

18. **Complex regional pain syndrome (CRPS):**
    a. Occurs with an identifiable nerve injury in Type I
    b. Is cured by amputation of the affected limb
    c. More commonly affects women
    d. Is excluded by the lack of an initiating noxious event in Type I
    e. Is accompanied by normal plain X-rays of the affected area in 30% of patients

19. **As regards the Vaughan Williams classification, the following is correct of anti-arrhythmic drugs:**
    a. Quinidine is Class Ia
    b. Amiodarone is Class III
    c. Procainamide is Class Ia
    d. Flecainide is Class Ib
    e. Bretylium is Class Ic

20. **Independent patient-related risk factors for postoperative vomiting (POV) in children include:**
    a. Anxiety
    b. Age over 3 years
    c. Previous history of motion sickness
    d. Obesity
    e. Previous history of postoperative vomiting

21. **Concerning latex allergy:**
    a. It is more common in asthmatics
    b. It is associated with allergy to kiwi fruit
    c. It is more commonly a type I hypersensitivity reaction
    d. Patients should be admitted the night before surgery
    e. Prophylactic corticosteroids are recommended

22. **A ventricular catheter used to measure intracranial pressure (ICP):**
    a. Is the gold standard
    b. Can be used to administer drugs
    c. Is placed in the fourth ventricle
    d. Uses the foramen of Munro as the reference point for the transducer
    e. Can be antibiotic-impregnated

23. **A young woman presents with a decreased conscious level and hypotension. Her urine output is 400–500 mL/h and she has a plasma sodium level of 156 mmol/L; the following is likely:**
    a. Syndrome of inappropriate ADH secretion (SIADH)
    b. Cerebral salt wasting syndrome
    c. Diabetes insipidus (DI)
    d. Urinary sodium >20 mmol/L
    e. Addisonian crisis

24. Postoperative complications of robotic laparoscopic surgery include:
    a. Airway oedema
    b. Paralytic ileus
    c. Delayed emergence from general anaesthesia
    d. Conjunctival burns
    e. Compartment syndrome of the lower limb

25. An asymptomatic patient presents for elective hernia repair with a 62 mmHg peak gradient across the aortic valve; the following is correct:
    a. This patient has critical aortic stenosis (AS)
    b. The valve area must be reduced by more than 50% to produce this gradient
    c. Cardiac ischaemia occurs commonly with normal coronary arteries
    d. A high left ventricular end-diastolic pressure (LVEDP) is ideal perioperatively
    e. Tachycardia should be avoided

26. Electroencephalogram (EEG) rhythms have the following properties:
    a. Wakefulness is characterized by β-wave activity
    b. β-waves have a higher frequency than δ-waves
    c. α-waves have the lowest frequency
    d. δ-waves can be normal in children
    e. θ-waves are seen in sleep

27. Blockade of the median nerve at the wrist results in:
    a. Weakness of opponens pollicis
    b. Weakness of adductor pollicis brevis
    c. Weakness of pronator teres
    d. Anaesthesia of the dorsal tip of the index finger
    e. Anaesthesia of the lateral palmar aspect of the ring finger

28. With regards to electrical safety, equipment design in the UK fulfils the following characteristics:
    a. Adherence to BS 5950
    b. Class I: double insulation
    c. Class III: conducting parts connected to earth
    d. Type B: maximum leakage <100 μA
    e. Type CF: maximum leakage <10 μA

29. The following colour-coding applies to gas cylinders in the UK:
    a. Helium: brown body with white shoulders
    b. CO_2: grey body with grey shoulders
    c. Air: grey body with black and white shoulders
    d. N_2O: blue body with blue shoulders
    e. Cyclopropane: orange body with white checked shoulders

30. An elderly patient is undergoing an elective hernia repair under general anaesthesia; Recommendations for Standards of Monitoring During Anaesthesia as set out by the Association of Anaesthetists of Great Britain and Ireland (AAGBI) state that:
    a. Airway pressure should be recorded
    b. A temperature probe must be available
    c. A single-handed anaesthetist cannot leave the patient during anaesthesia
    d. A stethoscope is no longer mandatory
    e. If the patient elects for regional anaesthesia, continued presence of the anaesthetist is still required

31. 2,3-Diphosphoglycerate (2,3-DPG) levels are increased in:
    a. High altitude
    b. Pregnancy
    c. Hyperthyroidism
    d. Acidosis
    e. Hypopituitarism

32. Blood lactate:
    a. Is a buffer
    b. Should be collected in a heparin fluoride tube
    c. Is assayed specifically for the D-isomer
    d. Provides assessment of regional perfusion
    e. Is hydrolysed by lactate dehydrogenase (LDH)

33. A fluid challenge:
    a. Can be adequately performed using packed red cells
    b. Resulting in a rise in central venous pressure (CVP) of <3 mmHg indicates an adequate circulating volume
    c. Resulting in a normal pulmonary artery wedge pressure (PAWP) represents euvolemia
    d. Should consist of 20 mL/kg of crystalloid in the septic patient
    e. Should be monitored using cardiac output rather than stroke volume

34. *Clostridium difficile:*
    a. Is a Gram-negative aerobe
    b. Spores are destroyed by alcohol hand gel
    c. Is a commensal in up to 60% of the general population
    d. Is eradicated by intravenous vancomycin
    e. Colonization can be asymptomatic

35. Meticillin-resistant *Staphylococcus aureus* (MRSA):
    a. Is a Gram-positive bacillus
    b. Is a facultative anaerobe
    c. Most commonly colonizes the respiratory tract
    d. Is destroyed by chlorhexidine hand wash
    e. Is sensitive to glycopeptide antibiotics

36. Regarding humidification:
    a. Ultrasonic nebulizers rely on the Bernoulli effect
    b. Fully saturated air at 20°C contains 17 g/m^3 water vapour at sea level
    c. At an altitude of 5000 feet, fully saturated air at 20°C contains less water vapour compared with sea level
    d. Back-pressure at the outlet will reduce efficiency of gas-driven nebulizers
    e. Droplets of 5 μm reach the tracheal region

37. The solutions below are correctly matched with respective sodium concentrations (in mmol/L):
    a. Bicarbonate 8.4%: 1000
    b. Glucose 5%: 30
    c. Hartmann's: 111
    d. 0.9% saline: 154
    e. Gelofusine: 154

38. Cricoid pressure:
    a. Should consist of 10 N at induction
    b. Should reach a maximum of 50 N
    c. Is discontinued if the patient actively vomits
    d. Is continued for laryngeal mask insertion during management of a difficult airway
    e. Risks airway obstruction when performed concurrently with a BURP manouvere

39. The jugular foramen transmits the following structures:
    a. Hypoglossal nerve
    b. Glossopharyngeal nerve
    c. Vagus nerve
    d. Internal jugular vein
    e. Middle meningeal artery

40. With respect to fentanyl, alfentanil demonstrates a:
    a. Shorter half-life
    b. Lower volume of distribution
    c. Lower fraction bound to plasma protein
    d. Lower lipid solubility
    e. Higher pK_a

41. N-acetylcysteine is administered via the following routes:
    a. Oral
    b. Intramuscular
    c. Nebulized
    d. Intravenous
    e. Subcutaneous depot

42. A young woman is brought into A&E with a history of aspirin overdose; she is tachypnoeic and unconscious with a GCS of 6 (E2 V2 M2). The following is correct:
    a. Serum salicylate levels do not determine prognosis
    b. Immediate management should include nasogastric tube placement and activated charcoal administration
    c. Urinary alkalinization is appropriate
    d. Haemofiltration is indicated for salicylate levels >3.3 mmol/L
    e. Hypoglycaemia is likely

43. Concerning diabetes mellitus:
    a. Diagnostic criteria include fasting plasma glucose of ≥ 6.0 mmol/L
    b. Diagnosis can be made using HbA_{1c} values
    c. For diagnosis of impaired glucose tolerance, random plasma glucose must be ≤ 11.1 mmol/L
    d. For major surgery, perioperative steroid cover is indicated
    e. It is the single biggest risk factor for spinal infection following epidural drug delivery

44. Appropriate drug treatment for a patient with an acute exacerbation of asthma includes:
    a. Ipratropium
    b. Theophylline
    c. Sodium cromoglycate
    d. Salbutamol
    e. Aminophylline

45. Concerning computed tomography (CT):
    a. It involves ionizing radiation
    b. It involves application of radiofrequency pulses
    c. 'Omnipaque' is an iodinated contrast agent
    d. 'Omnipaque' is a hyperosmolar contrast agent
    e. The biological effects of radiation are measured in Grays (Gy)

46. Serum urea and electrolytes should be measured in the following patients presenting for elective surgery:
    a. A hypertensive 61-year-old scheduled for middle ear drainage
    b. A 25-year-old on lithium therapy scheduled for tooth extraction
    c. An asthmatic 65-year-old scheduled for varicose veins surgery
    d. A 35-year-old on metolazone therapy scheduled for bronchoscopy
    e. A neonate presenting for herniorrhaphy

47. **Regarding blood gas analysis:**
    a. The pH will be lower if analysis is made at a lower temperature than the patient
    b. Standard bicarbonate is corrected for an abnormal partial pressure of CO_2 (P_{CO_2})
    c. Excess heparin will lower the pH of the sample
    d. The base excess is the amount of strong acid or base required to titrate a litre of blood to a pH of 7.4 and P_{CO_2} of 5.3 kPa at 37°C
    e. The Siggard–Andersen nomogram plots log arterial bicarbonate against plasma pH

48. **The Wilson scoring system:**
    a. Comprises four predictive factors
    b. Scores buck teeth
    c. Scores each factor on a three-point scale
    d. Is predictive of a difficult airway if the total score is greater than 4
    e. Scores weight

49. **A 25-year-old primigravida who is 10 weeks pregnant requires an appendicectomy and undergoes a rapid sequence induction using thiopentone and suxamethonium. She suffers from a prolonged period of paralysis after the operation, lasting more than 1 hour; the following statements apply:**
    a. She is likely to be heterozygous for cholinesterase genes
    b. Mivacurium administration at induction would have avoided this situation
    c. The normal genotype is Eu:Eu for cholinesterase
    d. Pregnancy may result in prolonged paralysis
    e. Dibucaine number increases with reduction of cholinesterase activity

50. **Concerning obstructive sleep apnoea (OSA):**
    a. Apnoea is defined as cessation of airflow for greater than 5 s
    b. Is defined as more than 10 episodes of apnoea or hypopnoea per hour of sleep
    c. An Apnoea Hypopnoea Index (AHI) of 5 is considered normal
    d. Grade 1 is defined by an AHI of 10–30
    e. Grade 4 patients are prone to cor pulmonale

51. **Activated protein C (APC):**
    a. Is a glycoprotein
    b. Recombinant form is administered continuously as an infusion over 48 hours
    c. Is vitamin K-dependent
    d. Is inactivated by thrombin
    e. Deficiency leads to a paradoxical bleeding diathesis

52. Signs of an anastomotic leak following transhiatal oesophagectomy include:
    a. Chylothorax
    b. Atrial fibrillation
    c. Wound crepitus
    d. Fever
    e. Wound drainage

53. The HELLP syndrome:
    a. Occurs in approximately 3% of pregnant women
    b. Shows reduced risk of development in smokers
    c. Presents preterm in 80% of sufferers
    d. Shows reduced perinatal mortality with maternal administration of dexamethasone
    e. Requires arterial hypertension as a prerequisite for diagnosis

54. The following statements are correct of statistical definitions:
    a. A false positive is a type I error
    b. A false negative rejects the null hypothesis when it is true
    c. A true positive is the ability of the test to be positive in the presence of the disease
    d. The positive predictive value is also known as precision rate
    e. Sensitivity is the ability to correctly identify people without a disease

55. The following agents are nephrotoxic:
    a. Amphotericin
    b. Captopril
    c. Furosemide
    d. Cimetidine
    e. Phenytoin

56. An increased alveolar–arterial (A–a) gradient is expected in:
    a. Ageing
    b. Cardiopulmonary bypass
    c. Tetralogy of Fallot
    d. A large ventricular septal defect
    e. Bronchoconstriction

57. Concerning the neonatal circulation:
    a. It changes from a parallel to a series system
    b. Permanent closure of the foramen ovale (FO) takes 4 hours
    c. The ductus arteriosus (DA) closes in response to decreasing prostaglandin E (PGE) levels
    d. The ductus venosus (DV) closes 4 weeks after birth
    e. Pulmonary artery pressure (PAP) decreases to adult values in 2 weeks

58. **Regarding preoxygenation:**
    a. Oxygen consumption ($\dot{V}O_2$) in the awake adult is approximately 3 mL/kg/min
    b. $\dot{V}O_2$ in the anaesthetized patient is approximately 3 mL/kg/min
    c. Mass movement of O_2 can maintain SaO_2 for over 1 hour
    d. Application of 100% O_2 via a patent airway prevents the development of acidosis
    e. $\dot{V}O_2$ in the term parturient is approximately 3 mL/kg/min

59. **Regarding severity scoring systems:**
    a. APACHE II is measured during the first 24 hours of admission
    b. SOFA has been validated for trauma patients
    c. WFNS Scale is used to assess outcome of head injury
    d. SAPS III predicts physiological status at ICU discharge
    e. MODS is performed on a daily basis

60. **When using intercostal chest drains:**
    a. Large-bore drains are more effective than small-bore drains for air drainage
    b. No evidence exists that clamping a drain at removal is beneficial
    c. Large-bore drains are effective for bronchopleural fistulae
    d. If applied, suction pressure should be -10 to -20 mmHg
    e. The most common point of insertion is in the mid-axillary line

61. **Concerning perioperative acute renal failure (ARF):**
    a. Incidence is increasing
    b. Is less likely with endovascular than an open repair of abdominal aortic aneurysms
    c. Pharmacological interventions are not effective in protecting renal function
    d. Low-dose dopamine does not offer clinically significant renal protection
    e. N-acetylcysteine is protective against radiocontrast nephropathy

62. **The listed murmurs are associated with the corresponding pathology:**
    a. Ejection: aortic stenosis
    b. Pansystolic: mitral regurgitation
    c. Pansystolic: ventricular septal defect
    d. Diastolic: mitral stenosis
    e. Continuous: patent ductus arteriosus

63. **The Fick principle can be used to measure:**
    a. Cardiac output
    b. Renal blood flow
    c. Diffusion across a membrane
    d. Cerebral blood flow
    e. Oxygen consumption

64. Cardioselective β-blockers include:
    a. Atenolol
    b. Labetalol
    c. Esmolol
    d. Propranolol
    e. Sotalol

65. Ideal characteristics of nerve stimulator devices for performing regional nerve blockade include:
    a. Constant-current output
    b. Constant-voltage output
    c. Current magnitude up to 5 A
    d. Square wave unipolar stimulus
    e. Stimulus duration of 1–2 ms

66. Concerning peribulbar anaesthesia:
    a. Complications include subarachnoid injection
    b. The inferolateral approach involves the junction of maxilla and zygoma
    c. The junction of the cornea and iris is called the limbus
    d. It carries less risk when axial length is >27 mm
    e. Medial approach is performed medial to the caruncle

67. A 32-year-old man undergoing a craniotomy in the sitting position develops a massive venous air embolism (VAE); the following statements regarding positioning the patient are correct:
    a. He should be placed in the Durant position
    b. Trendelenburg will exacerbate the symptoms of VAE
    c. He should be right lateral decubitus
    d. The aim is to drive the embolus through the right ventricle
    e. VAE cannot occur in the supine position

68. Complications seen following recovery from drowning include:
    a. Seizures
    b. ARDS
    c. Rhabdomyolysis
    d. Hyperthermia
    e. Pneumothorax

69. The following are correct for the LeFort classification system:
    a. Grade IV fractures are associated with base-of-skull fractures
    b. It applies to mandibular and maxillary fractures
    c. Grade I describes transverse fractures of mid-lower maxilla
    d. Grade II describes cribriform plate disruption
    e. Grade III describes fractures continuing from the top of the nose to the base of the maxilla

70. **A 50-year-old patient has undergone a laparotomy for intestinal obstruction; the following are likely:**
    a. Hypoglycaemia
    b. ACTH release from the anterior pituitary
    c. Sodium retention
    d. Hypokalaemia
    e. Cortisol levels >1500 μmol/L

71. **Glucose-6-phosphate dehydrogenase (G6PD) deficiency:**
    a. Confers resistance to malaria
    b. Is more common in females
    c. Is an autosomal recessive disorder
    d. Is a contraindication for suxamethonium
    e. Causes haemolysis in patients on ciprofloxacin therapy

72. **The filling ratio:**
    a. Is defined as the mass of gas in a cylinder divided by the mass of gas that would fill the cylinder
    b. Is defined as the mass of gas in a cylinder divided by the mass of liquid that would fill the cylinder
    c. Is applicable to substances below their critical temperature
    d. Is 0.75 for nitrous oxide in tropical climates
    e. Is 0.67 for nitrous oxide in temperate climates

73. **Bupivacaine:**
    a. Exhibits biphasic central nervous system effects
    b. Has a lower rate of systemic absorption when adrenaline is added
    c. Is highly protein-bound
    d. Has 80 mg/mL dextrose added to produce a 'heavy' version
    e. Has a direct vasodilatory effect

74. **A patient undergoing a thoracotomy with one-lung ventilation (OLV) becomes hypoxic; the following management is appropriate:**
    a. Insufflation of oxygen into the collapsed lung
    b. Application of continuous positive airway pressure (CPAP) to the collapsed lung
    c. Administration of a pulmonary vasodilator
    d. Application of 10–15 cmH$_2$O positive end-expiratory pressure (PEEP) to the collapsed lung
    e. Return to two-lung ventilation

75. **The Association of Anaesthetists of Great Britain and Ireland guidelines for management of suspected perioperative anaphylaxis include:**
    a. Adrenaline 50 μg intravenously for adults
    b. Chlorphenamine 20 mg intravenously
    c. Intravenous salbutamol for persistent bronchospasm
    d. Reporting of perioperative cases to the MHRA
    e. Administration of metaraminol if adrenaline infusion is unsuccessful

76. **Epidural analgesia in labour is associated with:**
    a. Increased rate of caesarean section
    b. Increased rate of instrumental vaginal delivery
    c. Increased duration of labour
    d. Back pain
    e. Maternal pyrexia

77. **The following is correct of the oesophageal Doppler:**
    a. FTc is cumulative flow time
    b. Peak velocity of aortic blood is a good estimate of myocardial contractility
    c. Stroke volume is the area under the waveform
    d. The aortic diameter is measured
    e. FTc is normally 330–360 ms

78. **The following are correct for hepatic encephalopathy:**
    a. Scoring consists of five grades
    b. Stupor is consistent with Grade 2
    c. Cerebral oedema is the leading cause of death
    d. Dietary protein restriction is recommended
    e. Definitive diagnosis is made with brain imaging

79. **Features indicative of a proximal bronchial carcinoma include:**
    a. Pleuritic chest wall pain
    b. Superior vena cava obstruction
    c. Hoarse voice
    d. Enophthalmos
    e. Haemoptysis

80. **Clinical features of hypocalcaemia include:**
    a. Tetany
    b. Hypotension
    c. Prolonged QT interval
    d. Convulsions
    e. Perioral paraesthesiae

81. **Examples of non-cutting spinal needles include:**
    a. Sprotte
    b. Quincke
    c. Whitacre
    d. Greene
    e. Tuohy

82. The following are correct of intravenous crystalloid solutions when compared with plasma:
    a. 0.9% sodium chloride is isosmolar
    b. 0.18% sodium chloride/glucose 4% is isosmolar
    c. 0.45% sodium chloride/glucose 5% is hypotonic
    d. 0.9% sodium chloride/glucose 5% is hyperosmolar and isotonic with reference to a cell membrane
    e. 10% glucose is hyperosmolar and hypotonic with reference to a cell membrane

83. According to the DeBakey classification for aortic dissections:
    a. There are five types
    b. Type II involves the distal part of the abdominal aorta
    c. Types III and IV are classified according to whether the dissection extends above and beyond the diaphragm
    d. Type I involves the ascending and descending aorta
    e. Type III is subdivided into A and B

84. Recognized side-effects of erythropoietin (EPO) include:
    a. Red cell aplasia
    b. Hypertension
    c. Heart failure
    d. Bronchoconstriction
    e. Altered coagulation

85. An infant presents for correction of a cleft palate; the following statements are correct:
    a. Continuous nasal discharge warrants postponement of surgery
    b. Intubation becomes more difficult with age in Pierre Robin sequence
    c. Polycythaemia is common
    d. Specific guidelines recommend optimal timing of surgery
    e. Low-grade infections preoperatively should not be treated with antimicrobial therapy

86. The following statements regarding WFNS grading system for subarachnoid haemorrhage (SAH) are correct:
    a. WFNS is an acronym for 'World Federation of Neuroscientists Scale'
    b. Grade 1 represents GCS 15 without any motor deficit
    c. Grade 1 is associated with over 80% recovery
    d. Grade 3 indicates the presence of a motor deficit
    e. Grade 5 indicates greatest severity on the scale

87. Dysphagia is a feature of:
    a. Diabetes
    b. Chagas' disease
    c. Scleroderma
    d. Plummer–Vinson syndrome
    e. Multiple sclerosis

88. **The following is correct for cerebral venous drainage:**
    a. The superior sagittal sinus drains into the left transverse sinus
    b. Deep structures drain into the internal cerebral vein on each side
    c. The external cerebral vein from each side combines to form the great cerebral vein
    d. The great cerebral vein is also called the vein of Galen
    e. All veins drain ultimately into the internal jugular veins on each side

89. **At an altitude of 10 000 feet:**
    a. Oxygen concentrators cannot be used
    b. Flowmeters set to a flow rate of 10 L/min will deliver a higher gas flow than dialled
    c. Barometric pressure is 40 kPa
    d. Venturi devices are inaccurate
    e. Gas viscosity is increased compared with sea level

90. **The total body water compositions listed are correct:**
    a. Preterm: 80%
    b. Neonate: 65%
    c. 1 year: 65%
    d. 3 years: 60%
    e. Adult: 40%

2. Practice Paper 2: Answers

1a. True
1b. False
1c. False
1d. True
1e. False
The Manley MP3 ventilator is a minute volume divider; it consists of two sets of bellows (a smaller time-cycling bellows receives fresh gas flow and empties into the main bellows), three unidirectional valves (one between bellows, the second between bellows and patient, the third between patient and an adjustable pressure-limiting (APL) valve), an APL valve and a reservoir bag.

2a. True
2b. False
2c. False
2d. True
2e. False
Prematurity is defined as live birth before 37 weeks' gestation from the first day of the last menstrual period. Before 32–34 weeks, surfactant synthesis is inadequate and preterm neonates are at risk of respiratory distress syndrome. Chemoreceptor responses are blunted and hypoxia results in a direct depression of the chemoreceptors causing apnoea and bradycardia. Apnoeas are defined as pathological when >20 s duration or <20 s but accompanied by bradycardia, cyanosis, pallor or hypotonia. Patent ductus arteriosus leads to left-to-right cardiac shunting with increased pulmonary blood flow and eventually pulmonary hypertension; cyanosis can then occur owing to reversal of shunt (Eisenmenger's syndrome).

Peiris K, Fell D. The prematurely born infant and anaesthesia. *Contin Educ Anaesth Crit Care Pain* 2009; **9**: 73–7.

3a. True
3b. False
3c. False
3d. True
3e. True
Upper GI bleeding is defined as bleeding arising from anywhere between the proximal oesophagus and the ligament of Treitz (duodenojejunal flexure). Acute upper GI bleeds have an incidence of 50–150 per 100 000. The mortality for patients admitted with a bleed is 10%; compared with 30% for those who develop bleeds during their hospital stay. The most common cause of bleeds in hospital is peptic ulcers (35–50%), followed by gastroduodenal erosions (8–15%), oesophagitis (5–15%) and varices (5–10%). The management of these patients in specialized units has reduced mortality from 11% to 5%. The severity is assessed by the Rockall score, which is based on age,

comorbidities, haemodynamic status, diagnosis and risk of re-bleeding as assessed endoscopically. Upper GI bleeding can be managed by:

- endoscopic injection with 1:10 000 adrenaline
- heat application by probes or multipolar coagulation (as effective as adrenaline)
- mechanical clips
- surgery
- angiographic embolization

Booth M. Upper gastrointestinal haemorrhage (non-variceal). In: Waldmann N, Soni N, Rhodes A, eds. *Oxford Desk Reference: Critical Care*. Oxford: OUP, 2008.

4a. False
4b. False
4c. False
4d. False
4e. True
Mortality from poisoning in children has been declining since 1976. Legislation for reducing pack sizes has had a significant impact on mortality. Blood carboxyhaemoglobin concentration ranges from 2–5% in neonates, since carbon monoxide is a by-product of protoporphyrin metabolism. Urinary alkalinization increases elimination of drugs with a low pK_a; this increases the ionized fraction presented to the tubular lumen, which prevents re-absorption. Aspirin use in children is associated with Reye's syndrome. Toxicity is related to amount ingested:

- <150 mg/kg is considered non-toxic
- 150–300 mg/kg leads to signs of mild to moderate toxicity
- >500 mg/kg is potentially life-threatening

Hawton K, Simkin S, Deeks J, et al. UK legislation on analgesic packs: before and after study of long term effect on poisonings. *BMJ* 2004; **329**: 1076–9.
Penny L, Moriarty T. Poisoning in children. *Contin Educ Anaesth Crit Care Pain* 2009; **9**: 109–13.

5a. True
5b. True
5c. False
5d. True
5e. False
Foreign bodies are the most common indication for bronchoscopy in the 1–3-year-old age group, and while foreign body aspiration can present as acute upper airway obstruction, it can be complicated by secondary pneumonia or abscess formation. Laryngeal haemangiomas are extremely rare; 85% present

before 6 months of age and typically have biphasic stridor without a fever. Other infective conditions are as follows:

Condition	Age group	Clinical syndrome	Most common cause
Croup	Peak age: 2 (6 months– 2 years)	Inspiratory stridor, respiratory distress barking cough, hoarseness	Parainfluenza, respiratory syncytial virus
Bacterial tracheiitis		Stridor, toxic, high fever, purulent secretions	*Staphylococcs aureus*, streptococci, *Haemophilus influenzae* type b
Epiglottitis	2–6 years	High fever, lethargy, inspiratory stridor, toxic	*Haemophilus influenzae* type b
Bronchiolitis	1–9 months	Fever, nasal discharge, dry cough	Respiratory syncytial virus

Advanced Life Support Group. *Advanced Paediatric Life Support: A Practical Approach*. Oxford: Wiley-Blackwell, 2004.
Spencer S, Yeoh BH, Van Asperen PP, et al. Biphasic stridor in infancy. *Med J Aust* 2004; **180**: 347–9.

6a. True
6b. False
6c. True
6d. False
6e. True
Abdominal gunshot wounds in unstable patients mandate exploratory laparotomy following the ABC approach of ATLS teaching. Fresh blood per rectum may indicate per-anal or rectal pathology and should always be investigated but does not warrant a laparotomy unless torrential bleeding occurs. Volvulus can be treated conservatively by decompression with rigid sigmoidoscopy, which is successful in 70–90% of patients; however, definitive surgery is necessary, since recurrence rates are high. If gangrene has occurred then laparotomy is indicated and decompression should not be performed. Although haemoperitoneum can be managed conservatively, in the context of blunt trauma this requires exploratory laparotomy.

Madiba TE, Thomson SR. The management of sigmoid volvulus. *J R Coll Surg Edinb* 2000; **45**: 74–80.
Marx JA, Isenhour JL. Abdominal trauma. In: Marx JA, ed. *Rosen's Emergency Medicine: Concepts and Clinical Practice*. St Louis, MO: Mosby, 2006.

7a. False
7b. True
7c. True
7d. False
7e. False
Primarily a disorder of osteoclasts, Paget's disease is characterized by massively increased bone turnover with three stages of disease progression: an osteoclastic bone resorption phase, an osteoclastic/blastic phase involving disorganized bone deposition and an exhaustive phase. It is more common in men and is rare before the age of 30 years. Bone pain is common, and hearing loss occurs when skull bones are involved. Classical biochemical findings are raised alkaline phosphatase with normal blood calcium and phosphate levels; osteoporosis is not a feature but can coexist. The new bone is metabolically active and arteriovenous connection can form leading to high-output cardiac failure.

Kumar P, Clark M. *Kumar and Clark's Clinical Medicine*, 7th edn. London: Saunders, 2009.

8a. False
8b. True
8c. True
8d. True
8e. True
The British Standard connector has a 15 mm diameter at the proximal end. An 8.5 mm diameter version exists for neonatal use. Ring, Adair and Elwyn (RAE) tubes have a preformed shape to fit the mouth or nose without kinking. Armoured tracheal tubes contain a spiral of metal wire or tough nylon and as such cannot be cut to length. Air-filled cuffs may ignite during laser surgery, so it is recommended that cuffs be filled with saline. A laryngectomy (Montadon) tube is a cuffed tube designed to facilitate positive-pressure ventilation in patients with a tracheostomy.

Al-Shaikh B, Stacey S. *Essentials of Anaesthetic Equipment*, 3rd edn. London: Churchill Livingstone, 2007.

9a. True
9b. False
9c. False
9d. False
9e. True
LASER is an acronym for 'light amplification by stimulated emission of radiation'. Airway fires are a recognized and potentially life-threatening complication of laser use, particularly in upper airway surgery. In the event of an airway fire during laser surgery, immediate management should consist of:

- Stopping the laser and flooding the area with 0.9% saline or sterile water
- Disconnecting the endotracheal tube (ETT) from the breathing system
- Immediately clamping the end of the ETT
- Withholding jet ventilation if in use

- Reinstituting ventilation when the fire is extinguished
- Removing debris with the use of a rigid sucker
- Replacement of the ETT using an exchange catheter; despite a normal appearance, a burnt ETT may risk blowing debris into the airway

Administration of 100% oxygen will support combustion; therefore FiO_2 is kept to a minimum during laser surgery.

Cook T, Cranshaw J. Airway fire. In: Allman KG, McIndoe AK, Wilson IH, eds. *Emergencies in Anaesthesia*, 2nd edn. Oxford: OUP, 2009.

10a. True
10b. False
10c. True
10d. True
10e. True

Prerequisites for VAE are a source of gas in communication with the venous system and a driving pressure difference; it is the volume of entrained air and the rate of accumulation that determine the morbidity, in addition to patient positioning. A significant VAE will lead to a rise in pulmonary arterial pressures owing to obstruction to flow. While the alveolar partial pressure of carbon dioxide ($PACO_2$) will fall abruptly, the arterial partial pressure, $PaCO_2$, will rise owing to the reduction in gas exchange and increase in physiological dead space. Tachyarrhythmias are common; the classical mill-wheel murmur is a machinery-like sound caused by blood mixing with air in the right ventricle and is a late sign. The chest X-ray is initially normal and may later show pulmonary oedema. Retinal gas bubbles are seen classically in arterial air embolism, these can result from transpulmonary shunting of VAE to the systemic circulation, known as a 'paradoxical' embolus.

Webber S, Andrzejowski J, Francis G. Gas embolism in anaesthesia. *Contin Educ Anaesth Crit Care Pain* 2002; **2**: 53–7.

11a. True
11b. True
11c. False
11d. True
11e. True

Tenon's capsule is a layer of thin connective tissue surrounding the globe, fusing anteriorly with the conjunctiva at the limbus and extending posteriorly to fuse with the dura of the optic nerve. It is a safe and reliable alternative to retrobulbar and peribulbar techniques, but is not without risk and globe perforation has been reported during dissection with Westcott's spring scissors. The risk of bleeding is lower than that of a peribulbar block, but akinesia is not as effective.

Frieman BJ, Friedberg MA. Globe perforation associated with subtenon's anesthesia. *Am J Ophthalmol* 2001; **131**: 520–1.

12a. True
12b. True
12c. False
12d. True
12e. True
Effects of hypothermia are as follows:

Mild (32–35°C)

- Ataxia and in coordination
- Confusion and disorientation
- Shivering

Moderate (<28–32°C)

- Stupor
- Metabolic acidosis and hyperkalaemia
- Hypovolaemia
- Cold diuresis
- Coagulopathy
- Dilated pupils (marked and minimally light responsive at 28–30°C)
- J-waves on ECG
- Arrythmias and ↓cardiac output

Severe (<28°C)

- Loss of consciousness
- Ventricular fibrillation and cardiac arrest
- Apnoea
- Isoelectric EEG at 18°C

Blanshard H, Bennett D. Metabolic and endocrine. In: Allman KG, McIndoe AK, Wilson IH, eds. *Emergencies in Anaesthesia*, 2nd edn. Oxford: OUP, 2009.

13a. True
13b. True
13c. False
13d. True
13e. True
Organophosphates are highly lipophilic toxic compounds that phosphorylate the esteratic site of acetylcholinesterase; this forms a very stable molecular structure, irreversibly inactivating the enzyme. The clinical syndrome of toxicity usually occurs 12–24 hours following exposure and is due to excess acetylcholine stimulating autonomic ganglia, post-ganglionic parasympathetic neurons and the neuromuscular junction. The array of symptoms include muscarinic effects such as lachrymation, salivation, miosis, bronchospasm and nodal conduction delay. Nicotinic effects lead to fasciculations, paralysis and cardiovascular instability; central nervous system effects include ataxia, slurred speech, seizures and loss of consciousness. In addition, altered responses to muscle relaxants occur. Specific treatment involves decontamination, atropinization and pralidoxime or obidoxime, which reactivate phosphorylated acetylcholinesterase. Prolonged ventilation may be necessary.

Karalliedde L. Organophosphorus poisoning and anaesthesia. *Anaesthesia* 1999; 54: 1073–88.

14a. True
14b. True
14c. True
14d. True
14e. True
BNP is a polypeptide named after its discovery in porcine brain. In humans it is released from cardiac ventricles in response to chamber stretch. Elevated levels may be due to:

Cardiac

- Heart failure (correlates with New York Heart Association [NYHA] and Goldman activity classifications)
- Diastolic dysfunction
- Acute coronary syndrome
- Hypertension
- Valvular heart disease
- Atrial fibrillation

Non-cardiac

- Acute pulmonary embolus
- Pulmonary hypertension
- Sepsis
- Chronic obstructive pulmonary disease (COPD) with cor pulmonale or respiratory failure
- Hyperthyroidism

Felker GM, Peterson JW, Mark DB. Natriuretic peptides in the diagnosis and management of heart failure. *CMAJ* 2006; **175**: 611–17.
Hobbs FDR, Davis RC, Roalfe AK, et al. Reliability of N-terminal pro-brain natriuretic peptide assay in diagnosis of heart failure: cohort study in representative and high risk community populations. *BMJ* 2002; **324**: 1498.
Singer M, Webb AR. *Oxford Handbook of Critical Care*, 3rd edn. Oxford: OUP, 2009.

15a. False
15b. True
15c. True
15d. False
15e. True
D-dimers are useful where there is a reasonable suspicion of PE. They should not be measured if clinical probability is high, or in probable massive PE. In suspected massive PE, CTPA should be performed within 1 hour. In the event of clinical deterioration or cardiac arrest with a probable massive PE, thrombolysis is recommended and should consist of alteplase 50 mg intravenously. In stable patients, where massive PE has been confirmed, alteplase 100 mg intravenously is given over 90 minutes; 80 IU/kg heparin can be given prior to CTPA. Leg ultrasound is useful in the detection of venous thromboembolism, not PE.

British Thoracic Society Guidelines. Management of suspected acute pulmonary embolus. *Thorax* 2003; **58**: 470–84.

16a. False
16b. True
16c. True
16d. False
16e. True

Epilepsy is a chronic neurological disorder characterized by recurrent seizures affecting approximately 50 million people worldwide. The majority of cases are idiopathic, but secondary causes include head injury, intracranial tumour and meningitis. It can be categorized by type of seizures:

- *Partial (focal)*: abnormal electrical activity that remains localized (focal); can be simple (no loss of consciousness) or complex (temporal lobe epilepsy)
- *Secondary generalized*: a partial seizure progresses to a generalized seizure
- *Generalized*: abnormal electrical activity affecting whole or part of the brain leading to loss of consciousness; includes tonic–clonic seizures and absences (occur mainly in children with a brief loss of consciousness or awareness)

Febrile convulsions most commonly affect children between the ages of 1–4 years and, while the risk is extremely low, affected children have a slightly higher incidence of epilepsy.

17a. True
17b. False
17c. True
17d. True
17e. False

Pulse oximetry is a non-invasive measurement of arterial blood oxygen saturation at the level of the arterioles; it is simple, accurate and rapid. SaO_2 is estimated by measuring the transmission of light through a pulsatile vascular tissue bed. It is accurate $\pm 2\%$ between 70% and 100%, readings below 70% are extrapolated. Causes of false low readings include:

- *Methaemoglobinaemia*: the iron atom of haem is in the ferric (Fe^{3+}) state; the affected haem positions of haemoglobin are less able to bind O_2, the unaffected haem causes the oxyhaemoglobin dissociation curve to shift to the left (prilocaine has a metabolite *ortho*-toluidine that may cause methaemoglobinaemia)
- *Methylene blue*
- *Indocyanine green*: an infrared-absorbing and fluorescent agent used for cardiac output measurement

Carboxyhaemoglobinaemia can occur after smoke inhalation. It results in a leftward shift of the oxyhaemoglobin dissociation curve and inhibits the cellular cytochrome oxidase system. Carboxyhaemoglobin is interpreted as oxyhaemoglobin and thus gives a false high reading. Bilirubinaemia is not a clinical problem with saturation measurement.

Al-Shaikh B, Stacey S. *Essentials of Anaesthetic Equipment*, 3rd edn. London: Churchill Livingstone, 2007.
Yentis S, Hirsch N, Smith G. *Anaesthesia and Intensive Care A to Z: An Encyclopaedia of Principles and Practice*, 4th edn. Oxford: Butterworth-Heinemann, 2009.

18a. False
18b. False
18c. True
18d. True
18e. True

The International Association for the Study of Pain has classified CRPS into two types:

- *Type I* (reflex sympathetic dystrophy): pain developing in the absence of an identifiable nerve injury
- *Type II* (causalgia): pain following major peripheral nerve injury

The following clinical characteristics are seen:

- *Sensory*: burning, disproportionate pain, allodynia, hyperalgesia, paraesthesiae
- *Autonomic*: swelling of the distal extremity, hyper- or hypohydrosis, vasodilatation or vasoconstriction, changes in skin temperature
- *Trophic*: thin shiny skin, nail and hair loss and osteoporosis
- *Motor*: weakness, incoordination, tremor

Pain may also be sympathetically maintained.

19a. True
19b. True
19c. True
19d. False
19e. False

The Vaughan Williams classification applies to antiarrhythmic drugs and is as follows:

Class I: sodium channel blockers (within myocardial cells)

- Ia: prolong action potential – disopyramide, quinidine, procainamide ('Double Quarter Pounder')
- Ib: shorten action potential – lidocaine, mexiletine ('Lettuce, Mayo')
- Ic: no effect on action potential – flecainide, propafenone ('Fries Please')

Class II: β-blockers, e.g. propranolol, atenolol
Class III: prolong action potential without affecting depolarization rate, e.g. amiodarone, bretylium
Class IV: calcium channel blockers, e.g. nifedipine, verapamil

20a. False
20b. True
20c. True
20d. False
20e. True

POV is twice as common in children as it is in adults, with an incidence of 13–42% in all paediatric patients. It is one of the leading causes of parental dissatisfaction and of unanticipated hospital admissions. Patient-related factors for the risk of developing POV include:

- *Age >3 years*: risk of POV increases markedly, rising steadily through to adolescence
- *Previous history of POV*
- *Previous history of motion sickness*
- *Postpubertal girls*: believed to be sex-hormone-related

Anxiety and obesity have not been confirmed to be related to POV. No data exist for smoking as a risk factor.

Association of Paediatric Anaesthetists of Great Britain and Ireland. *Guidelines for the Prevention of Post-Operative Vomiting in Children.* London: APAGBI, 2009. Available at: www.apagbi.org.uk/docs/Final%20APA%20 POV%20Guidelines%20ASC%2002%2009%20compressed.pdf.

21a. False
21b. True
21c. False
21d. False
21e. False
Natural rubber latex is produced from the sap of *Hevea brasiliensis* and allergy to latex proteins has emerged as an increasingly important occupational disease, affecting 7–13% of health-care workers, compared to 0.8% in non-health-care workers. Other groups at risk include rubber industry workers, individuals with certain fruit allergies (banana, kiwi, avocado) and patients with neural tube defects who have recurrent mucosal exposure to latex. The clinical presentation of latex allergy is most commonly due to type IV (delayed) hypersensitivity reaction, presenting with urticarial dermatitis hours or days after exposure to rubber additives. More serious reactions are IgE-mediated type I (immediate) hypersensitivity reactions to latex proteins, which can present with cutaneous, ocular or respiratory complications, or with systemic anaphylaxis. Patients' potential exposure to latex should be minimized and local guidelines should be in place to govern their perioperative management, with ward-based and theatre-based protocols. Patients should be pre-assessed and placed first on the operating list; prophylactic corticosteroids and antihistamines are not routinely recommended.

Royal College of Physicians. *Latex Allergy: Occupational Aspects of Management. A National Guideline.* London: RCP, 2008.
Richards M. Latex allergy. In: Allman K, Wilson I, eds. *Oxford Handbook of Anaesthesia*, 2nd edn. Oxford: OUP, 2006.
Faeley CA, Jones HM. Latex allergy. *Contin Educ Anaesth Crit Care Pain* 2002; 2: 20–3.

22a. True
22b. True
22c. False
22d. True
22e. True
Various devices are used to measure ICP: ventricular catheters, subdural bolts, intraparenchymal strain gauges and extradural catheters. The gold standard

remains the ventricular catheter, which is inserted through a right frontal burr hole into a lateral ventricle. In addition to measuring the intracranial pressure, it can be used for cerebrospinal fluid drainage or administering drugs, e.g. antibiotics. It can be connected to a saline manometer or a transducer that uses the foramen of Munro as the reference point. For ease of use, the external auditory meatus is often taken as the point of reference instead. Disadvantages of a ventricular catheter are its tendency for blockage, bleeding during insertion and infection. Currently antibiotic-impregnated catheters are commonly used.

Pattinson K, Wynne-Jones G, Imray CHE. Monitoring intracranial pressure, perfusion and metabolism. *Contin Educ Anaesth Crit Care Pain* 2005; 5: 130–3.

23a. False
23b. False
23c. True
23d. True
23e. False
The most likely diagnosis is DI or ingestion of osmotic diuretics. DI can be neurogenic or nephrogenic and untreated can lead to severe dehydration and hypotension. Her reduced conscious level may be a function of hypotension, hypernatraemia, or an underlying cause of DI, such as intracranial trauma (including subarachnoid haemorrhage), tumour or infection. Expected findings include hypernatraemia with high plasma and low urinary osmolality and an inappropriately high urinary sodium level. SIADH and cerebral salt wasting syndrome both lead to hyponatraemia; and while panhypopituitarism can lead to adrenal insufficiency and DI, Addison's disease is *primary* adrenal failure and, in the UK, is most often due to autoimmune destruction of the adrenal glands.

The following is an *aide-mémoire*:

Condition	Plasma sodium (mmol/L)	Urine sodium (mmol/L)	Plasma osmolality (mOsm/kg)	Urine osmolality (mOsm/kg)	Urine specific gravity
Normal	135–145	<10	285–295	600–1400	1.002–1.035
DI	↑	↑/normal	↑	↓	↓
SIADH	↓	↑/normal	↓	↑	↑
Cerebral salt wasting	↓	↑	↓	↑	↑

24a. True
24b. True
24c. True
24d. True
24e. True
The robotic system for laparoscopic surgery comprises a master console, a surgical manipulator and a visualization tower, allowing a three-dimensional

image of the surgical field. The patient is placed in the lithotomy position with a steep Trendelenburg (30−45°) tilt and pneumoperitoneum maintained over prolonged periods; complications include:

- Endotracheal tube migration
- Concealed intra-abdominal haemorrhage
- Conjunctival burns and oral ulceration due to acid reflux
- Compartment syndrome in lower limbs
- Cerebral oedema leading to delayed emergence
- Peripheral nerve compression

Irvine M, Patil V. Anaesthesia for robot-assisted laparoscopic surgery. *Contin Educ Anaesth Crit Care Pain* 2009; 9: 125−9.

25a. False
25b. True
25c. True
25d. False
25e. True
Severe AS is usually defined as an aortic valve area of ≤ 1.0 cm^2 because at this degree of stenosis the peak resting gradient often approaches 50 mmHg. Critical AS has varying definitions and incorporates the valve area (<0.7 cm^2) with the degree of symptoms. The gradient itself is not a good measure of severity per se, since in advanced severe disease the ventricle may fail and the gradient may decrease. Coronary perfusion relies on forward flow across the aortic valve and perfusion is governed by diastolic time (heart-rate-dependent) and the pressure difference between the aortic diastolic pressure and LVEDP; thus the higher the LVEDP, the higher the aortic diastolic pressure required to drive flow through the coronaries, as per the Hagen−Poiseuille formula. Patients often have left ventricular hypertrophy, which increases oxygen demand and makes ischaemia more likely; thus ideally afterload should be maintained to provide a driving pressure for coronary flow and tachycardia should be avoided as this shortens diastolic coronary filling and increases oxygen demand.

26a. True
26b. True
26c. False
26d. True
26e. True
An EEG is a recording of electrical activity within the brain transduced via scalp electrodes. Shape, distribution, incidence and symmetry of the readings are analysed. Rhythms include:

- *Alpha (α)-waves:* 8−10 Hz
- *Beta (β)-waves:* 13−30 Hz
- *Delta (δ)-waves:* 4 Hz
- *Theta (θ)-waves:* 4−8 Hz

Wakefulness is characterized by an EEG with dominant, low-amplitude, high-frequency β-wave activity. Sleep is characterized by a shift from β-wave to α-wave activity. θ-waves occur in early non-rapid eye movement (REM) sleep, δ-waves occur in deep non-REM sleep and may be normal in children.

Schupp M, Hanning CD. Physiology of sleep. *Contin Educ Anaesth Crit Care Pain* 2003; 3: 69–74.

Yentis S, Hirsch N, Smith G. *Anaesthesia and Intensive Care A to Z: An Encyclopaedia of Principles and Practice*, 4th edn. Oxford: Butterworth-Heinemann, 2009.

27a. True
27b. False
27c. False
27d. True
27e. True
The median nerve is formed from the medial and lateral cords of the brachial plexus within the lower axilla. Although it supplies the pronator teres, anaesthesia will not result from median nerve blockade at the wrist where it passes beneath the flexor retinaculum to supply the opponens pollicis, the abductor pollicis brevis and usually the flexor pollicis brevis. It also supplies the 1st and 2nd lumbricals and provides cutaneous innervation to the dorsal tips of the thumb, index and middle fingers and to the palmar aspects of these fingers to include the lateral aspect of the ring finger.

28a. False
28b. True
28c. False
28d. True
28e. True
BS (British Standard) 5724 refers to a document for comprehensive specification for safety of medical electrical equipment. BS 5950 relates to the structural use of steelwork in buildings.

Class I describes equipment with conducting parts connected to the earth, class II describes double insulation (so that no live parts are accessible to the user) and class III describes voltages below safety extra low voltage (SELV) <25 V AC or <60 V DC. Type B circuits have maximum leakage currents <100 μA, a type BF circuit is a floating version of a type B circuit and type CF circuits have a maximum leakage <10 μA and are designed for use in cardiac equipment.

29a. False
29b. True
29c. True
29d. True
29e. False

Substance	Body colour	Shoulder colour	Pin index
Oxygen	Black	White	2 and 5
Helium	Brown	Brown	n/a
CO_2	Grey	Grey	1 and 6
Air	Grey	White/black check	1 and 5
N_2O	Blue	Blue	3 and 5
Entonox	Blue	White/blue check	7
Cyclopropane	Orange	Orange	3 and 6

Al-Shaikh B, Stacey S. *Essentials of Anaesthetic Equipment*, 3rd edn. London: Churchill Livingstone, 2007.

30a. True
30b. False
30c. False
30d. False
30e. True
The AAGBI Recommendations for Standards of Monitoring During Anaesthesia and Recovery state that the anaesthetist must be present throughout the conduct of an anaesthetic, general or regional. Essential monitoring includes:

- pulse oximeter
- non-invasive blood pressure monitor
- electrocardiograph
- airway gases: oxygen, carbon dioxide and vapour
- airway pressure

The following must also be available:

- a nerve stimulator whenever a muscle relaxant is used
- a means of measuring the patient's temperature (not necessarily a probe)
- a stethoscope

Very occasionally, an anaesthetist working single-handedly may be called upon to perform a brief life-saving procedure nearby. Leaving an anaesthetized patient in these circumstances is a matter for individual judgement. If this should prove necessary, the surgeon must stop operating until the anaesthetist returns. Observation of the patient and monitoring devices must be continued by a trained anaesthetic assistant. Any problems should be reported to available medical staff.

Association of Anaesthetists of Great Britain and Ireland. *Recommendations for Standards of Monitoring During Anaesthesia and Recovery*, 4th edn. London: AAGBI, 2007. Available at: www.aagbi.org/publications/guidelines/docs/standardsofmonitoring07.pdf.

31a. True
31b. True
31c. True
31d. False
31e. False
2,3-DPG is a by-product of glycolysis; binding strongly to deoxygenated haemoglobin, it causes a rightward shift of the oxyhaemoglobin dissociation curve, favouring liberation of oxygen to tissues. Levels are affected thus:

Increased 2,3-DPG	Decreased 2,3-DPG
• Anaemia	• Acidosis
• Alkalosis	• Hypoposphataemia
• Chronic hypoxaemia	• Hypothyroidism
• High altitude	• Hypopituitarism
• Exercise	
• Pregnancy	
• Hyperthyroidism	
• Hyperphosphataemia	

32a. True
32b. True
32c. False
32d. True
32e. False
Whole blood lactate concentration is < 1.5 mmol/L and is analysed using enzyme-based methods specific for the L-isomer. It should be collected in heparin fluoride tubes to prevent coagulation and glycolysis, which generates lactate. Pyruvate is the final product of glycolysis and in aerobic conditions it enters the Krebs cycle, generating ATP; however, LDH catalyses the conversion of pyruvate to lactate and this can build up in anaerobic conditions such as tissue hypoxia. Levels can provide useful information on regional perfusion, such as the differential arterial–jugular bulb concentrations.

Singer M, Webb AR. *Oxford Handbook of Critical Care*, 3rd edn. Oxford: OUP, 2009.

33a. False
33b. False
33c. False
33d. True
33e. False
Packed red cells have a high haematocrit and do not adequately expand the plasma volume. An increase in CVP of ≥3 mmHg represents a significant increase and is probably indicative of an adequate circulating volume, although this may also be seen in vasoconstricted hypovolaemic patients. Furthermore, vasoconstriction may maintain normal CVP and PAWP. Cardiac output may remain unchanged despite an increase in stroke volume if the heart rate falls in response to a fluid challenge. The Surviving Sepsis Bundle recommends that

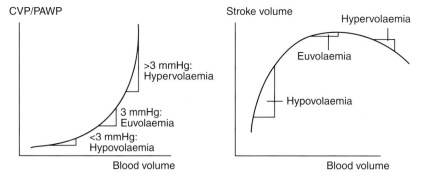

FIGURE 2.1 Response of central venous pressure (CVP)/pulmonary artery wedge pressure (PAWP) and stroke volume to a fluid challenge.

fluid boluses should consist of 20 mL/kg of crystalloid or 0.2–0.3 mg/kg of colloid equivalent given over 30 minutes. Responses of CVP/PAWP and stroke volume to a fluid challenge are illustrated in Figure 2.1.

Delinger RP, Leng MM, Cochet JM, et al. Surviving Sepsis Campaign: inter-national guidelines for management of severe sepsis and septic shock. *Crit Care Med* 2008; **36**: 296–327.
Singer M, Webb AR. *Oxford Handbook of Critical Care*, 3rd edn. Oxford: OUP, 2009.

34a. False
34b. False
34c. False
34d. False
34e. True
Clostridium difficile is a Gram-positive anaerobic spore-forming, toxin-producing rod that is present as a commensal in 1–3% of the population and risk of colonization increases with length of hospital stay (up to 20% of hospital patients). Alcohol hand gel is not effective in killing spores, thus handwashing techniques are paramount. It should be treated with oral metronidazole or oral vancomycin as intravenous administration does not achieve gut lumen minimum therapeutic concentration.

Aslam S, Musher DM. An update on diagnosis, treatment, and prevention of *Clostridium difficile*-associated disease. *Gastroenterol Clin North Am* 2006; 35: 315–35.

35a. False
35b. True
35c. False
35d. True
35e. True
MRSA is a strain of *S. aureus* resistant to β-lactam antibiotics, which include penicillins and cephalosporins. *S. aureus* is a Gram-positive coccus and a facultative anaerobe. MRSA colonizes the anterior nares most commonly, but

can colonize the throat and respiratory tract of healthy individuals. The Saving Lives Campaign was launched in 2005 to address and reduce the risk of healthcare-associated infections and include the *essential steps* of:

- hand hygiene
- use of personal protective equipment
- aseptic technique
- safe sharps disposal

Chlorhexidine has bacteriocidal and bacteriostatic activities and is effective in killing MRSA if used correctly, but is less effective against some Gram-negative organisms. MRSA is sensitive to glycopeptides, including vancomycin and teicoplanin.

www.clean-safe-care.nhs.uk.
www.dh.gov.uk/en/Publichealth/Healthprotection.

36a. False
36b. True
36c. False
36d. True
36e. True
Absolute humidity is the mass of water vapour present in a given volume of air and is a function of temperature not ambient pressure. Humidification can be achieved passively using heat and moisture exchange filters, or actively using water baths, hot water baths, cascade humidifiers, heated element humidifiers, or nebulizers, which can be gas-driven or ultrasonic. Gas-driven nebulizers rely on the Bernoulli effect whereby a stream of moving gas creates a pressure drop as it passes alongside the end of a tube, with one end of this tube in water; the negative pressure entrains water, which is broken up into droplets thus humidifying the stream of gas. Ultrasonic nebulizers are the most efficient, producing very stable droplets of 1 μm, which reach the alveoli.

37a. True
37b. False
37c. False
37d. True
37e. True

Solution	Sodium (mmol/L)
0.9% saline	154
Dextrose 4%/Saline 0.18%	30
Dextrose 5%	Nil
Hartmann's	131
Bicarbonate 8.4%	1000
Bicarbonate 1.26%	150
Haemaccel	145
Gelofusine	154

(*Continued*)

Solution	Sodium (mmol/L)
Hetastarch	154
Pentastarch	154
Albumin 4.5%	<160

5% dextrose contains 50 g of dextrose and no sodium.

38a. True
38b. False
38c. True
38d. False
38e. True
Before performing a rapid sequence induction, the cricoid cartilage should be identified on the awake patient and where possible the process explained. The original recommendation by Sellick was the application of 10 N just before induction, increased to 20–40 N as loss of consciousness ensues until the position of the endotracheal tube is confirmed and the cuff inflated. In the event of vomiting, the pressure must be released to avoid oeesophageal rupture. Cricoid pressure makes placement of a laryngeal mask airway difficult and in the management of a difficult airway the priority remains the oxygenation of the patient. Backward, upward, rightward pressure (BURP) is applied to assist in the management of a difficult airway but paradoxically could lead to airway obstruction.

Cook T, Cranshaw J. Airway. In: Allman KG, McIndoe AK, Wilson IH, eds. *Emergencies in Anaesthesia*, 2nd edn. Oxford: OUP, 2009.

39a. False
39b. True
39c. True
39d. True
39e. False
The foramen and transmitting structures from the base of the skull include:

Incisive canal

• Nasopalatine nerve
• Greater palatine artery

Greater palatine foramen

• Greater palatine nerve and vessels

Lesser palatine foramen

• Lesser palatine nerve and vessels

Foramen ovale

• Mandibular division of cranial nerve V

Foramen spinosum

• Middle meningeal artery

Foramen lacerum
Carotid canal

- Internal carotid artery
- Sympathetic fibres

Jugular foramen

- Internal jugular vein
- Cranial nerves IX, X and XI

Hypoglossal canal

- Cranial nerve XII

Condylar canal

- Vein from sigmoid sinus to vertebral veins of neck

Foramen magnum

- Junction of spinal cord and medulla
- Ascending spinal portion of cranial nerve XI
- Spinal vertebral arteries
- Branches C1–3 spinal nerves

Yentis S, Hirsch N, Smith G. *Anaesthesia and Intensive Care A to Z: An Encyclopaedia of Principles and Practice*, 4th edn. Oxford: Butterworth-Heinemann, 2009.

40a. True
40b. True
40c. False
40d. True
40e. False

	Fentanyl	Alfentanil
Volume of distribution (L/kg)	4	0.6
Clearance (mL min^{-1} kg^{-1})	13	6
Elimination half-life (min)	190	100
pK$_a$	8.4	6.5
Un-ionized at pH 7.4 (%)	9	89
Lipid solubility (from octanol–water coefficient)	600	90
Plasma protein-bound (%)	83	90

Peck TE, Hill SA, Williams M. *Pharmacology for Anaesthesia and Intensive Care*, 3rd edn. Cambridge: CUP, 2008.

41a. True
41b. False
41c. True
41d. True
41e. False
The acetylated form of the amino acid L-cysteine, N-acetylcysteine is a precursor for glutathione production. It is an antioxidant, scavenging oxygen radicals; it also boosts glutathione levels. Nitric oxide synthesis and cGMP levels are enhanced, which results in vasodilatation and inhibition of platelet aggregation. Its mucolytic function is a result of cleaving of disulfide bonds, reducing the length of mucoproteins and loosening secretions. Uses include:

- paracetamol poisoning
- non-paracetamol-induced liver failure
- radiocontrast induced nephropathy (particularly in those with pre-existing chronic renal impairment)
- myocardial ischaemia
- heavy metal poisoning (acts as chelating agent)

It is administered orally, intravenously or through a nebulizer.

Keays R, Barrett NA. N-acetylcysteine. In: Waldmann N, Soni N, Rhodes A, eds. *Oxford Desk Reference: Critical Care.* Oxford: OUP, 2008.

42a. True
42b. False
42c. True
42d. False
42e. False
Life-threatening toxicity is likely following intake of >7.5 g salicylate. Toxicity is complex as it consists of a metabolic acidosis with a respiratory alkalosis. The respiratory centre is directly stimulated, causing a respiratory alkalosis; oxidative phosphorylation is uncoupled owing to an inhibition of the Krebs cycle leading to inhibition of ATP-dependent reactions. Catabolic responses predominate, resulting in increased metabolic rate and oxygen consumption with increased carbon dioxide production, resulting in hyperthermia. Amino acid metabolism is inhibited while lipid metabolism is stimulated. Severe metabolic acidosis ensues with severe toxicity and respiratory compensation initially occurs. Loss of consciousness is uncommon but may occur owing to metabolic disturbances, but should raise suspicion of other toxin ingestion. Activated charcoal is indicated for the first 24 hours after ingestion, but nasogastric tube placement is hazardous in the unconscious patient with an unprotected airway. Alkalinization of the urine is more important than forced diuresis and urinary pH should be maintained at >7.0 with caution for potassium loss. Haemofiltration is indicated for salicylate levels >6.2 mmol/L or renal failure.

Singer M, Webb AR. *Oxford Handbook of Critical Care,* 3rd edn. Oxford: OUP, 2009.

43a. False
43b. False
43c. True
43d. False
43e. True
Diabetes mellitus is a multisystem disorder characterized by chronic hyper-glycaemia with disturbances of carbohydrate, fat and protein metabolism resulting from defects in insulin secretion, insulin action, or both. This leads to microvascular damage manifested by retinopathy, nephropathy and neuropa-thy. The 2006 WHO diagnostic criteria for diabetes mellitus are:

- Fasting plasma glucose: ≥ 7.0 mmol/L
- *or* 2 hours after 75 g oral glucose: ≥ 11.1 mmol/L

Diagnosis of intermediate hyperglycaemia: impaired glucose tolerance:

- Fasting plasma glucose: < 7.0 mmol/L
- *and* 2 hour after 75 g oral glucose: ≥ 7.8 but < 11.1 mmol/L

The above criteria identify a group at risk of premature death and increased incidence of microvascular damage and cardiovascular complications, such as ischaemic heart disease, peripheral vascular disease and stroke. Glycated haemoglobin (HbA$_{1c}$, A1C) is not currently a test suitable for the diagnosis of diabetes, but can be used to measure glycaemic control. Diabetes (followed by intravenous drug abuse) represents the most common risk factor for spinal infection following epidural administration.

Simpson KH, Al-Makadma YS. Epidural drug delivery and spinal infection. *Contin Educ Anaesth Crit Care Pain* 2007; 7: 112–15.
World Health Organization. *Definition and Diagnosis of Diabetes Mellitus and Intermediate Hyperglycaemia*. Geneva: WHO, 2006.

44a. True
44b. True
44c. False
44d. True
44e. True
The following drugs have bronchodilating properties:

- β$_2$-*adrenergic receptor agonists* (e.g. salbutamol): these stimulate adenylyl cyclase, leading to increased cAMP, affecting smooth muscle relaxation
- *Phosphodiesterase inhibitors* (e.g. aminophylline): mechanisms of action include non-specific phosphodiesterase inhibition, reducing breakdown of cAMP
- *Anticholinergic drugs* (e.g. ipratropium): vagolytic action at muscarinic receptors within the bronchial tree

Sodium cromoglycate is a mast cell stabilizer useful in the prophylaxis of hay fever and some forms of asthma.

45a. True
45b. False
45c. True
45d. False
45e. False
CT is an imaging technique in which X-rays are emitted from a source and pass through the patient (in the middle) to a detector at the opposite side. The X-rays pass through the patient at different angles as the source and detector are rotated about a single point; allowing generation of 3D images from a large series of X-rays taken from this single point of rotation. Magnetic resonance imaging (MRI) involves application of radiofrequency pulses to generate images. CT is considered a moderate to high radiation exposure technique and involves ionizing radiation (defined as radiation of sufficient energy to displace electrons from the atoms of cells and produce ions). The biological effects of radiation are measured in Sieverts (mSv), which is the derived SI unit of biological equivalence, while physical effects of absorbed radiation dose are measured in Grays (1 Gy is equal to absorption of 1 joule in the form of ionizing radiation by 1 kg of matter). Three factors control the degree of exposure of radiation to a subject: length of exposure, distance from source by the inverse square law and shielding whereby the radiation transmitted decreases exponentially with the thickness of the shield. Omipaque (Iohexol) is an iodinated contrast agent and is considered to be a 'low-osmolar contrast agent', although its osmolality ranges from 1.1 to 3 times that of blood; anaphylactic reactions and contrast nephropathy have been reported.

Brenner DJ, Hall EJ. Computed tomography – an increasing source of radiation exposure. *N Engl J Med* 2007; **357**: 2277–84.
Greenberger PA, Patterson R. Adverse reactions to radiocontrast media. *Prog Cardiovasc Dis* 1988; **31**: 239–48.

46a. True
46b. True
46c. True
46d. True
46e. False
For minor surgery, National Institute of Health and Clinical Excellence guidelines (2003) state that renal function measurement should be:

Considered for the following:

- ASA 1 patients >60 years
- ASA 2 patients with cardiovascular comorbidity
- ASA 2 patients with respiratory comorbidity >60 years
- ASA 3 patients with respiratory comorbidity

Recommended for the following:

- ASA 2 with renal comorbidity
- ASA 3 with cardiovascular or renal comorbidity

Lithium can cause diabetes insipidus, and thiazides can lead to hypokalaemia and hyponatraemia in addition to dehydration; hence electrolytes should be measured. Finally, renal function testing is not indicated in ASA I children <16 years presenting for minor or intermediate elective surgery such as herniorrhaphy.

National Institute for Health and Clinical Excellence Guidelines. *The Use of Routine Preoperative Tests for Elective Surgery*. London: NICE, 2003. Available at: guidance.nice.org.uk/CG3.

47a. False
47b. True
47c. True
47d. True
47e. False
Gas solubility increases with decreasing temperature; thus pH will increase (become more basic) as temperature decreases, since more CO_2 dissolves. Standard bicarbonate is the concentration of plasma bicarbonate when arterial P_{CO_2} has been corrected to 5.3 kPa at a temperature of 37°C with haemoglobin fully saturated; as this accounts for the respiratory component, it is therefore a measure of the metabolic component. The Siggard–Andersen nomogram plots log P_{aCO_2} against pH for calculating, by interpolation, the P_{CO_2}, the bicarbonate, the standard bicarbonate and the base excess.

Yentis S, Hirsch N, Smith G. *Anaesthesia and Intensive Care A to Z: An Encyclopaedia of Principles and Practice*, 4th edn. Oxford: Butterworth-Heinemann, 2009.

48a. False
48b. True
48c. True
48d. False
48e. True
The Wilson scoring system incorporates most of the difficult airway predictors. It consists of five predicting factors: weight, head and neck movement, jaw movement, receding mandible, and buck teeth. Each factor is scored on a three-point scale from 0 to 2. A total score of 2 or more is associated with an increased incidence of difficult intubation.

Vaughn RS. Predicting difficult airways. *Contin Educ Anaesth Crit Care Pain* 2001; **1**: 44–7.

49a. False
49b. False
49c. True
49d. True
49e. False
Plasma cholinesterase (pseudocholinesterase) is an enzyme that hydrolyses acetylcholine and many other chemicals (including mivacurium). Of particular

relevance to the anaesthetist is that it hydrolyses suxamethonium. Reduced activity of the enzyme causes prolonged paralysis. Causes are:

Inherited atypical cholinesterase

- Autosomal recessive inheritance. 95% of the population are homozygotes; 94% have Eu:Eu, two normal genes, 0.03% are 'atypical', 0.001% are 'silent' and 0.0001% are fluoride-resistant. 5% are heterozygotes
- Paralysis times are: normal: 1–5 minutes; atypical/silent: 2–4 hours; fluoride-resistant: 1–2 hours; heterozygotes: 10–20 minutes (this woman is unlikely to be a heterozygote)

Acquired deficiency

- Pregnancy, hepatic failure, malnutrition, burns

Inhibition by drugs

- Ecothiopate, cyclophosphamide

In pregnancy there is a marked (30%) reduction in cholinesterase levels, but this is counterbalanced by an increased volume of distribution. The dibucaine number is a measure of degree of inhibition of plasma cholinesterase and decreases with reduction of cholinesterase activity.

Walton NKD, Melachuri VK. Anaesthesia for non-obstetric surgery during pregnancy. *Contin Educ Anaesth Crit Care Pain* 2006; **6**: 83–5.
Yentis S, Hirsch N, Smith G. *Anaesthesia and Intensive Care A to Z: An Encyclopaedia of Principles and Practice*, 4th edn. Oxford: Butterworth-Heinemann, 2009.

50a. False
50b. False
50c. True
50d. True
50e. False

Apnoea is a complete cessation of airflow for more than 10 s and hypopnoea a reduction of >50% airflow for the same time. OSA is defined as the occurrence of more than five episodes per hour of sleep of either apnoea or hypopnoea. Classification is based on the AHI, which is the number of apnoeas or hypopnoeas per hour of sleep. In the absence of symptoms, an AHI of 2–5 is considered normal.

- *Grade 0* (AHI 0–10): typical heavy snorer, episodes of arousal
- *Grade 1* (AHI 10–30): moderately severe
- *Grade 2* (AHI 30–80): SpO_2 returns to baseline with arousal
- *Grade 3*: Sustained hypoxaemia; suggestive of hypoventilation; this group is at risk for development of cor pulmonale and cardiac disease

Williams JM, Hanning CD. Obstructive sleep apnoea. *Contin Educ Anaesth Crit Care Pain* 2003; **3**: 75–8.

51a. True
51b. False
51c. True
51d. False
51e. False
Protein C is a vitamin K-dependent serine protease enzyme, which is activated by thrombin to APC. It has antithrombotic, anti-inflammatory and pro-fibrinolytic properties, which is especially pertinent to the microcirculation. In the coagulation cascade, thrombin binds endothelial thrombomodulin, which then activates APC; APC must then associate with protein S before its anticoagulant effect is activated. Protein C deficiency is a rare genetic defect characterized by venous thrombosis and spontaneous abortions; it is a pro-coagulant state. APC cleaves factors Va and VIIIa. Drotrecogin alpha (Xigris) is a synthetic recombinant form of APC used in the treatment of severe sepsis. It is available for reconstitution in powder form, and is administered as multiple infusions over a total period of 96 hours; the maximum duration of one infusion is 12 hours.

Esmon CT. The normal role of activated protein c in maintaining homeostasis and its relevance to critical illness. *Crit Care* 2001; 5(Suppl 2): S7–12.

52a. False
52b. False
52c. True
52d. True
52e. True
A transhiatal approach to oesophagectomy involves an upper abdominal incision with trans-diaphragmatic access and subsequent cervical anastomosis, thus avoiding a thoracotomy. Anastomotic leaks present a major cause of morbidity and mortality following oesophagectomy, and common presenting signs include fever, leukocytosis, wound drainage, erythema, wound crepitus, swelling, pain and halitosis; in addition pleural effusions, pneumothoraces and mediastinitis can occur. Certain factors may make anastomotic leaks more likely to occur, such as malnutrition and perioperative steroid therapy. Postoperative atrial fibrillation can be associated with inadequate tissue per-fusion leading to anastomotic ischaemia and subsequent leak, thus constituting a potential cause rather than effect. Chylothorax is an uncommon compli-cation occurring in 1–2% and is due to disruption or surgical injury to the thoracic duct and more commonly follows transhiatal procedures.

Cooke DT, Lin GC, Lau CL, et al. Analysis of cervical esophagogastric anasto-motic leaks after transhiatal esophagectomy: risk factors, presentation, and detection. *Ann Thorac Surg* 2009; 88: 177–84.
Lerut T, Coosemans W, Decker G, et al. Anastomotic complications after esophagectomy. *Dig Surg* 2002; **19**: 92–8.

53a. False
53b. True
53c. True
53d. False
53e. False
HELLP syndrome is characterized by the presence of Haemolysis, Elevated Liver enzymes, and Low Platelets and complicates approximately 3% of pregnancies in pre-eclamptic and eclamptic women. The majority present preterm and smoking has been associated with an 80% reduction in the risk of developing HELLP. A Cochrane review has demonstrated no reduction in perinatal mortality due to respiratory distress syndrome, nor any reduction in maternal mortality following dexamethasone administration. Although most commonly associated with pre-eclampsia, HELLP syndrome can occur in the absence of hypertension and the latter is not a prerequisite for diagnosis.

Leeners B, Neumaier-Wagner P, Kus S, Rath W. Smoking and the risk of developing hypertensive diseases in pregnancy: what is the effect on HELLP syndrome. *Acta Obstet Gynecol Scand* 2006; 85: 1217–24.
Matchaba PT, Moodley J. Corticosteroids for HELLP syndrome in pregnancy. *Cochrane Database Syst Rev* 2009; (3): CD002076.

54a. True
54b. False
54c. True
54d. True
54e. False
A false positive is also known as a type I (or α) error, the error of rejecting the null hypothesis when it is true. A false negative is known as a type II (or β) error, the error of accepting the null hypothesis when it is not true. The null hypothesis states that no statistical difference exists in the variables studied between the groups.

In clinical testing:

- *True positive* (TP): the patient has the disease and the test is positive
- *False positive* (FP): the patient does not have the disease but the test is positive
- *True negative* (TN): the patient does not have the disease and the test is negative
- *False negative* (FN): the patient has the disease but the test is negative
- *Sensitivity* is the ability of the test to correctly identify those patients with the disease: sensitivity $= TP/(TP + FN)$
- *Specificity* is the ability to correctly identify those people without the disease: specificity $= TN/(TN + FP)$
- *Positive predictive value* (PPV) is known as the precision rate; it states how likely a patient is to have a disease, given a positive result: $PPV = TP/(TP + FP)$
- *Negative predictive value* (NPV) states how likely a patient is to not have a disease, given a negative result: $NPV = TN/(TN + FN)$

Lalkhen AG, McCluskey A. Clinical tests: sensitivity and specificity. *Contin Educ Anaesth Crit Care Pain* 2008; 8: 221–3.

55a. True
55b. True
55c. True
55d. True
55e. True
These drugs all cause nephrotoxicity. Glomerulonephritis has been reported as being due to gold, penicillamide, phenytoin, captopril and antibiotic therapy, including penicillins, rifampicin and sulphonamides. Penicillins, cephalosporins, thiazide diuretics, furosemide and cimetidine have led to the development of interstitial nephritis, while direct renal tubular toxicity (acute tubular necrosis) is caused by aminoglycosides, amphotericin and cyclosporin.

British Medical Association, Royal Pharmaceutical Society of Great Britain. *British National Formulary 58*. London: Pharmaceutical Press, 2009. Available at: bnf.org/bnf.

56a. True
56b. False
56c. True
56d. False
56e. False
The A−a gradient is used to assess alveolar−capillary gas exchange and diagnose the cause for hypoxia; a normal value is < 10 mmHg (0.5−1 kPa) and increases with normal ageing. An increased A−a gradient is found in causes of $\dot{V}/\dot{Q}$ mismatch and shunt, the latter uncorrected by additional inspired oxygen. In cardiopulmonary bypass, the alveolar partial pressure of oxygen ($P_{A}O_2$) will decrease as lung inflation ceases while the oxygenator maintains arterial oxygenation. Right-to-left shunts result in an increased gradient; in tetralogy of Fallot, preferential flow of mixed arterial and venous blood through the aortic valve leads to cyanosis and an increased gradient. Bronchoconstriction and hypoventilation are not causes, since the cause of hypoxia is independent of the alveolar−capillary interface.

57a. True
57b. False
57c. True
57d. False
57e. True
At birth the neonatal circulation changes from a parallel to a series system as a result of various changes. PAP decreases to adult values within 2 weeks, with most of the change occurring in the first 3 days. Left atrial pressure (LAP) rises owing to increased flow through the lungs. The FO closes when LAP exceeds right atrial pressure; permanent closure takes 4−6 weeks by the fusion of the septum secundum with the edges of the FO. The ductus arteriosus constricts in response to increasing $P_{a}O_2$ after the first breath and also in response to closure of the FO and decreasing PGE_1 and PGE_2 concentrations; physiological closure occurs in 10−15 hours and permanent closure in 2−3 weeks. DV closure occurs a few hours after birth, but the exact mechanism is unknown.

Power I, Kam P. *Principles of Physiology for the Anaesthetist*. London: Arnold Publishers, 2001.

58a. True
58b. True
58c. True
58d. False
58e. False

$\dot{V}o_2$ remains constant in the anaesthetized patient. A patent airway allows diffusion of O_2 into apnoeic lungs, producing 'apnoeic mass movement oxygenation'. This can maintain Sao_2 for up to 100 minutes. Application of O_2 via a patent airway in an apnoeic patient delays the onset of critical hypoxia but will not reverse hypoxaemia, or prevent hypercapnia developing and associated acidosis, which may become life-threatening. $\dot{V}o_2$ increases steadily throughout pregnancy and is 15–30% greater than normal at full term.

Sirian R, Wills J. Physiology of apnoea and the benefits of preoxygenation. *Contin Educ Anaesth Crit Care Pain* 2009; 9: 105–8.

59a. True
59b. True
59c. False
59d. False
59e. True

Acute Physiological and Chronic Health Evaluation (APACHE II) is a system used to classify disease severity. Points are given for initial values of 12 physiological measurements (listed below), age and previous health status to provide a general measure of severity of disease.

- temperature
- heart rate
- respiratory rate
- mean arterial pressure

- GCS
- sodium
- potassium
- creatinine

- haematocrit
- white cell count
- pH
- Po_2 or A–a gradient

Sequential Organ Failure Assessment (SOFA) is composed of scores for six organ systems: respiratory, cardiovascular, hepatic, coagulation, renal and neurological. Initially produced to describe organ dysfunction, it has subsequently been validated for a number of other situations, including trauma. The World Federation of Neurosurgical Societies (WFNS) Scale is used to predict outcome after aneurysmal subarachnoid haemorrhage (SAH). The WFNS SAH Scale is as follows:

Grade	GCS	Focal neurological deficit
0	15	Unruptured
1	15	Absent
2	13–14	Absent
3	13–14	Present
4	7–12	Present or absent
5	3–6	Present or absent

The Simplified Acute Physiological Score (SAPS III) assesses severity of illness and predicts vital status at hospital discharge based on ICU admission data. The Multiple Organ Dysfunction Score (MODS) was developed as a physiology-based tool to describe organ dysfunction as an ICU outcome. For each variable, the recorded value should be the first value of the day, rather than the worst value.

Antonelli M, Moreno R, Vincent JL, et al. Application of SOFA score to trauma patients. *Intensive Care Med* 1999; **25**: 389–94.

Drake CG, Hunt WE, Sano K, et al. Report of World Federation of Neurological Surgeons Committee on a Universal Subarachnoid Hemorrhage Grading Scale. *J Neurosurg* 1988; **68**: 985–6.

Knaus WA, Draper EA, Wagner DP, Zimmerman JE. APACHE II: a severity of disease classification system. *Crit Care Med* 1985; **13**: 818–29.

Marshall JC, Cook DJ, Christou NV, et al. Multiple Organ Dysfunction Score: a reliable descriptor of a complex clinical outcome. *Crit Care Med* 1995; **23**: 1638–52.

Moreno RP, Metnitz PG, Almeida E, et al. SAPS 3 – from evaluation of the patient to evaluation of the intensive care unit. Part 2: Development of a prognostic model for hospital mortality at ICU admission. *Intensive Care Med* 2005; **31**: 1345–55.

60a. False
60b. True
60c. True
60d. False
60e. True
Small-bore drains are as effective for air drainage and are more comfortable. Large-bore drains are required for drainage of collections of blood or pus. High-volume/low-pressure suction pumps are advocated for non-resolving pneumothoraces or after pleurodesis. If applied, suction pressure should be -10 to -20 cmH$_2$O through an underwater seal. The mid-axillary line (in the 'safe triangle') is the most common anatomical landmark used, avoiding scarring through muscle and breast tissue, or kinking if placed too posteriorly.

Paramasivam E, Bodenham A. Air leaks, pneumothorax, and chest drains. *Contin Educ Anaesth Crit Care Pain* 2008; **8**: 204–9.

61a. True
61b. False
61c. True
61d. True
61e. False
Perioperative ARF accounts for up to 25% of cases of hospital-acquired renal failure, with mortality of up to 6%. The Acute Dialysis Quality Initiative (ADQI) has formed a grading system for acute renal dysfunction. The acronym RIFLE defines grades of severity (R – risk; I – injury; F – failure) with two outcome variables (L – loss; E – end-stage) and has undergone evaluation in cardiac surgical and ICU patients. The incidence is increasing owing to increasing age and complexity of surgery. A 2005 Cochrane review of 37

randomized controlled trials concluded that there is no evidence that pharmacological interventions are effective in protecting renal function intraoperatively. Meta-analysis has concluded there is no role for low-dose dopamine for clinically significant renal protection. Phase II trials have shown lack of renal protective benefit of N-acetylcysteine.

Webb ST, Allen JSD. Perioperative renal failure. *Contin Educ Anaesth Crit Care Pain* 2008; 8: 176–80.

62a. True
62b. True
62c. True
62d. True
62e. True
Murmurs are transmitted sounds caused by turbulent flow of blood through an orifice. Systolic murmurs may be physiological; diastolic murmurs are always pathological. Murmurs can be classified as:

Systolic

Pansystolic: ventricular septal defect, mitral regurgitation, tricuspid regurgitation

Ejection: aortic stenosis or sclerosis, atrial septal defect

Diastolic

Mitral stenosis, aortic regurgitation

Continuous

Patent ductus arteriosus

63a. True
63b. True
63c. False
63d. True
63e. False
The Fick principle states that blood flow to an organ in unit time is equal to

$$\frac{\text{amount of marker taken up by the organ in unit time}}{\text{arteriovenous concentration difference of the substance}}$$

This can be used to determine blood flow to individual organs, e.g. cerebral (Kety–Schmidt technique) or renal blood flow. A variant of this principle using oxygen or carbon dioxide instead of the marker can be used to measure cardiac output. Fick's *law of diffusion* states that rate of diffusion across a semipermeable membrane is directly proportional to the concentration gradient across it.

64a. True
64b. False
64c. True
64d. False
64e. False
Atenolol, esmolol, bisoprolol and metoprolol demonstrate β_1-adrenorecep-
tor selectivity ('cardioselectivity'), although β_2-antagonism can be seen in high
doses.

Peck TE, Hill SA, Williams M. *Pharmacology for Anaesthesia and Intensive
Care*, 3rd edn. Cambridge: CUP, 2008.

65a. True
65b. False
65c. False
65d. True
65e. True
Nerve stimulator devices are used to locate peripheral nerves by producing
visible muscle contraction upon stimulation of the nerve innervating the
muscle. Ideal characteristics include:

- Constant-current output: $V = IR$, so current output must be constant
  despite changes in resistance of tissues, connectors and needles; in turn this
  means that the voltage is variable.
- Variable output control
- Linear output with digital display
- Square wave unipolar stimulus: this ensures accuracy and that all nerve
  fibres are stimulated simultaneously
- Two leads with clearly marked polarity
- Short pulse width 1–2 ms
- Frequency 1–2 Hz
- Small current 0.25–1 mA: less current is required when the negative lead is
  connected to the stimulator needle, since this elicits depolarization
- Battery indicator
- Good quality clips with low resistance

In addition, the device should be easily portable with detachable leads that
are easily sterilized.

Al-Shaikh B, Stacey S. *Essentials of Anaesthetic Equipment*, 3rd edn. London:
Churchill Livingstone, 2007.

66a. True
66b. True
66c. False
66d. False
66e. True
Peribulbar anaesthesia is indicated for surgery on the globe of the eye. The
limbus is the *sclerocorneal* junction. Risk of globe perforation increases with
axial length; if >27 mm extreme caution is warranted, a sub-Tenon's
block may be a safer option. Complications include subarachnoid injection,

perforation of the globe and extraocular muscle damage from intramuscular injection.

67a. True
67b. False
67c. False
67d. False
67e. False
VAE describes the introduction of air into the venous circulation. Risk factors include exposure of open veins or venous sinuses with subatmospheric pressure (open veins above the heart, central venous cannulation), procedures involving gas insufflation (laparoscopic surgery), laser surgery or exposure of large areas of tissue (mastectomy). If air enters the pulmonary circulation, the cardiac output may plummet and the circulation may fail. Management involves prompt identification, sealing the veins and flooding the wound to prevent further entry and increasing venous pressure to encourage the VAE out of the venous circulation. Venous pressure is increased by the administration of intravenous fluids, using a Trendelenburg position and positive end-expiratory pressure (PEEP). Combining the head-down tilt with a left lateral decubitus position (Durant's position) may be beneficial by trapping the air in the right atrium and preventing entry to the pulmonary circulation.

68a. True
68b. True
68c. True
68d. True
68e. True
The pathophysiology of submersion injury is related to reduced oxygen delivery to various organs, caused by 'wet drowning' (pulmonary aspiration of water) or 'dry-drowning' (laryngospasm without aspiration). Complications therefore occur in relation to the hypoxic injury on any organ system:

Central nervous system: cerebral oedema, hyperglycaemia, release of excitatory neurotransmitters, seizures, impaired cerebral autoregulation, autonomic dysfunction; worse with increasing age

Respiratory: 1–3 mL/kg fluid aspiration can impair gas exchange and alter surfactant function leading to acute respiratory distress syndrome (ARDS) or acute lung injury (ALI); pneumonia can also result

Cardiovascular: hypovolaemia, profound hypotension, myocardial dysfunction, arrhythmias, pulmonary hypertension due to vasoactive mediator release

Other: acidosis, rhabdomyolysis, acute tubular necrosis, disseminated intravascular coagulation, septicaemia

Verive MJ. *Near Drowning*. Available at: emedicine.medscape.com/article/ 908677-overview.

69a. False
69b. False
69c. True
69d. False
69e. False

In 1901 LeFort classified maxillary fractures after dropping heavy objects onto the faces of cadavers; there are only three categories:

I: Transverse fractures of the mid-lower maxilla
II: Triangular fractures from the top of the nose to the base of the maxilla
III: Severe fractures extending through the cribriform plate and zygoma. Often associated with base-of-skull fracture, they may result in a cerebrospinal fluid leak

Chesshire NJ, Knight DJW. The anaesthetic management of facial trauma and fractures. *Contin Educ Anaesth Crit Care Pain* 2001; **1**: 108–12.
Yentis S, Hirsch N, Smith G. *Anaesthesia and Intensive Care A to Z: An Encyclopaedia of Principles and Practice*, 4th edn. Oxford: Butterworth-Heinemann, 2009.

70a. False
70b. True
70c. True
70d. True
70e. False

The stress response is a neuroendocrine response following trauma or surgical insult consisting of an array of continuous and overlapping metabolic feedback processes:

Sympathoadrenal: elevated catecholamine levels released from the adrenal medulla lead to increased cardiac output and to tachycardia, and stimulate glucagon release
Neuroendocrine: hypothalamo–pituitary axis: corticotropin-releasing hormone (CRH), adrenocorticotropic hormone (ACTH, corticotropin) and antidiuretic hormone (ADH, vasopressin) release leads to sodium and water retention; renin–angiotensin stimulation leads to mineralocorticoid release – sodium/water retention and hypokalaemia; glucocorticoid release – cortisol levels can rise to >1500 nmol/L; this drives catabolism and anti-inflammatory activity; insulin resistance also occurs
Metabolic: catabolic processes predominate; lipolysis, protein breakdown, glycogenolysis and gluconeogenesis lead to hyperglycaemia
Immune: cytokine production – interleukins 1 and 6 (IL-1 and IL-6), tumour necrosis factor α (TNF-α); acute phase response

Desborough JP. The stress response to trauma and surgery. *Br J Anaesth* 2000; 85: 109–17.

71a. True
71b. False
71c. False
71d. False
71e. True
G6PD deficiency is the most common human enzyme deficiency worldwide and confers partial resistance to malaria. It is an X-linked recessive disorder, thus more commonly affecting males. G6PD catalyses the oxidation of glucose-6-phosphate while reducing NADP to NADPH within red blood cells, which in turn maintains glutathione in its reduced state. Reduced glutathione acts as a scavenger for oxidative metabolites and red cells are reliant upon G6PD for supply of NADPH; thus G6PD deficiency leads to haemolysis on exposure to certain oxidative stresses. These include drugs such as methylene blue, sulphones, quinolones (including ciprofloxacin), sulphonamides and antimalarials.

British Medical Association, Royal Pharmaceutical Society of Great Britain. *British National Formulary 58*. Section 9.1.5: G6PD deficiency. London: Pharmaceutical Press, 2009. Available at: bnf.org/bnf.

72a. False
72b. False
72c. True
72d. False
72e. False
Cylinders filled with liquid substances are under-filled, which allows for an increase in pressure caused by an increase in temperature. This minimizes the risk of pressure build-up and rupture. The filling ratio is defined as the mass of gas in the cylinder divided by the mass of water which would fill the cylinder. Applied to N_2O (and CO_2), filling ratios are 0.75 in temperate climates and 0.67 in tropical climates.

Davis PD, Kenny GNC. *Basic Physics and Measurement in Anaesthesia*, 5th edn. Oxford: Butterworth-Heinemann, 2003.

73a. True
73b. False
73c. True
73d. True
73e. True
Bupivacaine is an amide local anaesthetic that is used widely in anaesthetic practice. It is presented as 0.25% and 0.5% preparations and a 'heavy' 0.5% solution that contains 80 mg/mL of glucose. It has a maximum dose of 2 mg/kg, acts within 10–20 minutes and has a duration of action of 5–16 hours. In addition to local anaesthesia, it has profound cardiovascular effects; it is extremely cardiotoxic and binds to myocardial proteins, decreases peripheral vascular resistance and myocardial contractility. This has led to the discontinuation of its use in intravenous regional anaesthesia. In the central nervous system, it demonstrates a biphasic effect; initial excitation (lightheadedness, dizziness, fitting) is replaced by depression (drowsiness, coma). The addition

of adrenaline does not influence the rate of systemic absorption, since bupivacaine is highly lipid-soluble and has a direct vasodilatory effect. Bupivacaine is 95% protein-bound and has an elimination half-life of 0.3–0.6 hours.

Sasada M, Smith S. *Drugs in Anaesthesia and Intensive Care*, 3rd edn. Oxford: OUP, 2003.

74a. False
74b. True
74c. False
74d. False
74e. True

Hypoxia is a common complication of OLV. In the lateral thoracotomy position, under anaesthesia, the dependent lung is better perfused, while the non-dependent lung is better ventilated. Thus on institution of OLV, this ventilation/perfusion ($\dot{V}/\dot{Q}$) mismatch is partially reversed owing to an increase in pulmonary vascular resistance and hypoxic pulmonary vasoconstriction (HPV) of the non-ventilated lung; however, hypoxia remains common and may occur owing to equipment factors (tube malposition or circuit disconnection), surgical factors (great vessel compression) or patient factors (intrinsic disease). Management of hypoxia on OLV should include increasing the FiO_2 and ensuring adequate cardiac output; insufflation of O_2 into a collapsed lung will not reliably improve oxygenation and may in fact reduce HPV. Application of 5–10 cmH_2O CPAP with 100% O_2 is appropriate, as is partial re-inflation of the collapsed lung, but this must be coordinated with surgical activity as this may impair surgical access. Pulmonary vasodilators will worsen the hypoxia by increasing the $\dot{V}/\dot{Q}$ mismatch, diverting more blood to the non-ventilated lung. Finally if the situation does not improve, reinstitution of two-lung ventilation may become necessary.

The distribution of $\dot{V}/\dot{Q}$ from top to bottom of the lungs in an erect individual is illustrated in Figure 2.2.

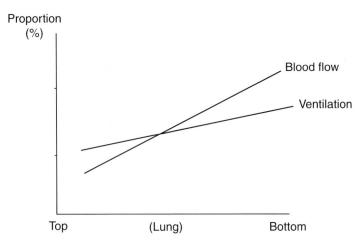

FIGURE 2.2   Distribution of ventilation and perfusion from top to bottom of the lungs in an erect individual.

75a. True
75b. False
75c. True
75d. False
75e. True

Recent guidelines stipulate that adrenaline may be administered intravenously providing the anaesthetist is appropriately trained and full resuscitation facilities are available, including vital monitoring. The dose of chlorphenamine is 10 mg intravenously. Cases should be reported to the Medicines Control Agency and AAGBI National Anaesthetic Anaphylaxis Database. Alternative vasopressors (such as metaraminol) are indicated should adrenaline fail to provide an adequate response.

Association of Anaesthetists of Great Britain and Ireland Guidelines. Suspected anaphylactic reactions associated with anaesthesia. *Anaesthesia* 2009; **64**: 199–211.

76a. False
76b. True
76c. True
76d. False
76e. True

Several randomized controlled trials (RCTs) and a meta-analysis of impact studies have demonstrated that an increase in epidural rates had no impact on operative delivery rates. A meta-analysis of RCTs comparing epidural with non-epidural analgesia during labour found that instrumental vaginal deliveries were more common in those receiving epidural analgesia. It was also found to prolong labour in both first and second stages by 42 and 14 minutes respectively.

50% of women experience back pain after childbirth; several RCTs confirm that no association exists between epidural analgesia and incidence of back pain. Epidural analgesia is associated with maternal pyrexia with an odds ratio of 4.0. The pyrexia appears to be independent of infection.

Howell CJ, Dean T, Luckling L, et al. Randomized study of long term outcome after epidural versus non-epidural analgesia during labour. *Br J Anaesth* 2002; **325**: 357–9.
McGrady E, Litchfield K. Epidural analgesia in labour. *Contin Educ Anaesth Crit Care Pain* 2004; **4**: 113–16.
Segal S, Su M, Gilbert P. The effect of a rapid change in availability of epidural analgesia on the caesarean delivery rate: a meta-analysis. *Am J Obstet Gynecol* 2000; **183**: 974–8.

77a. False
77b. True
77c. False
77d. False
77e. True

The oesophageal Doppler is based upon the Doppler principle, which is the change in frequency of sound waves as they are reflected from a moving object. This is utilized clinically to measure the velocity of blood flow in the descending aorta, which allows calculation of various parameters relating to cardiac function and filling status, including cardiac output and systemic vascular resistance. In the UK a nomogram is used (based on age, height and weight) to calculate the patient's aortic cross-sectional area; this is then multiplied by velocity of blood flow to calculate cardiac output. The Doppler waveform base is a function of left ventricular filling, heart rate and afterload. The flowtime corrected (FTc) to a heart rate of 60 is inversely related to the systemic vascular resistance. Most commonly a low FTc is caused by hypovolaemia, making a fluid challenge appropriate. Normal ranges are:

- FTc (330–360 ms): time of systolic aortic blood flow
- PV (90–120 cm/s at age 20 years; 70–100 cm/s at 50 years): an index of contractility

Anderson P, Hamilton M. Doppler. In: Waldmann N, Soni N, Rhodes A, eds. *Oxford Desk Reference: Critical Care.* Oxford: OUP, 2008.
Singer M. Oesophageal monitoring of aortic blood flow: beat by beat cardiac output monitoring. *Int Anesth Clin* 1993; **31**: 99–125.

78a. False
78b. False
78c. True
78d. False
78e. False
Hepatic encephalopathy describes the neurological sequelae of hepatic failure; precipitants include stress, surgery, trauma and infection. It is thought to be caused by reduced metabolism of ammonia, methionine and fatty acids leading to accumulation in the bloodstream. Four grades exist in the scoring system:

- *Grade 1*: confused, altered mood; EEG may be normal
- *Grade 2*: inappropriate, drowsy; EEG is abnormal
- *Grade 3*: stuporous but rousable, very confused, agitated
- *Grade 4*: coma, unresponsive to painful stimuli

Dietary protein restriction is not encouraged, since this promotes endogenous protein catabolism. Management can include enteral lactulose and neomycin to reduce ammonia production.

Singer M, Webb AR. *Oxford Handbook of Critical Care*, 3rd edn. Oxford: OUP, 2009.

79a. False
79b. True
79c. True
79d. True
79e. True
Lung cancer is the most common cause of cancer death in the UK; while incidence is increasing in women, it remains much more common in men. Bronchial carcinomas may be:

Non-small cell lung cancer (NSCLC)

- *Squamous carcinoma*: presents as endobronchial mass, grows slowly, late metastases

- *Adenocarcinoma*: peripherally located, medium growth, early metastases
- *Large cell carcinoma*: central or peripheral, early metastases

Small cell lung cancer (SCLC): central or peripheral, rapidly growing, highly malignant. Proximally located tumours typically produce symptoms of major airway obstruction and irritation:

- haemoptysis
- dyspnoea
- cough
- wheeze

- wheeze
- Pancoast's tumour
- pleural effusion
- superior vena cava obstruction

- stridor
- hoarseness
- Horner's syndrome (i.e. enophthalmos)

Peripherally located tumours are often asymptomatic, or present with pleural or chest wall invasion, or pleural effusion (causing progressive dyspnoea or pleuritic chest wall pain).

Chikwe J, Beddow E, Glenville B. *Oxford Specialist Handbooks in Surgery: Cardiothoracic Surgery*. Oxford: OUP, 2006.

80a. True
80b. True
80c. True
80d. True
80e. True
Calcium is critical for cell homeostasis, being involved in many processes, including neural transmission, haemostasis and coagulation, muscle contraction, secretory processes, and skeletal support. The normal concentration of plasma calcium (ionized and non-ionized) is 2.5 mmol/L and effects of hypocalcaemia are usually present when total calcium is below 2 mmol/L and are due to reduced level of ionized calcium. 99% of calcium is found in the bony skeleton. Features of hypocalcaemia begin with increased membrane excitability:

- paraesthesia
- muscle cramps

- spasm
- tetany

Tetany leads to the classic Chvostek (facial spasm on tapping the VIIth nerve) and Trousseau (carpopedal spasm on inflation of an arm tourniquet) signs. In severe cases it leads to:

- Respiratory insufficiency with bronchospasm and stridor
- Reduced myocardial contractility and congestive heart failure
- ECG changes including prolonged QT

- Irritability, confusion, extrapyramidal signs and convulsions may all occur
- Preterm labour may also occur (due to smooth muscle dysfunction)

Power I, Kam P. *Principles of Physiology for the Anaesthetist*, 2nd edn. London: Arnold Publishers, 2007.

81a. True
81b. False
81c. True
81d. True
81e. False

Spinal needles can be classified as:

Cutting type

- *Quincke*: short-bevelled cutting tip less often used because of its increased incidence of postdural puncture headache

Non-cutting type

- *Sprotte*: smooth-sided pointed tip with a wide lateral hole proximal to the tip
- *Whitacre*: pencil-tip-shaped with the hole just proximal to the tip
- *Greene*: oblique bevel with rounded edges

The Tuohy needle is not cutting and is not intended as a spinal needle.

Yentis S, Hirsch N, Smith G. *Anaesthesia and Intensive Care A to Z: An Encyclopaedia of Principles and Practice*, 4th edn. Oxford: Butterworth-Heinemann, 2009.

82a. True
82b. True
82c. True
82d. True
82e. True

Solution	Osmolality (mOsm/kg)	Osmolality (compared with plasma)	Tonicity
0.9% sodium chloride	308	Isosmolar	Isotonic
0.45% sodium chloride	154	Hyposmolar	Hypotonic
0.45% sodium chloride/ glucose 5%	432	Hyperosmolar	Hypotonic
5% glucose	278	Isosmolar	Hypotonic
10% glucose	555	Hyperosmolar	Hypotonic
0.9% sodium chloride/ glucose 5%	586	Hyperosmolar	Isotonic
0.18% sodium chloride/ glucose 4%	284	Isosmolar	Hypotonic
Hartmann's	278	Isosmolar	Isotonic

National Patient Safety Agency. *Rapid Responses Report: Reducing Risk of Hyponatraemia when administering Intravenous Infusions to Children*, NPSA/2007/22. London: NPSA, 2007.

83a. False
83b. False
83c. False
83d. True
83e. True
Although the simpler Stanford classification is more commonly used, the DeBakey classification divides aortic dissections into three types:

- Type I involves the ascending aorta, aortic arch and descending aorta
- Type II is confined to the ascending aorta only
- Type III is confined to the descending aorta distal to the left subclavian artery:
  - IIIa: dissections originating distal to the left subclavian artery but extending both proximally and distally, mostly above the diaphragm
  - IIIb: dissections originating distal to the left subclavian artery, extending only distally and possibly extending below the diaphragm

Hebballi R, Swanevelder J. Diagnosis and management of aortic dissection. *Contin Educ Anaesth Crit Care Pain* 2009; 9: 14–18.

84a. True
84b. True
84c. False
84d. False
84e. False
EPO is a glycoprotein produced in the peritubular endothelial cells of the kidney; it increases erythropoiesis. Recombinant EPO is used mainly in the treatment of anaemia in chronic renal insufficiency, but can also be used following chemo- or radiotherapy, in myelodysplasia, heart failure, and also in prematurity; it can also be used to stimulate erythropoiesis prior to auto-logous blood transfusion. Side-effects include hypertension, arteriovenous shunt thrombosis, red cell aplasia and flu-like symptoms; in addition, patients with chronic renal failure treated with EPO had significantly increased cardiovascular morbidity when haemoglobin was increased to > 13 g/dL.

Drüeke TB, Locatelli F, Clyne N, et al. Normalization of hemoglobin level in patients with chronic kidney disease and anemia. *N Engl J Med* 2006; 355: 2071–84.

85a. False
85b. False
85c. False
85d. False
85e. False
Cleft lip and palate (CLP) occur as a result of defects in palatal growth in the first trimester. Cleft lip can be diagnosed reliably at a routine 18–20-week

antenatal ultrasound scan; cleft palate is not clearly seen and is excluded after delivery of the baby. Most patients present with CLP alone, but there is association with many syndromes, including Pierre Robin sequence and Treacher Collins, Down's and fetal alcohol syndromes. Intubation typically becomes easier with age in Pierre Robin sequence and more difficult in Treacher Collins syndrome. No specific guidelines exist regarding timing for surgery, but after 3 months is typical, allowing anatomical and physiological maturation to occur. Continuous nasal discharge is common and not always associated with an infection; low-grade infections are best treated preoperatively to minimize airway complications and impaired wound healing.

Somerville N, Fenlon S. Anaesthesia for cleft lip and palate surgery. *Contin Educ Anaesth Crit Care Pain* 2005; 5: 76–9.

86a. False
86b. True
86c. True
86d. True
86e. True

The World Federation of Neurosurgical Societies (WFNS) Scale is used to predict outcome after aneurysmal SAH, as follows:

Grade	GCS	Focal neurological deficit
0	15	Unruptured
I	15	Absent
2	13–14	Absent
3	13–14	Present
4	7–12	Present or absent
5	3–6	Present or absent

Clinical evidence in over 1300 patients using the WFNS Scale suggested it is a good predictor of outcomes. Grade I SAH was associated with an 87.1% rate of recovery.

Sano K. Grading and timing of surgery for aneurysmal subarachnoid haemorrhage. *Neurol Res* 1994; 16: 23–6.
Teasdale GM. A universal subarachnoid scale: Report of a Committee of the World Federation of Neurosurgical Societies. *J Neurol Neurosurg Psychiatry* 1988; 51: 1457.

87a. True
87b. True
87c. True
87d. True
87e. True
Causes of dysphagia can be categorized into local and neuromuscular disorders. Local causes include diseases of the tongue and mouth, such as tonsillitis and candida, leading to odynophagia and dysphagia; local intrinsic causes include oesophageal strictures, malignancies, pharyngeal webs and foreign bodies; and local extrinsic causes include goitres and intrathoracic malignancies. Neuromuscular causes include motility disorders such as achalasia and bulbar palsies seen in brainstem infarction and multiple sclerosis. Plummer–Vinson syndrome presents as a triad of dysphagia due to oesophageal web, glossitis and iron-deficiency anaemia. Chagas' disease is a parasitic infection caused by *Trypanosoma cruzi*; dilatation of the digestive tract occurs, leading to secondary achalasia, dysphagia and severe malnutrition.

88a. False
88b. True
88c. False
88d. True
88e. True
The venous supply from the cerebrum and cerebellum drains into the dural sinuses. The superior sagittal sinus lies along the attached edge of the falx cerebri and usually drains into the right transverse sinus. The inferior sagittal sinus lies along the free edge of the falx and drains into the left transverse sinus. The transverse sinuses drain into the sigmoid sinuses and finally emerge as the internal jugular veins from the cranium. Deeper cranial structures drain into the two internal cerebral veins, which combine to form the great cerebral vein of Galen, which drains into the internal jugular vein. The cavernous sinuses lie on either side of the pituitary fossa and eventually drain into the transverse sinuses.

89a. False
89b. True
89c. False
89d. False
89e. False
At 10 000 feet, barometric pressure is 70 kPa. Oxygen concentrators can be used on aircraft and at altitude, although as minute ventilation increases, FiO_2 will decrease. Flowmeters are calibrated at sea level, thus at the lower barometric pressure encountered at 10 000 feet, high gas flows will cause the flowmeters to under-read owing to the lower gas density. The value of the dynamic viscosity coefficient is found to be a constant with pressure but the value depends on the temperature of the gas, being proportional to the square root of the absolute temperature; thus gas viscosity is likely to decrease because of the lower ambient temperatures at 10 000 feet.

Stonehill RB, Peoples AG. The accuracy of venturi masks at altitude. *Aviat Space Environ Med* 1982; 53: 818–21.

90a. True
90b. False
90c. True
90d. True
90e. False

	Preterm	Neonate	1 year	3 years	Adult
Weight (kg)	1.5	3	10	15	70
TBW (%)	80	78	65	60	60
ECF (%)	50	45	25	20	20
ICF (%)	30	35	40	40	40

TBW, total body water; ECF, extracellular fluid; ICF, intracellular fluid.

Cunliffe M. Fluid and electrolyte management in children. *Contin Educ Anaesth Crit Care Pain* 2003; 3: 1–4.

1. Fat embolism syndrome:
   a. Is more frequent in closed rather than open fractures
   b. Is caused by pancreatitis
   c. Can be diagnosed with urinary fat globules
   d. Has a mortality rate of 70%
   e. Is diagnosed using Schonfeld's criteria

2. An elderly patient presents for elective total hip replacement; the following statements are appropriate:
   a. The analgesic benefits of epidural over systemic analgesia are limited to the early postoperative period
   b. The hip joint is innervated by the femoral, sciatic, obturator and ilioinguinal nerves
   c. Lumbar plexus block will reliably block the sciatic nerve
   d. A '3-in-1' technique reliably blocks the lumbar plexus
   e. Complete anaesthesia of the hip joint requires sciatic nerve blockade

3. Concerning abdominal aortic aneurysms (AAA):
   a. Elective repair is required when diameter reaches 4.5 cm
   b. Higher rates of survival are associated with ruptures that are retroperitoneal
   c. When ruptured, aggressive fluid resuscitation is essential
   d. Aortic cross-clamping results in increased afterload
   e. Emergency repair has a 36% mortality in the UK

4. Features of severe pre-eclampsia include:
   a. Urinary protein: 500 mg/L
   b. Platelets: $<100 \times 10^9$/L
   c. Left iliac fossa pain
   d. Blood pressure: 140/95 mmHg
   e. Visual disturbances

5. von Willebrand's disease:
   a. Results in a prolonged bleeding time
   b. Is classified into two types
   c. Can be accompanied by a normal platelet count
   d. Is characterized by 'café-au-lait' spots
   e. Deteriorates during pregnancy

6. Features of *Mycoplasma pneumoniae* include:
   a. Rose spots
   b. Lung cavitation
   c. Cold agglutinins
   d. Myocarditis
   e. Predominance in the elderly

7. Concerning renal replacement therapy:
   a. Haemofiltration relies on the principle of diffusion
   b. Haemodialysis relies on the presence of a semipermeable membrane
   c. Haemodialysis can be intermittent
   d. Convective transport is independent of solute concentration gradients
   e. Haemodialysis is more efficient

8. Botulism:
   a. Is most commonly food-borne
   b. Is caused by an endotoxin from *Clostridium botulinum*
   c. Results in reversible binding of toxins to the neuromuscular junction
   d. Is characterized by a progressive ascending flaccid weakness
   e. Is uncommonly associated with parasympathetic symptoms

9. In a patient not suffering an acute myocardial infarction, elevated cardiac troponins may be encountered with:
   a. End-stage renal failure
   b. Poisoning
   c. Chemotherapy
   d. Pulmonary embolism
   e. Tachyarrhythmia

10. A 75-year-old patient undergoes a deep cervical plexus block prior to a carotid endarterectomy; signs indicative of sympathetic blockade include:
    a. Meiosis
    b. Exopthalmos
    c. Tachycardia
    d. Nasal stuffiness
    e. Anhydrosis

11. Concerning lymph drainage in the thorax:
    a. The thoracic duct passes through the aortic opening of the diaphragm
    b. The medial quadrants of the breast drain to the paraaortic nodes
    c. The thoracic duct drains all the lymph from the lower limbs and abdominal cavity
    d. A sentinel node is one that receives lymph drainage directly from a tumour
    e. The heart contains no lymphatics

12. Regarding insulin preparations:
    a. The half-life of intravenous soluble insulin is 5 minutes
    b. Protamine is used to increase solubility of insulin
    c. Zinc ions prolong the action of insulin
    d. Insulin glargine has a prolonged action
    e. Protamine–insulin preparations should not be administered intravenously

13. The Tuohy needle:
    a. Is commonly 16 G or 18 G
    b. Allows passage of a 21 G catheter in paediatric models
    c. Should be held fixed if withdrawing the catheter from beyond the tip during insertion
    d. Exists as 5, 10 and 15 cm models
    e. Bevel is called a Yale point

14. Concerning Synacthen stimulation testing:
    a. Post-Synacthen cortisol level of >550 nmol/L excludes adrenal atrophy
    b. An elevated basal adrenocorticotropic hormone (ACTH) level suggests secondary adrenocortical failure
    c. Exogenous dexamethasone renders the test invalid
    d. Normal basal cortisol is >170 nmol/L
    e. Chronic steroid use causes an inadequate rise in plasma cortisol

15. A newborn infant presents with central cyanosis, a harsh systolic murmur and pulmonary oligaemia; the following differential diagnoses apply:
    a. A large atrial septal defect (ASD)
    b. Tetralogy of Fallot
    c. Aortic coarctation
    d. Eisenmenger's syndrome
    e. Total anomalous pulmonary venous drainage (TAPVD)

16. The following are features of critical illness polyneuropathy (CIP):
    a. Nerve conduction studies reveal a severe reduction in velocities
    b. Absent reflexes are necessary for diagnosis
    c. Raised serum creatine kinase levels
    d. Mixed motor and sensory neuropathy
    e. An association with sepsis

17. The Surviving Sepsis Campaign Guidelines (2008) recommend:
    a. Fluid challenge of 1000 mL crystalloid or 300–500 mL colloid over 30 minutes
    b. Use of low-dose dopamine for renal protection
    c. Adults with severe sepsis and low risk of death should receive activated protein C
    d. Target tidal volumes of 6 mL/kg predicted body weight in patients with ARDS
    e. Administration of packed red cells if haemoglobin is ≤8.0 g/dL

18. **The following is correct of statistical analysis:**
    a. Standard error of the mean (SEM) is the square root of variance
    b. Student's *t*-test can be paired or unpaired
    c. Data skewed to the right is positive
    d. ANOVA test can be used when more than two groups exist
    e. Standard deviation is the spread of values around the median

19. **Perfluorocarbons as synthetic oxygen carriers:**
    a. Are based on the principles of Henry's law
    b. Have specific binding sites
    c. Are chemically inert
    d. Exhibit a linear oxygen dissociation relationship
    e. Are excreted via the lungs

20. **Highly trained athletes:**
    a. Develop hyperplasia of the myocardium
    b. Can be misdiagnosed with hypertrophic cardiomyopathy on echocardiogram
    c. With 'athletic heart syndrome' (AHS), commonly have deep T-wave inversion on ECG
    d. Have increased vagal tone
    e. Have second-degree heart block which resolves on exercise in one-third of individuals

21. **Regarding medical errors:**
    a. The majority are due to human error
    b. The most common type of error is 'knowledge-based'
    c. Boredom is a contributing factor for 'skill-based errors'
    d. A drug error is an example of a 'skill-based error'
    e. Latent errors are a form of human error

22. **Electroconvulsive therapy (ECT):**
    a. Consists of a pulsatile sine wave of 35 J
    b. Induces a tonic–clonic seizure
    c. Has a long parasympathetic phase
    d. Has a short sympathetic phase
    e. Should be preceded by administration of muscle relaxants

23. **When using CURB-65 as a severity assessment score for community-acquired pneumonia (CAP):**
    a. Confusion is a prognostic factor
    b. Urine output is a prognostic factor
    c. Maximal possible score is 5
    d. A score greater than 3 warrants ICU involvement
    e. It is predictive of mortality

24. Regarding Creutzfeldt–Jakob disease (CJD):
    a. Blood transfusion is the most common cause of the iatrogenic form
    b. Prion proteins are destroyed by formaldehyde
    c. Sterilization of contaminated equipment can only be achieved using ethylene oxide following disinfection
    d. Effective sterilization can be achieved by autoclaving at 138°C for 18 minutes following disinfection
    e. Cerebellar ataxia is a common early feature

25. A 70-year-old male is admitted to ICU following a laparotomy for a perforated duodenal ulcer; he has a history of ischaemic heart disease and is hypotensive. An oesophageal Doppler probe is inserted:
    a. A reduced aortic waveform height with rounded apex suggests left ventricular failure
    b. The flowtime corrected (FTc) is directly proportional to the systemic vascular resistance
    c. Normal range for peak velocity is 90–120 cm/s in this patient
    d. A fluid challenge would be an appropriate response for an FTc of 300 ms
    e. Inotropic therapy would be appropriate for this patient if the peak velocity is 40 cm/s

26. With regard to infections:
    a. The mortality associated with meticillin-resistant *Staphylococcus aureus* (MRSA) is higher than for meticillin-sensitive *S. aureus* (MSSA)
    b. The mortality associated with vancomycin-resistant enterococcus (VRE) is higher than for vancomycin-sensitive enterococcus (VSE)
    c. Selective decontamination of the digestive tract (SDD) has demonstrated a reduction in incidence of ventilator-acquired pneumonia
    d. Antibiotic cycling does not reduce mortality in ICU
    e. Restrictive antibiotic strategies have been shown to reduce mortality

27. The Wright respirometer:
    a. Is used for measuring forced expiratory volumes
    b. Consists of a vane moved by gas flow
    c. Has a vane that rotates in both directions
    d. Measures continuous flow accurately
    e. Produces an electrical output for analysis

28. Following a traction injury to the upper brachial plexus affecting the C5–6 nerve roots, the following is likely:
    a. Pronation of the forearm
    b. Loss of sensation over the medial surface of the arm
    c. Medial rotation of the arm
    d. Claw hand deformity
    e. Loss of arm abduction

29. The following factors reduce glomerular filtration rate (GFR):
    a. Vasodilatation of the efferent glomerular arterioles
    b. Angiotensin II
    c. Prostaglandins
    d. Hypotension
    e. Pregnancy

30. Carboprost is:
    a. A prostaglandin E_2 analogue
    b. Used for first-trimester abortion
    c. Administered intravenously
    d. Administered to a total dose of 8 mg
    e. Reported to cause bronchospasm

31. Concerning meta-analysis:
    a. It involves combining trials
    b. Power of trials are not increased
    c. Horizontal lines represent confidence intervals
    d. Lines on a forest plot must cross the line of equivalence to be considered 'significant'
    e. The size of the central mark on the plot represents power

32. Treatment goals recommended in the management of advanced heart failure include:
    a. Right atrial pressure <1 mmHg
    b. Mixed venous oxygen saturation $>60\%$
    c. Cardiac index >5 L min^{-1} m^{-2}
    d. Early institution of non-invasive ventilation for respiratory compromise
    e. Systemic vascular resistance $800-1200$ dyn s^{-1} cm^{-5}

33. Following an elective right hemicolectomy in a 70-year-old man:
    a. Nasogastric tubes are a cause of ileus
    b. Epidural analgesia reduces mortality
    c. Epidural analgesia reduces frequency of postoperative respiratory failure
    d. Early oral intake is contraindicated
    e. Clonidine can shorten the duration of ileus

34. According to the RIFLE classification of acute kidney injury:
    a. The risk class describes a >2 times increase in serum creatinine
    b. The risk class describes a urine output of <0.5 mL kg^{-1} h^{-1} for 6 hours
    c. The injury class describes a urine output of <0.5 mL kg^{-1} h^{-1} for 12 hours
    d. The system is predictive of mortality in hospital patients
    e. Acute kidney injury is defined as a 30% increase in creatinine from baseline in less than 48 hours

35. A 42-year-old patient on ICU admitted with respiratory failure has had a percutaneous tracheostomy inserted 3 days ago and has been successfully weaned from mechanical ventilation. You are alerted to her as she has suddenly become distressed, her oxygen saturations are 80%, her heart rate is 130/min and she is diaphoretic; you cannot hear breath sounds on her chest; initial management would include:
    a. Removal of the inner cannula
    b. Rapid sequence induction with endotracheal intubation
    c. Deflation of the tracheostomy tube cuff
    d. Removal of the tracheostomy and replacement with an endotracheal tube through the stoma site
    e. Removal of the tracheostomy and replacement with a smaller tracheostomy tube

36. A 24 kg child is booked for elective squint correction; the following breathing apparatus would be suitable:
    a. Bain circuit for spontaneous ventilation using fresh gas flow 100 mL kg^{-1} min^{-1}
    b. Magill system for controlled ventilation
    c. Humphrey ADE system for controlled ventilation with fresh gas flow of 3 L/min
    d. Humphrey ADE system for spontaneous ventilation
    e. The Lack system for spontaneous ventilation

37. Concerning sleep-related breathing disorders (SRBD) in children:
    a. 80% of sufferers have symptoms managed by adenotonsillectomy
    b. Adenotonsillectomy should be performed at specialist centres
    c. Repeated overnight arterial desaturations below 80% are indicative of severe obstructive sleep apnoea (OSA)
    d. If severe obstructive sleep apnoea is suspected, a chest radiograph is helpful
    e. When accompanied by weight <15 kg, further investigations are warranted

38. Methods to locate the epidural space include:
    a. Gutierrez's hanging drop technique
    b. Macintosh's indicator
    c. Ultrasonic localization
    d. Campbell–Howell method
    e. Odom's indicator

39. The National Patient Safety Agency Rapid Response Alert (2008) on reducing the risk of overdose following midazolam injection in adults:
    a. Reported approximately 500 patient safety incidents in one year
    b. Recommend the storage and use of high-strength midazolam is restricted to areas where use has been formally risk-assessed
    c. Require the use of flumazenil to be formally audited
    d. Recommend organizational policy for sedation
    e. Recommend overall responsibility be assumed by a senior clinician

40. The following is correct of antiemetic side-effects:
    a. Cyclizine decreases lower oesophageal sphincter tone
    b. Domperidone causes gynaecomastia
    c. Metoclopramide causes agitation
    d. All dopamine antagonists can cause dystonic reactions
    e. Ondansetron causes a bradycardia

41. Following deflation of a tourniquet applied to the lower limb for a period of 3 hours, there is:
    a. An increase in the serum lactate levels
    b. A rise in serum potassium levels, which peak after 30 minutes of deflation
    c. A rise in end-tidal CO_2, which peaks within 1 minute
    d. No association with irreversible muscle damage
    e. Increased fibrinolysis

42. The following are systemic effects of abdominal compartment syndrome (ACS):
    a. Reduced cardiac output
    b. Reduced pulmonary artery occlusion pressure (PAOP)
    c. Hypercapnia
    d. Reduced glomerular filtration rate (GFR)
    e. Increased intracranial pressure

43. Intra-aortic balloon pumps (IABPs):
    a. Are relatively contraindicated in patients with aortic regurgitation
    b. Are absolutely contraindicated in patients with abdominal aortic aneurysms
    c. Reduce left ventricular systolic pressure
    d. Are positioned just proximal to the origin of the subclavian artery
    e. Inflate immediately following end-diastole

44. Appropriate recruitment manoeuvres for patients in ICU:
    a. Include application of 30–40 cmH_2O continuous positive airway pressure (CPAP) for 40 s
    b. Include application of 20 cmH_2O CPAP for 20 minutes
    c. Have been demonstrated to improve survival in acute lung injury (ALI)
    d. Are most beneficial for patients ventilated for more than 3 days
    e. Consist of nocturnal pressure-supportive ventilation with spontaneous ventilation during daytime hours

45. The following statements regarding echocardiography are correct:
    a. Pulse repetition frequency is the number of pulses generated by the transducer in 1 minute
    b. Acoustic frequency is 3.5–7.5 MHz
    c. Transoesophageal technique utilizes higher frequencies than transthoracic
    d. The reflector in the Doppler method is the red cell
    e. It relies on piezoelectric transducers

46. A diver suddenly and fully immersed in cold water would be expected to have:
    a. Tachycardia
    b. A gasp reflex
    c. Apnoea
    d. Bradycardia
    e. Peripheral vasoconstriction

47. A 66-year-old man presents for emergency surgery with an intimal tear of his descending thoracic aorta; the following is correct:
    a. He has a type A aortic dissection
    b. He has a type B aortic dissection
    c. He is at risk of paraplegia
    d. A normal ECG is present in 50% of patients with coronary involvement
    e. This condition is usually preceded by an aortic aneurysm

48. Cook's modification of the Cormack and Lehane classification for difficult airway assessment describes the following:
    a. There are six grades
    b. Grades 3 and 4 are subdivided into A and B depending on the structures seen
    c. Grades 3B and 4 represent a 'difficult airway'
    d. Grades 2 and 3A indicate the requirement of a gum elastic bougie
    e. It is assessed on indirect laryngoscopy

49. A 34-year-old primigravida develops eclampsia in the second stage of labour; the following is correct:
    a. This is an indication for emergency caesarean section
    b. Spinal anaesthesia is absolutely contraindicated
    c. Immediate management is intravenous infusion of 4 g of magnesium sulphate
    d. Therapeutic levels of magnesium are in the range of 2–4 mmol/L
    e. In eclampsia one-third of fits occur postpartum

50. The following is correct of cardiac enzymes:
    a. Troponins are found only in cardiac muscle
    b. Serum troponin levels are independent of renal function
    c. CK-MB is a mitochondrial enzyme
    d. LDH-1 isoenzyme is found predominantly in cardiac muscle
    e. Raised troponin I is exclusively indicative of myocardial infarction (MI)

51. A 45-year-old man presents with lower back pain, urinary retention and perianal numbness developing within the last 3 hours; the following statements are correct:
    a. His condition is associated with the use of intrathecal 5% lidocaine
    b. He requires urodynamic studies urgently
    c. Spinal immobilization is not necessary
    d. Computed tomography is the imaging modality of choice
    e. Surgical correction should commence from within 12 hours of onset of symptoms

52. Treatment of poisoning with activated charcoal:
    a. Requires a charcoal : poison weight ratio of 2 : 1
    b. Is indicated for benzodiazepines
    c. Is indicated for lithium
    d. Is indicated for tricyclic antidepressants
    e. Is indicated for theophyllines

53. Pulmonary artery catheters (PACs):
    a. Allow direct measurement of cardiac output
    b. Calculate cardiac output using Fourier analysis
    c. Are inaccurate when measuring cardiac output in the presence of tricuspid regurgitation
    d. Have demonstrated benefit for critically ill patients
    e. Can be modified to allow pacing

54. Workplace exposure limits (parts per million, ppm) over 8 hours are:
    a. Halothane: 10
    b. Sevoflurane: 50
    c. Nitrous oxide: 50
    d. Isoflurane: 25
    e. Enflurane: 25

55. Coronary blood flow:
    a. Is approximately 80 mL/100 g/min
    b. Approximates 10% of total cardiac output at rest
    c. Is under predominant control of the autonomic nervous system
    d. Is related to the difference between aortic systolic pressure and left ventricular end-diastolic pressure (LVEDP)
    e. Is autoregulated

56. Signs of hypomagnesaemia include:
    a. Tremor
    b. Hyperreflexia
    c. Convulsions
    d. Shortened QT interval on the ECG
    e. T-wave flattening

57. **An increased functional residual capacity (FRC):**
    a. Necessitates a longer time for inhalational induction
    b. Occurs in the head-down position in patients with high thoracic spinal cord injury
    c. Is caused by application of PEEP
    d. Is found in asthmatics
    e. Is seen in the first trimester of pregnancy

58. **Drugs safe to use in porphyria include:**
    a. N_2O
    b. Phenytoin
    c. Bupivacaine
    d. Aspirin
    e. Etomidate

59. **A patient presents with a thyrotoxic crisis; appropriate management includes:**
    a. Dantrolene 1 mg/kg intravenously
    b. Propanolol 1–5 mg intravenously
    c. Aspirin 75 mg orally
    d. Potassium iodide 200–600 mg intravenously
    e. Thyroxine 0.1–0.2 mg orally

60. **The following statements are correct for dystrophia myotonica:**
    a. It is the most common of the myotonic syndromes
    b. Nerve block techniques abolish abnormal contractions
    c. Mitral valve prolapse occurs in up to 20% of patients
    d. Nerve stimulator use is mandatory
    e. Patients are more likely to require a caesarean section

61. **Concerning coning:**
    a. A unilateral constricted pupil is an early sign of uncal herniation
    b. Central herniation can result in decorticate posturing
    c. Central herniation can result in decerebrate posturing
    d. It may follow lumbar puncture
    e. Cheyne–Stokes respiration is a sign of cerebellar compression

62. **Vancomycin:**
    a. Is a glycopeptide
    b. Exerts bactericidal activity against Gram-positive and Gram-negative bacteria
    c. Can be administered orally
    d. Levels should be between 2 and 4 mg/L for therapeutic efficacy
    e. Causes 'red man syndrome' due to peripheral vasodilatation

63. **Regarding the ECG:**
    a. The normal axis is between $-30°$ and $+90°$
    b. δ-waves occur in Lown–Ganong–Levine syndrome
    c. Posterior myocardial infarction is diagnosed by dominant R-waves and ST depression in V1–V3
    d. Thrombolysis is indicated with 2 mm ST change in 1 limb lead
    e. Bifascicular block is characterized by left bundle branch block and left axis deviation

64. **The sciatic nerve:**
    a. Is formed from the anterior primary rami of L4–S3
    b. Divides into tibial and common peroneal nerves
    c. Division is commonly at its point of exit from the greater sciatic foramen
    d. Branches include the posterior cutaneous nerve of the thigh
    e. Can be blocked by anterior or posterior approaches

65. **The isobestic points of oxyhaemoglobin and deoxyhaemoglobin are:**
    a. 660 nm
    b. 590 nm
    c. 940 nm
    d. 805 nm
    e. 490 nm

66. **The following agents reduce intraocular pressure (IOP):**
    a. Topical adrenaline
    b. Acetazolamide
    c. Intravenous ketamine
    d. Propofol
    e. Intravenous atropine

67. **Regarding hypoxia:**
    a. It is defined as a PaO_2 <8 kPa
    b. Histotoxic hypoxia occurs in CO poisoning
    c. Stagnant hypoxia occurs in cyanide poisoning
    d. Ischaemic hypoxia occurs in cardiac failure
    e. Hypoxic hypoxia occurs in hypoventilation

68. **A 60-year-old male with a history of rheumatic fever presents for emergency abdominal surgery. At preoperative assessment, he is found to have a mid-diastolic murmur, atrial fibrillation and an enlarged left atrial appendage on chest X-ray; the following statements are appropriate:**
    a. Systemic vascular resistance should be kept low
    b. A transmitral pressure gradient of 20 mmHg during diastole is normal
    c. Diastolic pressure should be maintained
    d. Normal mitral valve area is 4–6 cm^2
    e. Left ventricular end-diastolic pressure (LVEDP) is a good indicator of preload

69. The trial outcomes listed are correct:
    a. MAGPIE: Decreased mortality with magnesium in pre-eclampsia
    b. MASTER: Decreased mortality with epidural analgesia for major abdominal surgery
    c. POISE: No difference in mortality with metoprolol vs placebo for non-cardiac surgery
    d. B-Aware: Bispectral index (BIS)-guided anaesthesia reduced awareness by over 50% in high-risk adults
    e. PAC-Man: Increased mortality in critically ill patient with use of pulmonary artery catheters (PACs)

70. Minitracheostomy:
    a. Is preferably performed through the higher tracheal rings
    b. Is the preferred method for emergency airway access
    c. Uses airway tubes typically sized 8 mm
    d. Incorporates a cuffed tube
    e. Is declining in use

71. A man is brought to A&E following a crush injury of both legs and pelvis; immediate investigations should include:
    a. Urine testing for myoglobin
    b. Arterial blood gas
    c. X-ray series of both legs
    d. Cross-matching 10 units of packed red cells
    e. Internal iliac arteriography

72. Concerning laryngoscope blades:
    a. Miller possesses a curved tip
    b. Polio Macintosh is mounted at 120° to the handle
    c. McCoy is hinged at the tip, allowing elevation of the tongue
    d. Macintosh blades are available as left-handed versions
    e. The Soper is a straight version of the Macintosh

73. Desflurane:
    a. Contains seven fluorine atoms
    b. Has a single chiral centre
    c. Has a blood : gas partition coefficient of 4.2
    d. Has the highest saturated vapour pressure (SVP) (at 20°C) of the halogenated anaesthetic volatile agents
    e. Sensitizes the myocardium to catecholamines

74. The following changes occur during whole blood storage:
    a. Decreased adenosine triphosphate (ATP) concentrations
    b. Progressive increase in potassium levels
    c. Increased free 2,3-diphosphoglycerate (2,3-DPG) concentration
    d. Addition of adenine increases shelf-life to 35 days
    e. Platelets are non-functional at 6 hours

75. **Malignant hyperthermia (MH):**
    a. Is inherited in an autosomal dominant fashion
    b. Can present with isolated rhabdomyolysis
    c. Exhibits anticipation
    d. Is not safely managed with administration of nitrous oxide
    e. Is confirmed by in vitro contraction of vastus muscle under separate exposure to halothane and theophylline

76. **Indications for an interpleural block include:**
    a. Fractured rib
    b. Chronic pancreatitis
    c. Laparoscopic cholecystectomy
    d. Mastectomy
    e. Shoulder surgery

77. **The coagulation disorders below are associated with the following laboratory test results:**
    a. Haemophilia A and normal thrombin time (TT)
    b. Haemophilia A and increased bleeding time
    c. Haemophilia B and increased activated partial thromboplastin time (APTT)
    d. Disseminated intravascular coagulation (DIC) and increased fibrinogen
    e. von Willebrand's disease and increased bleeding time

78. **Acute respiratory distress syndrome (ARDS) consists of:**
    a. A direct exogenous insult
    b. A fibroproliferative phase
    c. $Pao_2/Fio_2 \leq 300$ mmHg (40 kPa)
    d. Unilateral infiltrates on chest X-ray
    e. Mortality of 30–50%

79. **Common aetiologies of acute pancreatitis include:**
    a. Microlithiasis
    b. Trauma
    c. Chronic alcoholism
    d. Hypothermia
    e. Hypocalcaemia

80. **The following cannot be measured by spirometry:**
    a. Vital capacity (VC)
    b. Expiratory reserve volume (ERV)
    c. Residual volume (RV)
    d. Functional residual capacity (FRC)
    e. Total lung capacity (TLC)

81. Cancerning colloids:
    a. Gelofusine contains 124 mmol/L sodium
    b. Hetastarch has a half-life of 6–8 hours
    c. Starch-based colloids have higher rates of adverse reactions than gelatins
    d. Dextrans will lower the erythrocyte sedimentation rate (ESR)
    e. Molecular weight (MW) of gelofusine is 15–20 kDa

82. Turbulent flow is proportional to:
    a. Radius^4
    b. (Pressure gradient)$^{-1}$
    c. Reynolds number
    d. Length
    e. (Density of fluid)$^{-1}$

83. The stellate ganglion:
    a. Is part of the parasympathetic chain
    b. Lies either side of the vertebral column
    c. Is the fusion of 1st and 2nd thoracic ganglia
    d. Can be blocked at Chassaignac tubercle
    e. Blockade results in ptosis

84. The following are side-effects of propofol administration:
    a. Green hair
    b. Bradycardia
    c. Convulsions
    d. Acidosis
    e. Hypercholesterolaemia

85. Maternal death:
    a. Describes the death of a woman up to 48 hours after her pregnancy
    b. When 'indirect' describes death due to medical intervention
    c. Is most commonly due to pre-eclampsia
    d. When 'coincidental' describes death unrelated to pregnancy
    e. In the UK, the incidence is about 7 per 100 000 maternities

86. The positions in Generic Pacemaker Code (NBG) relate to the following functions:
    a. I – Chamber sensed
    b. II – Chamber paced
    c. III – Response to sensing
    d. IV – Programmability
    e. V – Shock chamber

87. A pressure of 10 bar is equal to:
    a. 145 lb/inch^2
    b. 100 kPa
    c. 10 200 cmH$_2$O
    d. 750 mmHg
    e. 7500 Torr

88. The following agents can be used for intravenous regional anaesthesia (IVRA):
    a. Bupivacaine
    b. Lidocaine
    c. Lidocaine with adrenaline
    d. Prilocaine
    e. Guanethidine

89. Fetal haemoglobin (HbF)
    a. Consists of two α and two β chains
    b. Binds 2,3-DPG less avidly than HbA
    c. Has a P$_{50}$ of 2.4 kPa
    d. Forms 50% of circulating haemoglobin at birth
    e. May persist

90. A sensorimotor neuropathy is a feature of:
    a. Charcot–Marie–Tooth disease
    b. Syringomyelia
    c. Leprosy
    d. Motor neuron disease
    e. Diphtheria

3. Practice Paper 3: Answers

1a. True
1b. True
1c. False
1d. False
1e. True

The term 'fat embolism' describes the presence of fat globules in lung parenchyma and the peripheral circulation after long bone injury (closed more frequently than open) or major trauma; it is often asymptomatic. Non-traumatic causes include pancreatitis, diabetes and osteomyelitis. A consequence is *fat embolism syndrome*, which produces a distinct pattern of clinical symptoms and signs. Clinical presentation is typically 24–72 hours after injury and is characterized by a triad of respiratory changes, neurological abnormalities and a petechial rash. Various diagnostic criteria exist, the most commonly used are Gurd's criteria and Schonfeld's criteria; the latter score petechiae, chest X-ray, hypoxaemia, fever, tachycardia and tachypnoea. The presence of fat globules in the urine is a non-specific finding following trauma. Mortality is 5–15%.

Gupta A, Reilly CS. Fat embolism. *Contin Educ Anaesth Crit Care Pain* 2007; 7: 148–51.

2a. True
2b. False
2c. False
2d. False
2e. True

A Cochrane systematic review concluded that epidural analgesia may be useful for postoperative pain relief following major lower limb joint replacements. However, the benefits may be limited to the early (4–6 hours) postoperative period. The hip joint is innervated by the femoral, sciatic and obturator nerves, with cutaneous innervation supplied by the lateral cutaneous nerve of the thigh (LCNT); thus, the sciatic nerve must be blocked for complete anaesthesia. A lumbar plexus block will reliably block the femoral and obturator nerves and the LCNT. The sciatic nerve (L4,5, S1,2,3) is derived from the sacral plexus and is thus not reliably blocked. A Winnie or '3-in-1' block attempts to block the femoral, obturator and LCNT with one injection; complete lumbar plexus block occurs in only 35% of patients.

Choi P, Bhandari M, Scott J, Douketis JD. Epidural analgesia for pain relief following hip or knee replacement. *Cochrane Database Syst Rev* 2003; (3): CD003071.

3a. False
3b. True
3c. False
3d. True
3e. True

The Multicentre Aneurysm Screening Study demonstrated a 53% reduction in mortality for patients who underwent elective surgery when an aneurysm diameter reached 5.5 cm. The UK Small Aneurysm Trial demonstrated no benefit in elective surgery for aneurysms under 5.5 cm diameter. Retroperitoneal rupture may result in a tamponade, which limits haemorrhage and is associated with better survival than intraperitoneal rupture, which usually results in cardiovascular collapse and death. Aggressive administration of fluids may result in increased mean arterial pressure, thrombus dislodgement and dilution of clotting factors and thus increased bleeding. Cross-clamping of the aorta results in increased left ventricular afterload and proximal hypertension. Following release of the clamp, there is a sudden decreased afterload and recirculation of ischaemic metabolites, which can result in ischaemia–reperfusion injury and arrhythmias. The 2005 NCEPOD enquiry reported a 6.2% mortality for open elective repairs and 36% for emergency abdominal aortic aneurysm repairs in the UK.

Leonard A, Thompson J. Anaesthesia for ruptured abdominal aortic aneurysm. *Contin Educ Anaesth Crit Care Pain* 2008; 8: 11–15.
Multicentre Aneurysm Screening Study Group. The multicentre aneurysm screening study into the effect of abdominal aortic aneurysm screening on mortality in men: a randomised controlled trial. *Lancet* 2002; 360: 1531–9.
National Confidential Enquiry into Patient Outcome and Death. *Abdominal Aortic Aneurysm: A Service in Need of Surgery?* London: NCEPOD, 2005.
The UK Small Aneurysm Trial Participants. Mortality results for randomised controlled trial of early elective surgery or ultrasound surveillance for small abdominal aortic aneurysms. *Lancet* 1998; 352: 1649–55.

4a. False
4b. True
4c. False
4d. False
4e. True

Pre-eclampsia is a multisystem disease, with severe pre-eclampsia affecting 5 per 1000 maternities in the UK. Pre-eclampsia is pregnancy-induced hypertension (PIH) in association with proteinuria (0.3 g in 24 hours) $\pm$ oedema. Virtually any organ system may be affected. Severe pre-eclampsia is defined as the presence of severe hypertension (diastolic BP ≥ 110 mmHg, or systolic BP ≥ 170 mmHg on more than two occasions) and proteinuria (> 1 g/L). In the absence of these, however, other clinical features suggestive of severe pre-eclampsia are:

- severe headache
- visual disturbance
- epigastric pain/vomiting
- clonus
- papilloedema

- liver tenderness
- platelet count $< 100 \times 10^9/L$
- abnormal liver enzymes (ALT or AST >70 IU/L)
- HELLP syndrome

It is important to remember that women may present with eclampsia without any prodromal symptoms.

Royal College of Obstetricians and Gynaecologists. *The Management of Severe Pre-Eclampsia/Eclampsia*, Guideline No. 10(A). London: RCOG, 2006.

5a. True
5b. False
5c. True
5d. False
5e. False
von Willebrand's disease is the most common inherited coagulation defect; usually as autosomal dominant transmission. It consists of an abnormality of the von Willebrand factor (vWF), which is a protein involved in platelet adhesion and carriage of factor VIII. It is classified into type I (quantitative reduction in vWF), type II (qualitative reduction of vWF) and type III (similar to I but a severe autosomal recessive form). Platelet counts may be normal. Partial thromboplastin time and bleeding time are prolonged. Before surgery, patients may benefit from administration of vWF concentrate or desmopressin (which increases levels of factor VIII and vWF); if these products are unavailable, fresh frozen plasma or cryoprecipitate can be given in an emergency. In pregnancy, factor VIII and vWF levels increase, but may fall soon after delivery.

'Café-au-lait' spots occur in neurofibromatosis (type I is named von Recklinghausen's disease).

Yentis S, Hirsch N, Smith G. *Anaesthesia and Intensive Care A to Z: An Encyclopaedia of Principles and Practice*, 4th edn. Oxford: Butterworth-Heinemann, 2009.

6a. False
6b. False
6c. True
6d. True
6e. False
Mycoplasma pneumoniae is a common cause of community-acquired pneumonia, predominantly affecting young adults. It has an insidious onset, presenting with a prodrome of headache and malaise, which often precedes chest signs by 1–2 weeks. Subsequent presentation includes persistent, dry cough, due to inhibition of ciliary movement by the bacterium, and low-grade fever. Often affecting the lower lobes, there is little correlation between clinical features and chest X-ray findings. Cold agglutinins occur in 50% and diagnosis is confirmed by a rising antibody titre. It can be complicated by myocarditis, pericarditis, erythema multiforme, haemolytic anaemia and myalgia or arthralgia. Rose spots are classical of *Chlamydia psittaci*; lung cavitation occurs rarely in *Legionella pneumophila*.

7a. False
7b. True
7c. True
7d. True
7e. True

Renal replacement therapy can be provided with haemodialysis (HD), haemofiltration (HF), a combination of these or peritoneal dialysis. Goals of treatment are solute and water clearance, correction of electrolyte and acid–base disturbances, and removal of toxins. Diffusion is the process of passive movement of substances along a concentration gradient and occurs across a semipermeable membrane in HD. The rate of diffusion is thus proportional to the concentration gradient, and this drives the process. HF relies on the principle of convective transport, where a solute is swept through a membrane by an ultrafiltrate (solvent drag). This is independent of solute concentrations; the membrane characteristics determine solute removal and transmembrane pressure serves to effectively push or pull a solute into the ultrafiltrate. Solute removal occurs more quickly in HD, which can be intermittent, whereas HF is a continuous form of renal replacement.

Hall NA, Fox AJ. Renal replacement therapies in critical care. *Contin Educ Anaesth Crit Care Pain* 2006; **6**: 197–202.

8a. True
8b. False
8c. False
8d. False
8e. False

Botulism is a rare and lethal disease caused by the exotoxins of the Gram-positive anaerobe *Clostridium botulinum*, typically found in soil and dust. Toxins are classed A–E; A, B or E account for almost all human cases. It can be transmitted thus:

- food-borne (most common, especially with canned foods)
- wound botulism
- intestinal colonization (seen in infants)
- deliberate (bioterrorism)
- accidental (through therapeutic use)

The toxin binds *irreversibly* to the presynaptic membrane of cholinergic neurons. Symptoms include gastrointestinal disturbance, sore throat, fatigue, dizziness, paraesthesias, cranial involvement and a progressive *descending* flaccid weakness; parasympathetic symptoms are common.

Wenham T, Cohen A. Botulism. *Contin Educ Anaesth Crit Care Pain* 2008; **8**: 21–5.

9a. True
9b. True
9c. True
9d. True
9e. True

Cardiac muscle contains a contractile complex with contractile proteins (actin and myosin) and regulatory proteins (troponin and tropomyosin). The troponin complex consists of three single-chain polypeptides: troponins T, I and C. Cardiac troponins (cTn) have been recommended as the biomarker of choice in the diagnosis of myocardial infarction by the Joint European Society of Cardiology and American College of Cardiology Committee. There are a variety of causes for a raised cTn in the absence of coronary artery disease:

Demand ischaemia (mismatch between myocardial oxygen demand and supply, in the absence of flow-limiting coronary artery stenosis)

- Sepsis/systemic inflammatory response syndrome
- Hypotension
- Hypovolaemia
- Tachyarrhythmias
- Left ventricular hypertrophy

Myocardial ischaemia

- Prinzmetal's angina (vasospasm)
- Cerebrovascular accident (CVA), intracranial haemorrhage (over-activity of the autonomic nervous system)

Direct myocardial cell injury

- Trauma, myocarditis, pericarditis, toxins

Myocardial strain

- Congestive heart failure, pulmonary embolism, extreme exercise

Chronic renal insufficiency

- End-stage renal failure

Wolfe Barry JA, Barth JH, Howell SJ. Cardiac troponins: their use and relevance in anaesthesia and critical care medicine. *Contin Educ Anaesth Crit Care Pain* 2008; 8: 62–6.

10a. True
10b. False
10c. False
10d. True
10e. True

Horner's syndrome is caused by interruption of the sympathetic innervation to the head; it may be due to lesions along the pathway, intentional cervical sympathectomy or inadvertent sympathetic blockade. It consists of partial ptosis, meiosis, apparent enophthalmos, lack of sweating (anhydrosis) and nasal stuffiness on the ipsilateral side.

Yentis S, Hirsch N, Smith G. *Anaesthesia and Intensive Care A to Z: An Encyclopaedia of Principles and Practice*, 4th edn. Oxford: Butterworth-Heinemann, 2009.

11a. True
11b. False
11c. True
11d. True
11e. False
The thoracic duct drains all the lymph from the lower limbs, abdominal and pelvic cavities, left thorax, left head and neck, and left upper limb; it passes through the aortic opening in the diaphragm and drains the cisterna chyli. The medial breast drains into internal mammary nodes via intercostal spaces, while the lateral quadrants drain into anterior axillary nodes. The heart contains extensive networks of lymph vessels throughout the epicardium, myocardium and endocardium.

12a. True
12b. False
12c. True
12d. True
12e. True
Human insulin is produced by recombinant DNA technology, and available preparations can be categorized into short-, intermediate- and long-acting. Soluble insulin is short-acting and is ideal for use in diabetic emergencies; it has an onset of action within 30 minutes subcutaneously, and following intravenous administration its effect disappears within 30 minutes. Intermediate- and long-acting preparations are formulated with protamine and zinc to reduce solubility and prolong the action of insulin. Onset of action is usually 1–2 hours and duration ranges from 16 to 35 hours.

British Medical Association, Royal Pharmaceutical Society of Great Britain. *British National Formulary 58*. Section 6.1.1: Insulins. London: Pharmaceutical Press, 2009. Available at: bnf.org/bnf.

13a. True
13b. True
13c. False
13d. True
13e. False
Tuohy needles are commonly used for epidural insertion in the UK. During insertion, the needle should be removed with the catheter to avoid risk of transection by the oblique bevel (named the Huber point). The 10 cm model is most commonly used, but 5 and 15 cm models exist.

14a. True
14b. False
14c. False
14d. True
14e. False

The Synacthen test is used to assess adrenocortical function. Failure of blood cortisol to rise above a certain level indicates adrenal insufficiency. For the short Synacthen test, a basal serum cortisol is taken; 250 μg of tetracosactide (Synacthen, an analogue of ACTH) is then administered and blood cortisol is analysed at 30 and 60 minutes following injection. Healthy individuals should have a basal serum cortisol of >170 nmol/L with diurnal variation, cortisol levels should rise to >500 nmol/L (peak normally 800–1000 nmol/L) at either 30 or 60 minutes, with an increase of at least 200 nmol/L. The long Synacthen test involves an intramuscular depot injection of tetracosactide with subsequent cortisol analysis at exactly 30 minutes and 1, 2, 4, 7 and 24 hours. In Addison's disease, plasma cortisol fails to rise above reference levels, but in secondary causes (i.e. chronic steroid use), delayed but normal responses are seen. Increased ACTH levels are seen in primary (Addison's) adrenocortical insufficiency.

Dorin RI, Qualls CR, Crapo LM. Diagnosis of adrenal insufficiency. *Ann Intern Med* 2003; **139**: 194–204.

15a. False
15b. True
15c. False
15d. False
15e. False

Tetralogy of Fallot consists of a ventricular septal defect, pulmonary outflow obstruction (stenosis), right ventricular hypertrophy and an overriding aorta; this leads to central cyanosis as blood flows from right to left and deoxygenated blood is ejected systemically. A harsh systolic murmur of pulmonary stenosis occurs and pulmonary oligaemia results. A left-to-right shunt occurs in an ASD, with increased pulmonary blood flow; Eisenmenger's syndrome can result in the long term, but presents in later childhood and not in the neonatal period. Coarctation will lead to upper limb hypertension, weak femoral pulses and a harsh murmur often radiating to the back, but pulmonary oligaemia and central cyanosis are not features. Finally, TAPVD is a rare cyanotic defect that presents very soon after birth and relies upon a patent foramen ovale or atrioventricular septal defect for the infant's survival. Presentation depends on the degree of pulmonary venous obstruction, but severe cyanosis and respiratory distress occur, with a split 2nd heart sound and a systolic flow murmur; heart failure can also occur.

16a. False
16b. False
16c. False
16d. True
16e. True
CIP often presents as difficulty weaning from mechanical ventilation and occurs in 70–80% of patients with sepsis or multi-organ dysfunction; it occurs in 25–63% of those who are mechanically ventilated for > 1 week. Primary axonal degeneration of motor and sensory fibres occur leading to a mixed motor and sensory neuropathy, with motor signs predominating. Electro-physiological studies show reduced amplitude of nerve action potentials but a relative preservation of nerve conduction velocities and latencies; needle electromyography shows fibrillation potentials. Muscle biopsy is necessary to distinguish between CIP and critical illness myopathy. Plasma creatine kinase levels are normal or near-normal and absent reflexes are not a prerequisite for diagnosis.

Maramattom BV, Wijdicks EFM. Acute neuromuscular weakness in the intensive care unit. *Crit Care Med* 2006; 34: 2835–41.
Visser LH. Critical illness polyneuropathy and myopathy: clinical features, risk factors and prognosis. *Eur J Neurol* 2006; 13: 1203–12.

17a. True
17b. False
17c. False
17d. True
17e. False
The 2008 Surviving Sepsis Guidelines use the Grades of Recommendation, Assessment, Development and Evaluation (GRADE) system to guide assessment of quality of evidence from high (A) to very low (D) and to determine the strength of recommendation. A strong recommendation is a '1', and a weak recommendation is a '2'. Fluid therapy includes resuscitation with crystalloids or colloids (1B), targetting a CVP ≥ 8 mmHg (≥ 12 if mechanically ventilated) (1C), fluid challenges as stated (1D). Vasopressors are used to maintain mean arterial pressures >65 mmHg (1C), with noradrenaline and dobutamine being the initial agents of choice (1C). Vasopressin may be added to noradrenaline (2C), but there is no role for low-dose dopamine for the purpose of renal protection (1A).

Recombinant human activated protein C (rhAPC) should be considered in adult patients with sepsis-induced organ dysfunction with clinical assessment of high risk of death (typically APACHE II ≥ 25 or multi-organ failure) if there are no contraindications. Adults with a low risk of death should not receive rhAPC (1A). Tidal volumes of 6 mL/kg should be targeted in patients with acute lung injury or ARDS (1B), with an initial upper limit plateau pressure of ≤ 30 cmH$_2$O (1C).

Packed red cells should be given when haemoglobin decreases to <7.0 g/dL to target a haemoglobin between 7.0 and 9.0 g/dL in adults (1B). A higher level may be required in special circumstances (e.g. myocardial ischaemia, severe hypoxaemia, acute haemorrhage, cyanotic heart disease or lactic acidaemia).

Delinger RP, Leng MM, Cochet JM, et al. Surviving Sepsis Campaign: International guidelines for management of severe sepsis and septic shock. *Crit Care Med* 2008; **36**: 296–327.

18a. False
18b. True
18c. True
18d. True
18e. False
In data that are normally distributed (parametric), the mean, mode and median are equal. Frequently, data are not normally distributed (non-parametric); the distribution may be skewed to the right (positive) or to the left (negative) or be bimodal. The standard deviation (SD) is the square root of the variance, the SEM is the SD divided by the degrees of freedom. Variance, SD and SEM are all related to the mean. Tests for parametric data include Student's t-test and ANOVA (and their paired counterparts). Non-parametric data tests include Mann–Whitney U, Wilcoxon signed rank, Friedman's and Kruskal–Wallis.

Rowbotham DJ. Basic statistics. In: Pinnock C, Lin S, Smith T, eds. *Fundamentals of Anaesthesia*, 3rd edn. Greenwich, UK: Greenwich Medical Media Ltd, 2009.

19a. True
19b. False
19c. True
19d. True
19e. True
Perfluorocarbons are chemically inert compounds composed of a carbon skeleton containing fluorine atoms, which confer stability. They are infused as an intravenous emulsion because of their hydrophobic nature and exhibit a linear oxygen dissociation relationship; hence oxygen release is directly pro-portional to oxygen partial pressure. Henry's law is applicable, since they have no specific oxygen binding sites and dissolution relies on physical solubi-lization; they also dissolve other gases such as carbon dioxide and inhaled anaesthetics. The emulsion droplets are taken up by the reticuloendothelial cells and transported as lipids to the lungs, where perfluorocarbons are exhaled. They also contribute to greenhouse pollution.

Spiess B. Perfluorocarbon emulsions: one approach to intravenous artificial respiratory gas transport. *Ann Anaesthesiol* 1994; **11**: 103–13.

20a. False
20b. True
20c. False
20d. True
20e. False
The AHS is a collection of structural and functional changes occurring in highly exercise-trained individuals, particularly with endurance training. Highly trained athletes develop myocardial hypertrophy with increased myocardial mass and wall thickness and increased chamber size. Maximal stroke volume and cardiac output increase and athletes have lower resting heart rates owing to increased vagal tone. The cardiac hypertrophy can be mistaken as hyper-trophic cardiomyopathy on echocardiography, but the athelete's heart shows symmetrical hypertrophy that regresses on de-conditioning and no diastolic dysfunction, with a normal left atrial cavity size. Up to one-third of highly trained athletes have first-degree heart block, which often improves with exercise, and Mobitz I is sometimes seen in AHS but Mobitz II is rare. In AHS the ECG commonly shows ST elevation due to early repolarization; T-wave changes are common and can be bizarre, including peaked, inverted or biphasic T-waves in precordial leads; deep inverted T-waves can occur, but are rare and should prompt exclusion of cardiac pathology.

Topoll EJ, Califf RM. The athelete's heart. In: *Textbook of Cardiovascular Medicine*, Vol 355. Philadelphia: Lippincott Williams & Wilkins, 2006.

21a. True
21b. False
21c. True
21d. True
21e. False
The widely accepted classification by Reason divides errors into three subtypes:

- *Skill-based error*: most frequently due to subconscious actions occurring as a result of tiredness, boredom and stress (drug errors, forgetting to switch on a ventilator)
- *Rule-based error*: application of an incorrect or inadequate rule to a given situation, classically a misdiagnosis (failing to perform an anaesthetic machine check, failing to implement guidelines)
- *Knowledge-based error*: occurring as a result of incorrect or incomplete information and the loss of situational awareness (allowing patient hypothermia to develop without realizing significance)

In any safety mechanism there are *active* errors (or failures) that occur at the point of contact between a human and some part of a system, and *latent* errors ('accidents waiting to happen') which refer to a failure of design or organization which allow harm to occur.

Mallory S, Weller J, Bloch M, Maze M. The individual, the system, and medical error. *Contin Educ Anaesth Crit Care Pain* 2009; **3**: 179–82.
Reason JT. *Human Error*. Cambridge: CUP, 1990.
Reason J. Human error: models and management. *BMJ* 2000; **320**: 768–70.

22a. False
22b. True
22c. False
22d. False
22e. True
The National Institute for Health and Clinical Excellence recommends that ECT be used to achieve short-term improvement of severe symptoms after an adequate trial of other treatment options or when the condition is potentially life-threatening, in individuals with:

- severe depressive illness
- catatonia
- prolonged/severe manic episode

It consists of a pulsatile *square* wave that discharges at $\sim$35 J to one or both cerebral hemispheres. Following a brief tonic–clonic convulsion, there is a short-lived parasympathetic phase that consists of vagal stimulation, which may result in asystole. This is followed by a longer sympathetic phase, consisting of increased heart rate, blood pressure, myocardial and cerebral oxygen consumption. Bolam was a patient who underwent ECT without muscle relaxants or body restraints and suffered a severe fracture of the pelvis. The '*Bolam vs Friern Hospital Management Committee*' (1957) became an English tort law case for the appropriate standard of reasonable care in negligence cases – 'The Bolam Test'. Suxamethonium $\sim$0.5 mg/kg is often given to avoid these injuries.

Bolam vs Friern Hospital Management Committee 1957 (1 WLR 583).
National Institute for Health and Clinical Excellence. *The Clinical Effectiveness and Cost Effectiveness of Electroconvulsive Therapy (ECT) for Depressive Illness, Schizophrenia, Catatonia and Mania.* London: NICE, 2003. Available at: guidance.nice.org.uk/TA59.
Royal College of Anaesthetists. *Guidance for ECT provided in Remote Sites.* London: RCOA, 2003.

23a. True
23b. False
23c. True
23d. True
23e. True
CURB-65 is a set of clinical criteria validated for prediction of mortality in CAP and recommended by the British Thoracic Society in the assessment of severe pneumonia. There are five core prognostic factors in CURB-65, which assess the clinical severity of CAP:

- Confusion (Abbreviated Mental Test Score <8)
- Urea >7 mmol/L
- Respiratory rate $\geq$30/min
- Blood pressure (<90 mmHg systolic or $\leq$60 mmHg diastolic)
- Age >65 years

Each is assigned a score of 1, thus giving a maximal value of 5. Additional prognostic factors that do not contribute to the score are hypoxaemia with PaO_2 <8 kPa regardless of FiO_2 and bilateral or multilobar involvement on chest X-ray. Pre-existing adverse factors include coexisting illness, congestive cardiac failure, coronary disease and diabetes.

A score of 0–1 warrants outpatient management. A score of 2 should be assessed clinically and considered with additional factors. It may warrant inpatient stay. A score of 3 is high-risk and warrants ICU involvement.

Sadashivaiah JB, Carr B. Severe community-acquired pneumonia. *Contin Educ Anaesth Crit Care Pain* 2009; **9**: 87–91.

24a. False
24b. False
24c. False
24d. True
24e. True
Creutzfeldt–Jakob disease (CJD) is a progressive neurodegenerative disease caused by transmission of prion proteins and is a form of transmissible spongiform encephalopathy. Types include the numerically most common sporadic, followed by variant, iatrogenic and genetic forms. Iatrogenic CJD is extremely rare and most commonly occurred following use of human growth hormone preparations, but also use of contaminated neurosurgical equipment, dura mater and corneal grafts.

Effective disinfectants: sodium hydroxide, sodium hypochlorite, guanidine thiocyanate, phenol.

The National Creutzfeldt–Jakob Disease Surveillance Unit (NCJDSU). Website: www.cjd.ed.ac.uk.
Rutala WA, Weber DJ. Creutzfeldt–Jakob disease: recommendations for cleaning and sterilization. *Clin Infect Dis* 2001; **32**: 1348–56.

25a. True
25b. False
25c. False
25d. True
25e. True
The oesophageal Doppler is based upon the Doppler principle, which is the change in frequency of sound waves as they are reflected from a moving object. This is utilized clinically to measure the velocity of blood flow in the descending aorta, which allows calculation of various parameters relating to cardiac function and filling status, including cardiac output and systemic vascular resistance. The Doppler waveform base is a function of left ventricular filling, heart rate and afterload. The flowtime corrected (FTc) to a heart rate of 60 is inversely related to the systemic vascular resistance. Most commonly a low FTc is caused by hypovolaemia, making a fluid challenge appropriate. In the face of hypotension and a low peak velocity, left ventricular failure is likely and inotropic support may be indicated. Normal ranges are:

- FTc (330–360 ms): time of systolic aortic blood flow
- PV (90–120 cm/s at age 20 years; 70–100 cm/s at 50 years): an index of contractility

Singer M. Oesophageal monitoring of aortic blood flow: beat by beat cardiac output monitoring. *Int Anesth Clin* 1993; **31**: 99–125.

26a. False
26b. False
26c. True
26d. False
26e. True
There is no significant excess mortality associated with either MRSA or VRE; however, in both cases infections are associated with longer ICU and hospital stays. SDD, antibiotic cycling and restrictive antibiotic strategies have all been demonstrated to reduce mortality in ICU patients. Meta-analysis for SDD demonstrated reduction in lower airway infections and mortality. The aim of SDD is to prevent or treat, if present, oropharyngeal or gastrointestinal presence of potentially pathogenic microorganisms, leaving intact the indigenous flora, which is protective. Quarterly empiric antibiotic rotational schedules in a surgical and trauma ICU reported decreased infections and overall mortality. In another study, antibiotics were stopped if Gram–stain was negative or failure to culture significant bacterial growth from samples obtained at bronchoalveolar lavage; these restrictive antibiotic strategies led to a significant reduction in mortality for patients with ventilator-acquired pneumonia.

Blunt MD, Viira DJ, Brown N, et al. The implications of methicillin resistant *Staphlococcus aureus* (MRSA) in the general intensive care unit. *Lancet* 1998; ii: 1197.
Fagon JY, Chastre J, Wolf M, et al. Invasive and non-invasive strategies for management of suspected ventilator-associated pneumonia: a randomised trial. *Ann Intern Med* 2000; **132**: 621–30.
Raymond DP, Pelletier SJ, Crabtree TD, et al. Impact of a rotating empiric antibiotic schedule on infectious mortality in an intensive care unit. *Crit Care Med* 2001; **29**: 1101–8.
Varley AJ, Williams H, Fletcher S. Antibiotic resistance in the ICU. *Contin Educ Anaesth Crit Care Pain* 2009; **9**: 114–18.
van Saene HKF, Peters AJ, Ramsay G, et al. All great truths are iconoclastic: selective decontamination of the digestive tract moves from heresy to level one truth. *Int Care Med* 2003; **29**: 677–90.

27a. False
27b. True
27c. False
27d. False
27e. False
Tidal volumes can be measured using a Wright respirometer, which relies on unidirectional rotation of a vane by gas flow; the movement of the vane produces a mechanical reading. Continuous flow causes inaccuracies in measurement and it does not produce an electrical output for analysis or recording. At low tidal volumes, the respirometer has a tendency to underestimate; at high volumes, it overestimates owing to inertia.

Davis PD, Kenny GNC. *Basic Physics and Measurement in Anaesthesia*, 5th edn. Oxford: Butterworth-Heinemann, 2003.

28a. True
28b. False
28c. True
28d. False
28e. True
Traction injuries to the upper brachial plexus can occur with excessive opposite movement of the head away from the shoulder and will affect nerves originating from the C5–6 roots. The following muscles will be affected: supraspinatus, infraspinatus, subclavius, biceps brachii, part of brachialis, coracobrachialis, deltoid and teres minor. This results in Erb–Duchenne ('waiter's tip') palsy and the affected arm is medially rotated owing to action of the unaffected pectoralis major and pronated owing to biceps paralysis, with loss of sensation over the lateral portion of the arm.

Snell RS. *Clinical Anatomy for Medical Students*, 6th edn. Boston: Little, Brown, 2000.

29a. True
29b. False
29c. False
29d. True
29e. False
GFR is the volume of fluid filtered from the glomerular capillaries into Bowman's capsule per unit time. This is influenced by renal blood flow, oncotic and hydrostatic forces, and basement membrane characteristics. Vasoconstriction of the afferent arteriole and vasodilatation of the efferent arteriole will lower GFR. Angiotensin II causes vasoconstriction of the efferent arteriole, leading to preservation of GFR, and prostaglandins cause afferent arteriolar vasodilatation. Hypotension will lead to a reduction in renal perfusion pressure and blood flow, lowering GFR. In pregnancy, GFR increases by up to 50% by the end of the first trimester.

Ronco C, Bellomo R, Kellum JA. *Critical Care Nephrology*, 2nd edn. London: Saunders, 2008.

30a. False
30b. False
30c. False
30d. False
30e. True
Carboprost (Hemabate) is a $PGF_{2\alpha}$ analogue used as a uterotonic agent for management of postpartum haemorrhage caused by uterine atony refractory to conventional therapy of uterine massage and intravenous oxytocin preparations, and induction of *second*-trimester abortion. It is administered intramuscularly in 250 μg doses and can be repeated up to a total dose of 2 mg. Side-effects include nausea, vomiting, diarrhoea, hyperthermia, flushing and bronchospasm (due to contractile effects on smooth muscle), and is therefore contraindicated in asthma.

31a. True
31b. False
31c. True
31d. False
31e. False
A meta-analysis combines data from randomized controlled trials, scoring each according to their methodology. Results are pooled to increase the number of subjects and power. A forest plot (see Figure 3.1) shows separate randomized controlled trial results on one graph. The horizontal lines represent confidence intervals, the size of the central mark represents sample size. Lines that cross the 'line of equivalence' are statistically 'non-significant'.

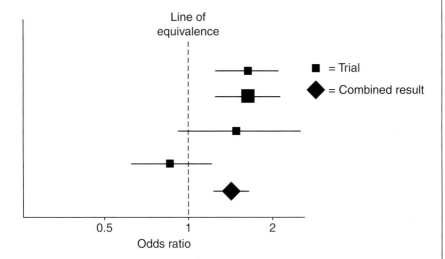

FIGURE 3.1   Forest plot for meta-analysis.

Yentis S, Hirsch N, Smith G. *Anaesthesia and Intensive Care A to Z: An Encyclopaedia of Principles and Practice*, 4th edn. Oxford: Butterworth-Heinemann, 2009.

32a. False
32b. True
32c. False
32d. True
32e. True
The aim of treating advanced heart failure is two-pronged; first to treat symptoms (mainly pulmonary congestion) and to treat the underlying pathology. Clinical trials have demonstrated that continuous positive airway pressure (CPAP) reduces the need for intubation compared with standard therapy. There have been important trials leading to evidence-based guidelines in managing the condition.

Treatment goals are:

Clinical

- Eliminate peripheral and pulmonary oedema
- Systolic arterial pressure >90 mmHg
- Improve renal and liver function
- Maintain adequate oxygenation

Haemodynamic

- Right atrial pressure <8 mmHg
- Pulmonary capillary wedge pressure <16 mmHg
- Mixed venous oxygen saturation >60%
- Cardiac index >2 L min^{-1} m^{-2}
- Systemic vascular resistance between 800–1200 dyn s^{-1} cm^{-5}

Scottish Intercollegiate Guidelines Network. *Management of Chronic Heart Failure: A National Guideline*. Edinburgh: SIGN, 2007.

The Task Force on Acute Heart Failure of the European Society of Cardiology. Executive summary of the guidelines on the diagnosis and treatment of acute heart failure. *Eur Heart J* 2005; **26**: 384–416.

Valchanov K, Parameshwar J. Inpatient management of advanced heart failure. *Contin Educ Anaesth Crit Care Pain* 2008; **8**: 167–71.

33a. True
33b. False
33c. True
33d. False
33e. True

Nasogastric tubes may prolong paralytic ileus and predispose to pulmonary aspiration; use is not routinely indicated for mid-to-lower abdominal procedures. The MASTER Trial (Multicentre Australian Study of Epidural anaesthesia) assigned 915 patients undergoing major abdominal surgery to receive intraoperative epidural anaesthesia with postoperative epidural analgesia, or intravenous opioids. Mortality was low in both groups and only one of eight categories of morbid endpoints (respiratory failure) occurred less frequently in patients managed with an epidural technique.

A 2006 Cochrane review showed no obvious advantage in keeping patients 'nil by mouth' following gastrointestinal surgery. The review supported the early commencement of enteral feeding. Clonidine via the intravenous and epidural routes can shorten the duration of ileus and improve pain control after colorectal procedures.

Andersen HK, Lewis SJ, Thomas S. Early enteral nutrition within 24 h of colorectal surgery versus later commencement of feeding for postoperative complications. *Cochrane Database Syst Rev* 2006; (4): CD004080.

Kitching AJ, O'Neill SS. Fast-track surgery and anaesthesia. *Contin Educ Anaesth Crit Care Pain* 2009; **9**: 39–43.

Nelson RL, Edwards S, Tse B. Prophylactic nasogastric decompression after abdominal surgery. *Cochrane Database Syst Rev* 2007; (2): CD004929.

Rigg JR, Jamrozik K, Myles PS, et al. Epidural anaesthesia and analgesia and outcome of major surgery: a randomised trial. *Lancet* 2002; **359**: 1276–82.

Wu CT, Jao SW, Borel CO, et al. The effect of epidural clonidine on perioperative cytokine response, postoperative pain, and bowel function in patients undergoing colorectal surgery. *Anesth Analg* 2004; **99**: 502–9.

34a. False
34b. True
34c. True
34d. True
34e. False
The Acute Dialysis Quality Initiative Working Group has developed the RIFLE criteria, a consensus definition for acute kidney injury (AKI). The acronym RIFLE defines grades of severity (R – risk; I – injury; F – failure) with two outcome variables (L – loss; E – end-stage) and has undergone evaluation in cardiac surgical and ICU patients.

Severity	Urine output	Glomerular filtration rate (GFR)
Risk	<0.5 mL kg^{-1} h^{-1} for 6 hours	Serum creatinine >1.5x baseline or GFR decrease >25%
Injury	<0.5 mL kg^{-1} h^{-1} for 12 hours	Serum creatinine >2x baseline or GFR decrease >50%
Failure	<0.3 mL kg^{-1} h^{-1} for 24 hours, or anuria for 12 hours	Serum creatinine >3x baseline, GFR decrease >75% or serum creatinine ≥4 mg/dL with an acute rise >0.5 mg/dL
Outcome		
Loss	Persistent acute renal failure = complete loss of kidney function >4 weeks requiring renal replacement therapy (RRT)	
End-stage kidney disease	Need for renal replacement therapy >3 months	

Bellomo R, Ronco C, Kellum JA, et al. Acute renal failure – definition, outcome measures, animal models, fluid therapy and information technology needs: the Second International Consensus Conference of the Acute Dialysis Quality Initiative (ADQI) Group. *Crit Care* 2004; **8**: R204–12.

Lopes JA, Fernando P, Jorge S, et al. Acute kidney injury in intensive care unit patients: a comparison between the RIFLE and the Acute Kidney Injury Network classifications. *Crit Care* 2008; **12**: R110.

35a. True
35b. False
35c. True
35d. False
35e. False
Temporary tracheostomies have become a more commonly performed intervention in the UK in recent years. This is partly as a result of the availability of percutaneous techniques, which allow the intensivist to perform the tracheostomy themselves. Indications include:

• upper airway obstruction
• avoidance of the complications of prolonged tracheal intubation
• severe neurological injury with a requirement to maintain an airway
• facilitation of weaning from mechanical ventilation and discharge from ICU

The scenario above is one of a non-patent airway and the priority is to re-establish the airway in the safest possible manner. Well-formed tracks from the skin to the tracheal stoma are not considered formed until 72 hours after surgical tracheostomy, or 7 days after a percutaneous technique. Thus any attempt to place a tube through the stoma is potentially hazardous. In the first instance, the tube should be considered blocked and simple manouevres (such as removing the inner cannula, passing a suction catheter and deflating the tracheostomy tube cuff) may allow passage of oxygen. If these do not work then the tracheostomy must be considered 'displaced', and if the patient cannot breathe through their mouth then the tracheostomy must be removed. If the patient can breathe spontaneously through their stoma site then this may be considered sufficient and oxygen applied. Failing this, the stoma should be occluded to see if the patient can breathe through their mouth. If neither of these is possible then artificial ventilation must be commenced and endotracheal intubation will become necessary.

Intensive Care Society. *Standards for the Care of the Adult Patient with a Temporary Tracheostomy*. London: ICS, 2008. Available at: www.ics.ac.uk.

36a. False
36b. False
36c. True
36d. True
36e. False
The Magill breathing system is a Mapleson A, comprising an adjustable pressure-limiting (APL) valve at the patient end and a reservoir bag at the machine end; it is efficient for spontaneous ventilation requiring a fresh gas flow (FGF) equal to alveolar minute volume ($70 \text{ mL kg}^{-1} \text{ min}^{-1}$), but is not efficient for controlled ventilation and not suitable for paediatric practice, since the expiratory valve adds resistance and gives a large apparatus dead space; it also adds weight to the patient end. The Lack system is a coaxial version of the Magill and is thus not suitable for paediatrics. The Bain Mapleson D system is efficient for controlled ventilation, but for spontaneous ventilation it requires a FGF of $150-200 \text{ mL kg}^{-1} \text{ min}^{-1}$; it is not recommended for use in children <20 kg. The Humphrey ADE system is a versatile system that can

perform as a Mapleson A, D or E and can be used in paediatrics for controlled or spontaneous ventilation, offering little resistance from the APL valve and a low internal resistance with smooth 15 mm tubing; it can also be connected to a ventilator (Penlon Nuffield 200).

Doyle E. *Paediatric Anaesthesia.* Oxford: OUP, 2007.

37a. True
37b. False
37c. True
37d. True
37e. True
Adenotonsillectomy may be performed in a district general hospital for the majority of children. Severe OSA is described by polysomnographic indices including Obstructive Index > 10; Respiratory Disturbance Index > 40; O_2 saturations nadir $< 80\%$. A chest X-ray and 12-lead ECG may be helpful in identifying pulmonary hypertension, which may ultimately lead to right heart failure. Further investigations should be performed for the following indications:

- diagnosis of OSA unclear
- age < 2 years
- weight < 15 kg
- Down's syndrome
- cerebral palsy
- residual symptoms after adenotonsillectomy

- hypotonia or neuromuscular disorders
- craniofacial abnormalities
- mucopolysaccharidosis
- obesity
- significant comorbidity

Royal College of Anaesthetists. *Tonsillectomy and Adenoidectomy in Children with Sleep Related Breathing Disorders.* Consensus Statement of a UK Multidisciplinary Working Party. London: RCOA, 2008.

38a. True
38b. True
38c. True
38d. False
38e. True
Various methods have been used to locate the epidural space, most of which rely on the subatmospheric pressure present. These include:

- Loss of resistance to air or saline (most common technique)
- Gutierrez's method: a hanging drop of saline on the hub of a needle is drawn in as the epidural space is entered (more reliable in thoracic than lumbar region)
- Odom's indicator: a fine-bore glass tube filled with saline and a bubble that moves in response to a drop in pressure
- Macintosh's extradural space indicator: a small rubber balloon filled with air connected to an adaptor causing it to deflate on entering the epidural space
- Macintosh's spring-loaded needle
- Ultrasonic localization
- Oxford epidural space detector

The Campbell–Howell method is a rebreathing technique used for indirect CO_2 measurement.

39a. True
39b. True
39c. True
39d. True
39e. True
The following recommendations were published by the National Patient Safety Agency following 498 incidents where the wrong dose of midazolam was administered to adults undergoing conscious sedation:

- High-strength midazolam should be stored in areas where the use of this concentration has been formally risk-assessed (intensive care, theatres, palliative care wards)
- All other areas should have only low-strength midazolam
- Therapeutic protocols for midazolam should be made clear
- All practitioners involved directly or indirectly in sedative procedures should have the knowledge, skills and competence required
- Flumazenil should be available in these areas and its use audited
- Organizational policy should be drawn up and a senior clinician be assigned the responsibility

National Patient Safety Agency. *Rapid Responses Report: Reducing Risk of Overdose with Midazolam Injection in Adults.* London: NPSA, 2008. Available at: www.nrls.npsa.nhs.uk/resources/type/alerts/?entryid45=59896&p=2.

40a. False
40b. True
40c. True
40d. True
40e. True
Emesis is a common consequence of anaesthesia and surgery, despite advances in pharmacological and non-pharmacological methods of avoiding postoperative nausea and vomiting. Cyclizine increases lower oesophageal sphincter tone and has mild anticholinergic effects (explaining the increased heart rate on intravenous injection). Ondansetron has a favourable side-effect profile, but can cause headache, flushing, constipation and bradycardia. All dopamine antagonists can cause dystonic reactions; domperidone increases prolactin levels and may cause galactorrhoea and gynaecomastia; metoclopramide may precipitate the neuroleptic malignant syndrome, sedation or agitation when given intramuscularly. Antiemetics can be classified as:

- *Dopamine antagonists*
  - Phenothiazines: chlorpromazine
  - Butyrophenones: droperidol, domperidone
  - Benzamides: metoclopramide
- *Anticholinergics*: hyoscine, atropine, glycopyrrolate
- *Antihistamines*: cyclizine
- *5-HT$_3$ antagonists*: ondansetron, granisetron
- *Miscellaneous*: steroids, cannabinoids, benzodiazepines, propofol

Peck TE, Hill SA, Williams M. *Pharmacology for Anaesthesia and Intensive Care*, 3rd edn. Cambridge: CUP, 2008.

41a. True
41b. False
41c. True
41d. False
41e. True
Tourniquets provide a bloodless surgical field, but can cause significant morbidity through tissue ischaemia distal to application and direct pressure injuries to underlying structures. Upon inflation, there is a progressive rise in $P\text{CO}_2$ and fall in $P\text{O}_2$ within muscle cells, with a decline in ATP and creatine phosphate stores, which are exhausted after 2 and 3 hours respectively. The serum lactate rises (by 2 mmol/L) following deflation owing to reperfusion of the ischaemic limb and serum potassium levels peak at 3 minutes (an increase of 0.3 mmol/L). There is increased finbrinolytic activity following deflation, owing to release and circulation of tissue plasminogen activator. Irreversible muscle damage can occur following inflation times of 2–3 hours.

Deloughry JL, Griffiths R. Arterial tourniquets. *Contin Educ Anaesth Crit Care Pain* 2009; 9: 56–60.
Seeber P, Shander A. *Basics of Blood Management.* Oxford: Wiley-Blackwell, 2007.

42a. True
42b. False
42c. True
42d. True
42e. True
Compartment syndrome develops when a compartment, defined by bony, muscular or fascial layers, becomes subject to elevated pressure. Normal intra-abdominal pressure (IAP) is between zero and slightly subatmospheric. ACS has been graded according to IAP into:

- *Grade I*: 10–15 mmHg
- *Grade II*: 16–25 mmHg
- *Grade III*: 26–35 mmHg
- *Grade IV*: >35 mmHg

ACS causes a direct pressure injury, leading to reduced organ perfusion, tissue ischaemia and organ dysfunction:

Cardiovascular: ↓Left ventricular afterload
↓Venous return leading to ↓cardiac output
↑Pulmonary and systemic vascular resistance
↓Myocardial contractility
↑Central venous pressure and PAOP
Respiratory: ↑Intrathoracic pressure
↓$Pa\text{O}_2/Fi\text{O}_2$ ratio
↓Pulmonary and chest wall compliance causing hypercapnia

Renal:	↓ Renal plasma flow and GFR
	↑ Antidiuretic hormone and renin release
Central nervous system:	↑ Intracranial pressure

Burch JM, Moore EE, Moore FA, Franciose R. The abdominal compartment syndrome. *Surg Clin North Am* 1996; **76**: 833–42.

Hopkins D, Gemmell LW. Intra-abdominal hypertension and the abdominal compartment syndrome. *Contin Educ Anaesth Crit Care Pain* 2001; **1**: 56–9.

43a. False
43b. False
43c. True
43d. False
43e. False

IABPs are used as circulatory assist devices in critically ill cardiac patients (see Figure 3.2). They are sited most commonly via the femoral artery, to lie within the descending thoracic aorta, 2–3 cm *distal* to the origin of the subclavian artery. Indications include acute myocardial infarction, cardiogenic shock and left ventricular (LV) failure. The goal is to improve ventricular function and improve the myocardial oxygen supply : demand ratio. LV coronary blood flow occurs in diastole; thus the IABP inflates during diastole and deflates just before the onset of systole. It increases the pressure difference between aortic and LV diastolic pressure, which drives flow within the coronary arteries as per the Hagen–Poiseuille formula. The aims are:

- ↓ LV systolic pressure and end-diastolic pressure
- ↓ LV wall tension
- ↑/→ coronary artery blood flow
- ↓ afterload and ↑ cardiac output

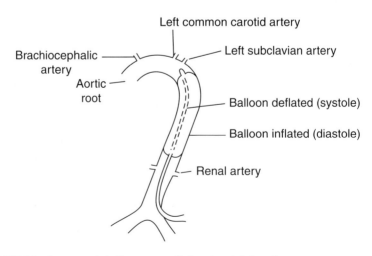

FIGURE 3.2   Intra-aortic balloon pump (inflated and deflated).

Absolute contraindications include aortic regurgitation, aortic dissection, chronic end-stage heart failure and aortic stents. Relative contraindications include severe peripheral vascular disease, arterial reconstruction, tachyar-rhythmias, sepsis, aortic abdominal aneurysm and severe coagulopathy.

Krishna M, Zacharowski K. Principles of intra-aortic balloon pump counterpulsation. *Contin Educ Anaesth Crit Care Pain* 2009; 9: 24–8.

44a. True
44b. False
44c. False
44d. False
44e. False
Intrapulmonary shunt in perfused but unventilated alveoli is the mechanism underlying hypoxaemia in ALI and acute respiratory distress syndrome (ARDS). A successful recruitment manoeuvre (RM) is designed to reach an opening pressure to open 'derecruited', atelectatic lung regions that, with the addition of positive end-expiratory pressure (PEEP) after the manoeuvre may improve both PaO_2 and CO_2 exchange, reflecting increased alveolar venti-lation. The response to an RM is a function of many factors, including phase and extent of lung injury, level of PEEP, potential for recruitment and RM technique used. Patients with 'high potential for recruitment' are those ventilated for not more than 48–72 hours; those ventilated for more than 3 days are considered 'low potential'. To date, no study has demonstrated an improved survival using these measures in ALI or ARDS.

Mackay A, Al-Haddad M. Acute lung injury and acute respiratory distress syndrome. *Contin Educ Anaesth Crit Care Pain* 2009; 9: 152–6.
Mascia L, Zanierato M, Ranieri M. Recruitment manoeuvres. In: Waldmann N, Soni N, Rhodes A, eds. *Oxford Desk Reference: Critical Care*. Oxford: OUP, 2008.

45a. False
45b. True
45c. True
45d. True
45e. True
Ultrasound waves are formed when a voltage is applied across a substance with piezoelectric properties. Pulse repetition frequency is the number of pulses generated by the transducer in 1 s. Acoustic frequency is 3.5–7.5 MHz. Transthoracic echocardiography (TTE) uses low-frequency transducers of 2–4 MHz, transoesophageal echocardiography (TOE) requires less penetration for better resolution at 3.5–7.5 MHz. The reflector in the Doppler method is the red cell, which allows measurement of blood flow velocity.

Moppett I, Shajar M. Transoesophageal echocardiography. *Contin Educ Anaesth Crit Care Pain* 2001; 1: 72–5.
Roscoe A, Strang T. Echocardiography in intensive care. *Contin Educ Anaesth Crit Care Pain* 2008; 8: 46–9.

46a. False
46b. False
46c. True
46d. True
46e. True
The diving reflex is an adaptive mechanism seen in aquatic mammals, but also exists in humans. It occurs upon immersion of the face in cold water; afferents are transmitted via the trigeminal (VI division) nerve leading to vagal stimulation. The following phases occur:

- apnoea
- bradycardia
- peripheral vasoconstriction
- blood redistribution and shift in deep dives

The reflex is oxygen-conserving and allows mammals to stay under water for longer periods. Debate has arisen as to the exact mechanisms involved, but it may be due to the cooling effect leading to lower oxygen requirements, as seen in hypothermia. The reflex forms the basis of facial immersion used to terminate supraventricular tachycardias.

Golden FC, Tipton MJ, Scott RC. Immersion, near drowning and drowning. *Br J Anaesth* 1997; 79: 214–25.
Mathew PK. Diving reflex. Another method of treating paroxysmal supraventricular tachycardia. *Arch Intern Med* 1981; 141: 22–3.

47a. False
47b. True
47c. True
47d. False
47e. True
The incidence of aortic dissection is approximately 1:100 000, with a male-to-female ratio of up to 5:1 and is rare below the age of 40 years. The DeBakey classification has been largely superseded by the Stanford classification, which is as follows:

- *Type A*: involves the ascending aorta
- *Type B*: does not involve the ascending aorta

Limb ischaemia develops in approximately 13% while paraplegia occurs in 2.5%. ECG findings may be consistent with acute myocardial infarction, but is normal in up to one-third of individuals with coronary involvement.

European Society of Cardiology. Diagnosis and management of aortic dissection. Recommendations of the Task Force on Aortic Dissection. *Eur Heart J* 2001; 22: 1642–81.
Melchior T, Hallam D, Johansen BE. Aortic dissection in the thrombolytic era: early recognition and optimal management is a prerequisite for increased survival. *Int J Cardiol* 1993; 42: 1–6.

48a. False
48b. False
48c. True
48d. False
48e. False
Cook's modification of the Cormack and Lehane classification system is based upon direct laryngoscopy; there are still four grades, but grades 2 and 3 are subdivided further as follows:

Easy:

- *Grade 1*: entire vocal cords
- *Grade 2A*: posterior portion of the vocal cords plus some portion of laryngeal inlet

Restricted (elastic bougie required):

- *Grade 2B*: posterior rim of the vocal cords with no inlet
- *Grade 3A*: epiglottis

Difficult (airway adjuncts required):

- *Grade 3B*: some soft palate but no epiglottis
- *Grade 4*: hard palate only

49a. False
49b. False
49c. False
49d. True
49e. True
Eclampsia is a life-threatening complication of pregnancy, characterized by tonic–clonic seizures caused by hypertensive disease of pregnancy. UK incidence is approximately 1 per 2000, while pre-eclamptic toxaemia (PET) affects about 2–3% of pregnancies. PET is currently the second leading cause of direct maternal death (tied with sepsis). Eclampsia is not an indication for emergency caesarean section: priority must be resuscitation, stabilization of the mother and termination of fits. Immediate management is the ABC approach with 100% oxygen and left lateral tilt in the prepartum woman.

The MAGPIE trial studied 10 141 patients with pre-eclampsia; incidence of convulsions and mortality were reduced with magnesium versus placebo; thus intravenous magnesium sulphate is the first-line treatment of eclamptic convulsions, with a therapeutic range of 2–4 mmol/L (4 g loading dose given over 15–20 minutes, then 1–2 g per hour as a continuous infusion). Most fits occur in the third trimester and up to 40% postpartum. Regional anaesthesia is not contraindicated unless there is a coagulopathy. Complications include cerebrovascular accident, cerebral oedema, aspiration and complications of pre-eclampsia, with coagulopathy, cardiac failure, pulmonary oedema and fetal and maternal deaths. It is important to remember that women may present with eclampsia without any prodromal symptoms.

Duley L, Carroli G, Farrell B, et al. Do women with pre-eclampsia, and their babies, benefit from magnesium sulphate? The MAGPIE Trial: A randomised placebo-controlled trial. *Lancet* 2002; **359**: 1877–90.

Lewis G, ed. The Confidential Enquiry into Maternal and Child Health (CEMACH). *Saving Mothers' Lives: Reviewing Maternal Deaths to make Motherhood Safer – 2003–2005*. The Seventh Report on Confidential Enquiries into Maternal Deaths in the UK. London: CEMACH, 2007. Available at: www.cmace.org.uk/getattachment/05f68346-816b-4560-b1b9-af24fb633170/Saving-Mothers'-Lives-2003-2005_ExecSumm.aspx.

Royal College of Obstetricians and Gynaecologists. *Management of Severe Pre-Eclampsia and Eclampsia*, Guideline No. 10(A). London: RCOG, 2006. Available at: www.rcog.org.uk/womens-health/clinical-guidance/management-severe-pre-eclampsiaeclampsia-green-top-10a.

50a. False
50b. False
50c. False
50d. True
50e. False

CK-MB: Creatine kinase is a cytosolic enzyme occurring as three different isoenzymes. CK-MB is found predominantly in cardiac muscle (30%). It rises 3–12 hours after MI, peaks at 24 hours and falls 2–3 days (normal <190 IU/L).

AST: Aspartate aminotransferase rises after 12 hours post-MI and peaks at 1–2 days (normal <35 IU/L).

LDH: Lactate dehydrogenase is a cytosolic enzyme that catalyses the conversion of lactate to pyruvate. Five isoenzymes are known and LDH-1 is predominant in cardiac muscle. It rises within 24 hours of an MI, reaches a peak within 3–6 days, and returns to baseline within 8–12 days.

Troponins are components of striated but not smooth muscle and there are three types: T, I and C. Troponins T and I are only found in cardiac muscle and levels are absolutely indicative of myocardial damage but can be raised by causes other than MI, such as myocarditis or cardiac trauma. Serum levels increase within 3–12 hours from the onset of chest pain, peak at 24–48

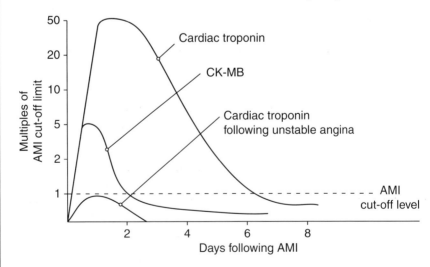

FIGURE 3.3 Cardiac markers. AMI: acute myocardial infarction, CK-MB: creatine kinase, muscle and brain isoenzyme.

hours and return to baseline over 5–10 days. In renal failure, levels can be sustained. Cardiac troponin markers are illustrated in Figure 3.3.

Khan IA, Tun A, Wattanasauwan N, et al. Elevation of serum cardiac troponin I in noncardiac and cardiac diseases other than acute coronary syndromes. *Am J Emerg Med* 1999; **17**: 225–9.

51a. True
51b. False
51c. False
51d. False
51e. False
Cauda equina syndrome (CES) results from sacral and lumbar nerve root dysfunction within the lumbar vertebral canal. A variety of clinical features may arise when root dysfunction occurs, but the term 'cauda equina syndrome' is reserved for bladder, bowel or sexual dysfunction and perianal or 'saddle' numbness. The most common cause is herniation of central lumbar discs, particularly at L4/5 and L5/S1. Less common causes include trauma, infections and metastatic processes. The use of intrathecal hyperbaric 5% lidocaine through small-bore needles has been implicated in multiple cases of CES. This is postulated to be as a result of less turbulence through the small needle resulting in pooling of toxic concentrations of lidocaine around cauda equina nerve roots. Management consists of:

- urgent surgical referral
- MRI as the imaging modality of choice
- surgical decompression via discectomy (if caused by disc herniation)

Patients with urinary retention have a poor outcome. Meta-analysis supports the view that early surgery is related to better results with incomplete CES. The case is less certain for CES with retention.

DeLong WB, Polissar N, Neradilak B. Timing of surgery in cauda equina syndrome with urinary retention: meta-analysis of observational studies. *J Neurosurg Spine* 2008; **8**: 305–20.
Lavy C, James A, Wilson-MacDonald A, Fairbank J. Cauda equina syndrome. *BMJ* 2009; **338**: b936.

52a. False
52b. True
52c. False
52d. True
52e. True
Activated charcoal is processed to provide a highly porous surface area. 1 g of activated charcoal has a surface area of 500 m^2 consisting of micropores that bind certain substances by van der Waals forces, adsorbing drugs taken in overdose and reducing absorption. It is estimated to reduce absorption of poisonous substances by 60%. A charcoal : poison weight ratio of 10 : 1 is required and is very useful for the adsorption of benzodiazepines, theophylline, tricyclics, anticonvulsants and phenothiazines. It does not bind effectively

with alcohols, glycols, strong acids and bases or to inorganic compounds such as lithium, arsenic, lead and iron.

Singer M, Webb AR. *Oxford Handbook of Critical Care*, 3rd edn. Oxford: OUP, 2009.

53a. True
53b. False
53c. True
53d. False
53e. True
PACs allow direct measurement of right atrial, right ventricular, pulmonary artery and pulmonary artery wedge pressures and cardiac output via thermodilution using the Stewart–Hamilton equation. Causes of inaccuracy include:

- intracardiac shunts
- excessively slow bolus of cold injectate
- thermistor impingement against vessel wall
- tricuspid regurgitation

The PAC-Man Trial, a multicentre British study that randomly assigned 1041 critically ill patients to management with or without a PAC, demonstrated no clear evidence of benefit or harm associated with use.

Harvey S, Harrison DA, Singer M, et al. Assessment of the clinical effectiveness of pulmonary artery catheters in management of patients in intensive care (PAC-Man): a randomised controlled trial. *Lancet* 2005; **366**: 472–7.

54a. False
54b. False
54c. False
54d. False
54e. False
Workplace exposure limits have been approved by the Health and Safety Commission. The Control of Substances Hazardous to Health (COSHH) Regulations 2002 impose requirements by reference to a list. Time-weighted averages (TWAs) are collected. No safe exposure limit has been ascertained for sevoflurane or desflurane. Abbott Laboratories have recommended an exposure limit of 20 ppm for sevoflurane.

Volatile agent	Long-term 8-hour TWA	
	ppm	mg/m³
Halothane	10	82
Isoflurane	50	383
Enflurane	50	383
Nitrous oxide	100	183

Health and Safety Executive. *Control of Substances Hazardous to Health (COSHH)*. London: HSE, 2002.

55a. True
55b. False
55c. False
55d. False
55e. True
Coronary blood flow approximates 5% of cardiac output and its value is 80 mL/100 g/min ($\sim$250 mL/min). Myocardial oxygen consumption is approximately 9.7 mL/100 g/min (29 mL/min). Flow to subendocardial regions of the left ventricle occurs during diastole; therefore duration of diastole (i.e. heart rate), affects blood flow inversely. Flow is also governed by the following factors, as per the Hagen–Poiseuille equation:

- ΔP: pressure difference between aortic diastolic pressure and LVEDP
- r: radius of coronary arteries, which is governed by autoregulation, stenoses/spasm, drugs (vasoconstrictors and vasodilators); the autonomic nervous system has very little direct influence
- η: blood viscosity (haematocrit)

56a. True
56b. True
56c. True
56d. False
56e. True
Plasma magnesium levels are normally between 0.8 and 1.1 mmol/L. Hypomagnesaemia can be caused by inadequate intake, inadequate gut absorption or excessive gut or renal losses. Symptoms and signs include tremor, weakness, irritability, ataxia, confusion or personality change, hyperreflexia, and tonic–clonic convulsions. ECG changes are non-specific, but include ST depression, broad and flattened T-waves, U-waves, loss of voltage, and a prolonged QT interval. It is commonly associated with hypocalcaemia and hypokalaemia.

57a. True
57b. False
57c. True
57d. True
57e. False
FRC is defined as the volume remaining in the lungs at the end of normal tidal expiration and consists of the expiratory reserve volume plus the residual volume. A small FRC leads to rapid arterial desaturation following apnoea, compounded by higher metabolic rates seen in pregnancy and paediatric practice; positive end-expiratory pressure (PEEP) will increase FRC. Conversely, inhalational induction of anaesthesia will take longer with a large FRC. FRC is reduced in the supine and head-down positions, while *forced vital capacity* is greater in the head-down position in patients with high spinal injuries owing to the effects of gravity.

58a. True
58b. False
58c. True
58d. True
58e. False

Porphyria describes a heterogeneous group of diseases characterized by defects in the enzymes involved in the biosynthesis of haem, resulting in the over-production and excretion of intermediate compounds (porphyrins). Barbiturates, phenytoin and sulphonamides are definite precipitants. Etomidate, lignocaine and chlordiazepoxide are implicated in laboratory studies. A full list of unsafe drugs can be found in the British National Formulary.

British Medical Association, Royal Pharmaceutical Society of Great Britain. *British National Formulay 58*. Section 9.8.2: Drugs unsafe for use in acute porphyrias. London: Pharmaceutical Press, 2009.
Yentis S, Hirsch N, Smith G. *Anaesthesia and Intensive Care A to Z: An Encyclopaedia of Principles and Practice*, 4th edn. Oxford: Butterworth-Heinemann, 2009.

59a. True
59b. True
59c. False
59d. True
59e. False

Thyrotoxic crisis ('thyroid storm') is a medical emergency that presents in thyrotoxic patients, precipitated by an intercurrent illness, emergency surgery and trauma. It is rarely encountered, because of effective antithyroid therapy. Presentation is with hyperpyrexia ($>41\,^{\circ}C$), tachycardia, hypotension, heart failure, jaundice, confusion, agitation and coma. Management involves prompt recognition, supportive therapy and treating the precipitating cause. Management consists of:

- ABC with 100% O_2
- Rehydration with crystalloid to compensate for large insensible losses
- Treating hyperpyrexia with tepid sponging and paracetamol; aspirin is not used, since it displaces thyroid hormone further from protein-binding sites
- β-blockade: propranolol is given in 1 mg increments up to 10 mg. The goal is a heart rate below 90/min
- Hydrocortisone 200 mg four times daily treats adrenal insufficiency and reduces thyroxine release and peripheral conversion to triiodothyronine
- Dantrolene can be used to prevent the action of calcium ions, which is initiated by the thyroid hormones in the sarcoplasmic reticulum
- Anti-thyroid medication: carbimazole or propylthiouracil may be used

Mortality, even with prompt diagnosis, is estimated to be 20–50%.

Farling PA. Thyroid disease.*Br J Anaesth* 2000; **85**: 15–28.
Blanshard H, Bennett D. Metabolic and endocrine. In: Allman KG, McIndoe AK, Wilson IH, eds. *Emergencies in Anaesthesia*, 2nd edn. Oxford: OUP, 2009.
Burch HB, Wartofsky L. Life-threatening thyrotoxicosis. Thyroid storm. *Endocrinol Metab Clin North Am* 1993; **22**: 263–77.

60a. True
60b. False
60c. True
60d. False
60e. True
Dystrophia myotonica is an autosomal dominant condition exhibiting anticipation, presenting in the second or third decade and involving persistent contraction of skeletal muscles following stimulation. It is the most common of the myotonic syndromes, with an incidence of 5 per 100 000. Clinical features include progressive atrophy of skeletal, cardiac and smooth muscle, which leads to deterioration of respiratory function and cardiomyopathy. There is degeneration of cardiac conduction fibres causing dysrhythmias and a tendency for mitral valve prolapse in 20% of patients. Progressive bulbar palsy can lead to aspiration. The condition may deteriorate in pregnancy; Caesarean sections are more common owing to uterine muscle dysfunction. The triggers for contracture during a general anaesthesia are suxamethonium, nerve stimulator use and neostigmine. Regional anaesthesia does not prevent muscle contractures, although direct local anaesethetic infiltration to the muscles may be effective.

Teasdale A. Neuromuscular disorders. In: Allman KG, Wilson IH, eds. *Oxford Handbook of Anaesthesia*, 2nd edn. Oxford: OUP, 2006.

61a. False
61b. True
61c. True
61d. True
61e. False
Coning is defined as the herniation of intracranial structures secondary to raised intracranial pressures following exhaustion of compensatory mechanisms. Herniation may be supratentorial (central or uncal) or infratentorial. Uncal herniation often presents with a unilateral dilated pupil as a result of compression of cranial nerve III against the tentorial edge leading to disruption of parasympathetic nerve supply to the pupil. Central herniation can result in decorticate and later, decerebrate posturing in addition to Cheyne–Stokes respiration as midbrain compression occurs. Lumbar puncture and increased intracranial pressure can result in infratentorial coning.

Williams M, Dominic Bell MD, Moss E. Brainstem death. *Contin Educ Anaesth Crit Care Pain* 2003; 3: 161–6.

62a. True
62b. False
62c. True
62d. False
62e. False
Vancomycin is a complex glycopeptide containing vancosamine and several amino acid moieties. It is active against most aerobic and anaerobic Gram-positive bacteria. Intravenous dosing is 500 mg–1 g, 12-hourly (15 mg/kg in children, 8-hourly). Side-effects include renal impairment, ototoxicity, blood dyscrasias and phlebitis. Rapid infusion can result in 'red man syndrome' characterized by flushing due to histamine release; also hypotension, pruritus,

dyspnoea and cardiac arrest. Plasma levels are monitored and should be < 10 mg/L pre-dose with a peak of < 30 mg/L 2 hours post-dose. Vancomycin is not absorbed orally.

British Medical Association, Royal Pharmaceutical Society of Great Britain. *British National Formulary 58.* Section 5.1.7: Vancomycin. London: Pharmaceutical Press, 2009.

63a. True
63b. False
63c. True
63d. False
63e. False

The ECG is the surface recording of the electrical activity of the heart. Its display is recorded onto an oscilloscope. The normal axis is −30° to +90°, which arises owing to the mean electrical vectors occurring during ventricular depolarization and can be assessed by initially looking at leads I (0°) and aVF (+90°). The δ-wave occurs in Wolff–Parkinson–White syndrome, where conduction occurs through an aberrant atrioventricular connection (the bundle of Kent) and is absent in Lown–Ganong–Levine syndrome. The PR interval is abnormally short in both conditions. ECG criteria for thrombolysis are:

- 1 mm ST change in ≥2 contiguous limb leads
- 2 mm ST change in ≥2 contiguous chest leads
- new left bundle branch block (LBBB)

Bifascicular block is characterized by right bundle branch blocks (RBBB) and left axis deviation.

Hampton J. *The ECG Made Easy*, 7th edn. New York: Churchill-Livingstone, 2008.
Massel D. Observer variability in ECG interpretation for thrombolysis eligibility: experience and context matter. *J Thromb Thrombolysis* 2003; **15**: 131–40.

64a. True
64b. True
64c. False
64d. False
64e. True

The sciatic nerve (L4–S3) divides into tibial and common peroneal nerves, from two-thirds down the thigh to the popliteal fossa, although it may divide anywhere in the thigh. The posterior cutaneous nerve of the thigh is not a branch, but runs close and may be blocked along with it. Anterior (Beck), posterior (Labat), lateral and lithotomy approaches have all been described.

65a. False
65b. True
65c. False
65d. True
65e. False

The term *isobestic point* refers to a particular wavelength at which the absorbances of two or more sets of substances are equal. For oxyhaemoglobin and deoxyhaemoglobin, the isobestic points are 590 and 805 nm.

66a. True
66b. True
66c. False
66d. True
66e. False
Topical adrenaline vasoconstricts conjunctival vessels, dilates the pupil and reduces IOP (normally 10–15 mmHg); it also reduces aqueous humor production while increasing drainage. Acetazolamide reduces IOP by inhibition of carbonic anhydrase, which leads to a reduction in aqueous humor production. All volatile and intravenous anaesthetic agents reduce IOP, with the exception of ketamine. Intravenous atropine has no significant effect on IOP but topically administered may cause it to rise, especially in glaucomatous eyes.

Murgatoyd H, Bembridge J. Intraocular pressure. *Contin Educ Anaesth Crit Care Pain* 2008; 8: 100–3.

67a. False
67b. True
67c. False
67d. True
67e. True
Hypoxia is a deficiency of oxygen at the tissue level. It is influenced by tissue oxygen demand (which is increased in trauma, surgery, burns or sepsis, amongst many other causes), oxygen supply and cellular utilisation. Type I respiratory failure is defined as PaO_2 <8 kPa with normo- or hypocapnoea. Hypoxia may be classified as:

- *Hypoxic hypoxia* (hypoxaemia): PaO_2 <12 kPa; reduced FiO_2, hypoventilation, diffusion impairment, shunt or $\dot{V}/\dot{Q}$ mismatch
- *Anaemic hypoxia*: reduced haemoglobin causes reduced tissue oxygen delivery
- *Stagnant (ischaemic) hypoxia*: reduced tissue blood flow secondary to reduced cardiac output or obstruction to capillary flow
- *Histotoxic (cytotoxic) hypoxia*: inability to utilize oxygen at the tissue level; cyanide or carbon monoxide poisoning

McLellan SA, Walsh TS. Oxygen delivery and haemoglobin. *Contin Educ Anaesth Crit Care Pain* 2004; 4: 123–6.

68a. False
68b. False
68c. True
68d. True
68e. False
When mitral valve area falls to 2.5 cm^2, peak early diastolic ventricular filling rate falls and diastasis is lost. Ideal conditions include:

- Low to normal heart rate
- Maintain sinus rhythm
- Maintain systemic vascular resistance (SVR)
- Avoid venodilatation/venous congestion

During exercise, however, heart rate increases and flow is maintained by a transmitral pressure gradient. With a smaller area, the gradient becomes present at rest and mean left atrial pressure rises. Normal mitral valve area is 4–6 cm^2. Symptomatic mitral stenosis patients have valve areas of 0.75–1.25 cm^2 and pressure gradients as high as 20–30 mmHg during diastole. Chronic left atrial hypertension results in increased pulmonary capillary pressures which can lead to pulmonary congestion and hypertension. Considerations for anaesthetic management of a patient with mitral valve stenosis should take into account fixed mitral flow. LVEDP is used to estimate left ventricular preload, but is inaccurate in the presence of mitral stenosis.

Gibson DG. Valve disease. In: Warrell DA, Cox TM, Firth JD, eds. *Oxford Textbook of Medicine*, 5th edn. Oxford: OUP, 2010.

69a. True
69b. False
69c. False
69d. True
69e. False

MAGPIE (Magnesium Sulphate for the Prevention of Eclampsia) studied 10 141 patients with pre-eclampsia; incidence of convulsions and mortality were reduced with magnesium versus placebo. Major morbidity (organ failure, ICU admission and length of stay) was not affected to a statistically significant degree. MASTER (Multicentre Australian Study of Epidural Anaesthesia; $n = 915$) evaluated epidural versus intravenous opioid analgesia for major abdominal surgery in high-risk patients. The study found no difference in mortality or major morbidity except respiratory failure (which was less frequent in the epidural group) between groups; the epidural group had superior postoperative analgesia. POISE (Perioperative Ischaemic Evaluation Study; $n = 8357$) randomized patients scheduled for non-cardiac surgery and not already on β-blocker therapy to β-blockade with metoprolol or placebo. The primary endpoints (cardiovascular death, myocardial infarction and cardiac arrest) occurred less frequently in the metoprolol group; however, total mortality was increased. B-Aware ($n = 2463$) found BIS reduced the risk of awareness by 82% in adults at a high risk of intraoperative awareness. PAC-Man ($n = 1041$) demonstrated no difference in hospital mortality associated with use of a PAC. See the chapter on 'Relevant Studies for the Final FRCA: Trials'.

Deveraux PJ, Yang H, Yusuf S, et al. POISE Study Group. Effects of extended-release metoprolol succinate in patients undergoing non-cardiac surgery (POISE Trial): a randomised controlled trial. *Lancet* 2008; 371: 1839–47.

Duley L, Carroli G, Farrell B, et al. Do women with pre-eclampsia, and their babies, benefit from magnesium sulphate? The MAGPIE Trial: A randomised placebo-controlled trial. *Lancet* 2002; 359: 1877–90.

Harvey S, Harrison DA, Singer M, et al. Assessment of the clinical effectiveness of pulmonary artery catheters in management of patients in intensive care (PAC-Man): a randomised controlled trial. *Lancet* 2005; 366: 472–7.

Myles PS, Leslie K, McNeil J, et al. Bispectral index monitoring to prevent awareness during anaesthesia: the B-Aware randomised controlled trial. *Lancet* 2004; 363: 1757–63.

Rigg JRA, Jamrozik K, Myles PS, et al. Epidural anaesthesia and analgesia and outcome of major surgery: a randomised controlled trial. *Lancet* 2002; 359: 1276–82.

70a. False
70b. False
70c. False
70d. True
70e. True
Minitracheostomy describes the insertion through the cricothyroid membrane of a non-cuffed tube, usually sized 4 mm; this small size has led to a decline in its use in many centres. Benefits include clearance of secretions and avoiding the requirement for endotracheal intubation. Relative contraindications include coagulopathy or abnormal neck anatomy.

Bodenham A. Tracheostomy. In: Waldmann N, Soni N, Rhodes A, eds. *Oxford Desk Reference: Critical Care*. Oxford: OUP, 2008.

71a. False
71b. True
71c. False
71d. True
71e. False
Crush syndrome, also known as Bywaters' syndrome, involves direct pressure injury to muscle tissue leading to myocyte damage and disruption of vascular supply. Ischaemia and increased cell permeability lead to release of potassium, myoglobin and intracellular enzymes, causing traumatic rhabdomyolysis and subsequent acute renal failure. The crush syndrome is a reperfusion injury, occurring following release of pressure. Immediate priority is resuscitation and stabilization of the injured patient according to ATLS guidelines. Blood gas analysis will provide information on gas exchange, blood lactate, haemoglobin concentration and life-threatening hyperkalaemia.

Malinoski DJ, Slater MS, Mullins RJ. Crush injury and rhabdomyolysis. *Crit Care Clin* 2004; **20**: 171–92.

72a. True
72b. False
72c. False
72d. True
72e. True
Left-sided Macintosh blades are used for patients with right-sided facial deformities that make the use of a standard right-sided blade difficult. The polio blade is mounted at an angle of 135° to the handle and was originally designed to intubate patients in a negative-pressure ventilator ('iron lung'). Magill and Miller are both straight blades, but Miller blades possess a curved tip and flatter flange and web. The McCoy blade is similar to the Macintosh except that it is hinged at the tip; operation of a lever allows elevation of the epiglottis, making it useful for difficult intubation and for patients with immobilized cervical spines.

Yentis S, Hirsch N, Smith G. *Anaesthesia and Intensive Care A to Z: An Encyclopaedia of Principles and Practice*, 4th edn. Oxford: Butterworth-Heinemann, 2009.

73a. False
73b. True
73c. False
73d. True
73e. False
Desflurane is a halogenated ether presented without preservative. Desflurane contains six fluorine atoms and, unlike halothane, does not sensitize the myocardium to catecholamines but does have irritant properties and does increase airway secretions. It undergoes the least hepatic metabolism of all the volatile agents (0.02%). Increased fluorination of the carbon skeleton increases the SVP but reduces the stability and boiling point of the agent; hence it is stored in a specialized microprocessor controlled vaporizer (Tec Mk 6) in which it is heated and stored under pressure (2 atm, representing its SVP at 39°C) and added to the fresh gas flow stream.

Peck TE, Hill SA, Williams M. *Pharmacology for Anaesthesia and Intensive Care*, 3rd edn. Cambridge: CUP, 2008.

74a. True
74b. True
74c. False
74d. True
74e. False
One unit of whole blood is between 405 and 495 mL in volume and is most commonly prepared with CPD or CPD-A (citrate–phosphate–dextrose with adenine), or with SAG-M (saline–adenine–glucose and mannitol). Blood is stored at 2–6°C and addition of adenine increases shelf-life to 35 days, while mannitol reduces red cell fragility. Biochemical changes occur due to altered red cell metabolism and as storage time increases, the following occurs:

- ↓ATP due to continued glucose metabolism
- ↑Lactic acid production and ↓pH
- ↓2,3-DPG levels reaching zero at 14 days in CPD-A
- ↑K^+ levels reaching 30 mmol/L by 28 days
- Leftward shift of the oxyhaemoglobin dissociation curve (Valtis–Kennedy effect due to ↓2,3-DPG)
- Citrate–calcium chelation leading to in vivo anticoagulation and alkalosis
- ↑Spherocytosis as storage time increases and in vivo red cell destruction

Stored platelets last for 3–5 days.

Yentis S, Hirsch N, Smith G. *Anaesthesia and Intensive Care A to Z: An Encyclopaedia of Principles and Practice*, 4th edn. Oxford: Butterworth-Heinemann, 2009.

75a. True
75b. True
75c. False
75d. False
75e. False
The triggers for MH are all volatile anaesthetics (not nitrous oxide) and succinylcholine. For treatment of MH, dantrolene is available as dantrolene

sodium 20 mg and mannitol 3 mg; mannitol is added to solubilize the dantrolene and diuresis is an extra benefit. Further mannitol can be administered if urine output is satisfactory. Diagnosis is confirmed by in vitro contraction of vastus muscle under separate exposure to halothane, and caffeine. When compared with normal muscle, the tension in MH-positive and susceptible patients increases at lower halothane and caffeine concentrations.

Halsall PJ, Hopkins PM. Malignant hyperthermia. *Contin Educ Anaesth Crit Care Pain* 2003; 3: 5–9.

76a. True
76b. True
76c. False
76d. True
76e. False
This block is indicated as analgesia for breast surgery, upper abdominal surgery (open cholecystectomy), chronic pancreatitis and fractured ribs. Laparoscopic cholecystectomy may cause shoulder pain due to subdiaphragmatic gas, thus is not effectively covered by this block. The patient is positioned laterally and a 16 G Tuohy needle is connected to a column of saline via a one-way valve. It is introduced at 45° to the skin at the posterior angle of the upper border of the fourth to the sixth rib, thus avoiding the neurovascular bundle. A loss-of-resistance technique is employed and free flow of saline indicates entry into the space between parietal and visceral pleurae. Local anaesthetic is injected directly or via an epidural catheter, threaded 8–10 cm into the space, ensuring a closed system throughout. The effect is due to paravertebral spread.

77a. True
77b. False
77c. True
77d. False
77e. True
Both haemophilia A and B lead to increased APTT due to deficiency of factors VIII:C and IX respectively, while the TT and bleeding time are normal. Patients with von Willebrand's disease usually have a normal platelet count with an increased bleeding time, due to factor VIII:vWF deficiency. DIC is characterized by platelet and factor consumption with low fibrinogen levels and increased International Normalized Ratio (INR), APTT and TT.

Purday J. Haematological disorders. In: Allman KG, Wilson IH, eds. *Oxford Handbook of Anaesthesia*, 2nd edn. Oxford: OUP, 2006.

78a. False
78b. True
78c. False
78d. False
78e. True

Acute lung injury (ALI) is a syndrome of inflammation and increased permeability of lung tissue. Diagnostic features of ALI are:

- PaO_2/FiO_2 $\leq$300 mmHg (40 kPa) regardless of level of positive end-expiratory pressure (PEEP)
- bilateral infiltrates on chest X-ray
- pulmonary artery wedge pressure (PAWP) <18 mmHg
- acute onset of respiratory failure

ARDS is the most severe form of ALI. The diagnostic criteria are similar, except that PaO_2/FiO_2 is $\leq$200 mmHg (26 kPa). ARDS consists of three phases: exudative (oedema and haemorrhage), proliferative (organization and repair) and fibrotic. The initial insult may be direct (chest trauma, smoke inhalation) or distant (peritonitis, burns). Mortality is 30–50% for ARDS uncomplicated by other organ failure.

Singer M, Webb AR. *Oxford Handbook of Critical Care*, 3rd edn. Oxford: OUP, 2009.

79a. True
79b. True
79c. True
79d. True
79e. False

Acute pancreatitis describes an autodigestive process. Proteolytic enzymes cause haemorrhagic necrosis of parenchymal tissue. Listed are the common aetiologies of acute pancreatitis ('*GET SMASHED*'):

- *G*: Gallstones (macrolithiasis or microlithiasis)
- *E*: EtOH (ethanol: chronic alcoholism)
- *T*: Trauma
- *S*: Steroids
- *M*: Mumps
- *A*: Autoimmune diseases (e.g. sclerosing cholangitis)
- *S*: Scorpion bites
- *H*: Hypercalcaemia, hypothermia
- *E*: ERCP (endoscopic retrograde cholangiopancreatography)
- *D*: Drugs (azathioprine, valproate, thiazides, furosemide)

Hypocalcaemia often accompanies and complicates acute pancreatitis, but is not a cause.

Young SP, Thompson JP. Severe acute pancreatitis. *Contin Educ Anaesth Crit Care Pain* 2008; 8: 125–8.

80a. False
80b. False
80c. True
80d. True
80e. True

A spirometer can measure the following values (normal values for a 70 kg man):

- tidal volume (TV): volume of gas inspired or expired during normal breathing (500 mL)
- inspiratory reserve volume (IRV): maximum volume of gas inspired from the normal end-inspiratory position (2500 mL)
- expiratory reserve volume (ERV): maximum volume expired from the normal end-expiratory position (1500 mL)
- inspiratory capacity (TV + IRV): 3000 mL
- vital capacity (TV + IRV + ERV): 4500 mL

Lung volumes that cannot be measured via spirometry, but require plethysmography, N_2 washout or helium dilution are:

- residual volume (RV): volume of gas remaining in the lungs after maximal expiration (1200–1500 mL)
- total lung capacity (VC + RV): volume of gas in the lung after maximal inspiration (6000 mL)
- functional residual capacity (RV + ERV): volume of gas in the lungs at resting end-expiratory level (3000 mL standing and 2000 mL supine).

Lung volumes are illustrated in Figure 3.4.

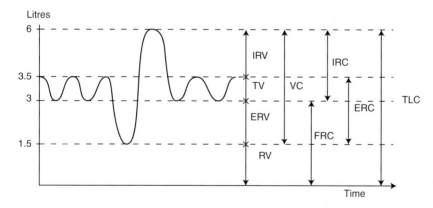

FIGURE 3.4   Lung volumes: IRV, inspiratory reserve volume; TV, tidal volume; ERV, expiratory reserve volume; RV, residual volume; VC, vital capacity; FRC, functional residual capacity; IRC, inspiratory reserve capacity; ERC, expiratory reserve capacity; TLC, total lung capacity.

Atkinson RS, Rushman GB, Davies NJH. *Lee's Synopsis of Anaesthesia*, 13th edn. Oxford: Butterworth-Heinemann, 2005.

81a. False
81b. False
81c. False
81d. True
81e. False
Colloids are suspensions of particles unable to pass freely across a semi-permeable membrane; they are divided into:

- *Gelatins*: with MW of 30−35 kDa and intravascular half-life of 2−4 hours
- *Hydroxyethylstarches*: composed of etherified amylopectin and have intravascular persistence of 24−36 hours and varying MW (>50 kDa)
- *Dextrans*: glucose polymers with MW of 40, 70 and 110 (withdrawn) kDa; they reduce blood viscosity, thereby lowering ESR, but may affect blood crossmatching and renal function

82a. False
82b. False
82c. False
82d. False
82e. True
Turbulent flow is proportional to:

- $Radius^2$
- $\sqrt{(Pressure\ gradient)}$
- $(Length)^{-1}$
- $(Density\ of\ fluid)^{-1}$

Reynolds number (Re) is a dimensionless quantity that describes the relationship between tube and fluid characteristics and the velocity at which turbulent flow occurs; when Re >2000, turbulent flow occurs.

83a. False
83b. True
83c. False
83d. True
83e. True
The stellate ganglion is part of the cervical sympathetic chain, lying either side of the vertebral column. It is the fusion of the inferior cervical and 1st thoracic ganglion and is present in 80% of individuals. It provides much of the sympathetic nerve supply to the head, neck and upper extremities. The Chassaignac tubercle is the transverse process of C6 and is palpated level with the cricoid cartilage; successful blockade results in Horner's syndrome − ptosis, meiosis and anhydrosis. Indications for blockade include:

- complex regional pain syndrome
- phantom limb pain
- Raynaud's syndrome (where circulation is improved)

84a. True
84b. True
84c. False
84d. True
84e. False
Propofol is a phenol derivative that is presented as a 1 or 2% lipid emulsion. Complications of use include the *propofol infusion syndrome*, which is characterized by intractable bradycardia, acidosis, rhabdomyolysis and renal failure with prolonged infusions. It exhibits anticonvulsant properties and although involuntary movements are associated with its use, no evidence of epileptiform activity exists. Prolonged infusion can lead to hypertriglyceridaemia. Quinol metabolites confer green discolouration to urine and hair. Pain on injection also occurs.

Rowe K, Fletcher S. Sedation in the intensive care unit. *Contin Educ Anaesth Crit Care Pain* 2008; 8: 50–5.
Sasada M, Smith S. *Drugs in Anaesthesia and Intensive Care*, 3rd edn. Oxford: OUP, 2003.

85a. False
85b. False
85c. False
85d. True
85e. True
The ICD9 definition of maternal death is as follows:

- A maternal death is defined as any death that occurs during or within 1 year of pregnancy, ectopic pregnancy or abortion and that is directly or indirectly related to these conditions
- A *direct* maternal death is a death resulting from obstetric complications of the pregnancy state from interventions, omissions or incorrect treatment or from a chain of events resulting from any of the above
- An *indirect* maternal death is defined as a death resulting from previously existing disease, or from disease that developed during pregnancy and that was not due to direct obstetric causes but was aggravated by the physiological effects of the pregnancy
- A *coincidental* death is death that occurs from unrelated causes that happen to occur in the pregnancy or puerperium
- A *late* death is defined as a death that occurs between 42 days and 1 year after abortion, miscarriage or delivery

Lewis G, ed. The Confidential Enquiry into Maternal and Child Health (CEMACH). *Saving Mothers' Lives: reviewing maternal deaths to make motherhood safer – 2003–2005*. The Seventh Report on Confidential Enquiries into Maternal Deaths in the UK. London: CEMACH, 2007. Available at: www.cmace.org.uk/getattachment/05f68346-816b-4560-b1b9-af24fb633170/Saving-Mothers'-Lives-2003-2005_ExecSumm.aspx.

86a. False
86b. False
86c. True
86d. True
86e. False
Pacemakers have a generic code – NBG, which is derived from the NASPE (North American Society of Pacing and Electrophysiology), BPEG (British Pacing and Electrophysiology group) and is generic. The code is as follows:

I   Chamber paced (O – none, A – atrium, V – ventricle, D – dual)
II   Chamber sensed (O, A, V, D)
III   Response to sensing (O – none, T – trigger, I – inhibit, D – dual)
IV   Programmability (O – none, P – simple, M – multi,
       C – communicating, R – rate modulation)
V   Antitachycardia function (O – none, P – pacing, S – shock, D – dual)

The first three letters describe antibradycardic functions, the fourth describes programmability (including rate modulation) and the fifth describes antitachycardia functions.

Diprose P, Pierce JMT. Anaesthesia for patients with pacemakers and similar devices. *Contin Educ Anaesth Crit Care Pain* 2001; **1**: 166–70.

87a. True
87b. False
87c. True
87d. False
87e. True
The SI unit of pressure is the pascal (Pa), which is equal to 1 N/m^2. In anaesthetic practice, it is more common to use the kilopascal (kPa). The following units are approximately equal:

* 1 atmosphere (atm)
* 1 bar
* 100 kPa
* 1020 cmH_2O
* 750 mmHg
* 750 Torr
* 14.5 $lb/inch^2$

Davis PD, Kenny GNC. *Basic Physics and Measurement in Anaesthesia*, 5th edn. Oxford: Butterworth-Heinemann, 2003.

88a. False
88b. True
88c. False
88d. True
88e. False
Lidocaine and prilocaine are the local anaesthetics of choice for intravenous regional anaesthesia (Bier's block). Adrenaline should never be added, owing

to its vasoconstrictive effects and potential for end-organ damage and also its attendant cardiovascular effects. Bupivacaine is contraindicated owing to potential for refractory cardiac toxicity. Guanethidine inhibits noradrenaline release and is used for sympatholytic nerve blocks in the management of chronic and neuropathic pain states, but is not an anaesthetic agent.

89a. False
89b. True
89c. True
89d. False
89e. True
HbF consists of two α and two γ chains. Lower 2,3-DPG (diphosphoglycerate) levels results in a leftward shift of the oxyhaemoglobin dissociation curve, which results in a decreased PO_2 and favours O_2 transfer from mother to fetus. HbF forms 80% of circulating haemoglobin at birth and is replaced by HbA within 3−5 months. It may persist in haemoglobinopathies.

90a. True
90b. True
90c. True
90d. False
90e. True
All are causes of sensorimotor neuropathies except motor neuron disease, which is characterized by degeneration of the ventral horns of the spinal cords and atrophy of the ventral roots, presenting with mixed upper and lower motor neuron signs. Charcot−Marie−Tooth disease is a hereditary disorder featuring distal limb wasting and muscle atrophy with varying degrees of sensory loss. Syringomyelia is caused by tubular cystic cavities forming within the spinal cord and give rise to sensorimotor and autonomic neuropathies. *Mycobacterium leprae* infection (leprosy) is a common cause of neuropathy in developing countries and most commonly affects peripheral nerves and skin, with sensory neuropathies predominating. Finally, diphtheria results from the exotoxin produced by *Corynebacterium diphtheriae*, which can lead to a demyelinating neuropathy in non-immunized individuals who develop infection.

Kumar P, Clark M. *Kumar and Clark's Clinical Medicine*, 7th edn. London: Saunders, 2009.

4. Practice Paper 4: Questions

1. The following are exclusion criteria for paediatric day case surgery:
   a. Post-conceptual age <60 weeks
   b. Uninvestigated cardiac murmur
   c. Sickle cell disease
   d. Laparoscopic surgery
   e. Diabetes

2. Recognized side-effects of ondansetron include:
   a. Constipation
   b. Tachycardia
   c. Chest pain
   d. Seizures
   e. Transient blindness

3. The following cause a leftward shift of the oxyhaemoglobin dissociation curve:
   a. Hypothermia
   b. Reduced blood pH
   c. Hyperphosphataemia
   d. Carbon monoxide poisoning
   e. Methaemoglobinaemia

4. Hypothermia:
   a. Results in cutaneous vasoconstriction
   b. Results in cutaneous vasodilatation
   c. Increases heart rate
   d. Can result in ventricular fibrillation below $28°C$ core body temperature
   e. Results in increased oxygen delivery ($\dot{D}O_2$)

5. Lung compliance decreases with:
   a. Pulmonary fibrosis
   b. Emphysema
   c. Pulmonary vascular engorgement
   d. Age
   e. Pulmonary oedema

6. The Centers for Disease Control and Prevention classification for HIV patients states:
   a. There are four broad groups of patients
   b. Asymptomatic infection describes Group I
   c. Persistent generalized lymphadenopathy occurs in Group II
   d. Symptomatic HIV infection describes Group IV
   e. Acute seroconversion occurs a few years after infection

7. A 58-year-old man presents with acute variceal haemorrhage; the following statements are correct:
   a. Mortality is reduced by β-blockade
   b. Terlipressin has been shown to reduce mortality
   c. The most common cause is primary biliary cirrhosis
   d. Band ligation is superior to sclerotherapy in reducing recurrence of bleeding
   e. Rupture of varices occur when portal pressure is ≥ 8 mmHg

8. Concerning intracranial pressure (ICP) waveforms:
   a. They consist of three peaks named A, B and C waves
   b. A-waves are always pathological
   c. The presence of B-waves after a head injury is a poor sign
   d. A-waves last 5–20 minutes
   e. C-waves are of little clinical significance

9. A previously well 75-year-old woman with type 2 diabetes mellitus presents with delirium, malaise and weakness; arterial blood gas analysis shows pH 7.28, Pao_2 10.5 (Fio_2 60%), $Paco_2$ 3.6 kPa, K^+ 6.5 mmol/L, glucose 38 mmol/L. The following is correct:
   a. Ketosis is expected
   b. Diuretic therapy is indicated
   c. This is caused by insulin deficiency
   d. The anion gap is expected to be very high
   e. Anticoagulation is indicated

10. Regarding magnetic resonance imaging (MRI):
   a. Superconducting magnets contain wires with an electrical resistance of zero
   b. The superconductor coil of wire is kept at a temperature of 0°C
   c. Liquid helium is used to produce superconductivity
   d. Clinical magnets have a field strength of 0.1–3 Tesla
   e. Gadolinium compounds do not pass through the blood–brain barrier

11. The liver:
   a. Has portal tracts comprising branches of the hepatic artery, hepatic vein and bile duct
   b. Receives the majority of its blood supply from the hepatic artery
   c. Receives 20% of cardiac output
   d. Produces vitamin K-dependent clotting factors: II, VII, IX and XII
   e. Contributes 4% of the total body albumin pool per day

12. Lidocaine:
   a. Has a pK_a of 8.1
   b. Is not removed by haemodialysis
   c. Is an amide
   d. Is a Class 1c antiarrhythmic
   e. Is 95% protein-bound in the plasma

13. Glucagon:
    a. Is secreted by α-cells of the pancreas
    b. Inhibits adenylate cylcase secretion
    c. Has a half-life of 60 minutes
    d. Secretion is increased during stress
    e. Stimulates secretion of insulin

14. A 42-year-old man presents for excision of a phaeochromocytoma; surges in blood pressure would be expected:
    a. At endotracheal intubation
    b. During tumour manipulation
    c. On venous ligation
    d. On induction of anaesthesia
    e. During the immediate postoperative period

15. Regarding delirium in intensive care:
    a. Incidence is >60%
    b. It is predictive of increased mortality
    c. Haloperidol is first-line drug treatment
    d. Benzodiazepines are first-line drug treatment
    e. Haloperidol is a cause of neuroleptic malignant syndrome

16. A man presents to A&E with ethylene glycol poisoning; the following are expected:
    a. Decreased anion gap
    b. Increased osmolar gap
    c. Type B lactic acidosis
    d. Administration of enteral charcoal
    e. Urate crystals in the urine

17. Concerning disease-modifying anti-rheumatoid drugs:
    a. Gold causes bone marrow depression
    b. Sulfasalazine causes bradycardia
    c. Penicillamine causes hepatitis
    d. Cyclosporin causes gingival hypertrophy
    e. Hydroxychloroquine causes permanent retinopathy

18. The following statements are correct for scoliosis:
    a. The most common form is neuromuscular
    b. Preoperative spirometry would be expected to reveal a restrictive lung defect
    c. The Cobb angle involves perpendicular lines from the inner surfaces of upper and lower, maximally tilted, vertebrae
    d. A curvature of greater than $10°$ is considered abnormal
    e. Surgery is indicated if the curvature is greater than $25°$ in children

19. When using peripheral nerve stimulators:
    a. A current of 15–40 mA is applied to the ulnar nerve
    b. The negative electrode is placed proximally on a limb
    c. Successful ulnar stimulation results in contraction of the abductor pollicis brevis muscle
    d. The duration of stimulus is less than 0.2 ms
    e. The stimulus should consist of a square wave

20. Concerning brachial plexus injuries in the supine anaesthetized patient:
    a. C8 and T1 nerve roots are prone to injury by compression against the scapula and cervical vertebrae
    b. The arm should not be abducted beyond 90°
    c. The hand should preferably be supine
    d. The head should be turned to the opposite side of the abducted arm
    e. The ulnar nerve is most prone to injury in the ulnar groove

21. Contents of the anterior mediastinum include the:
    a. Thymus gland
    b. Thyroid gland
    c. Aortic arch
    d. Internal mammary artery
    e. Vagus nerves

22. Esmolol:
    a. Is a negative inotrope
    b. Has intrinsic sympathomimetic activity
    c. Is highly lipid-soluble
    d. Has active metabolites
    e. Is cardioselective for the β_1 receptor

23. Intraocular pressure (IOP) is reduced by:
    a. Propofol
    b. Thiopentone
    c. Ketamine
    d. Benzodiazepines
    e. N_2O

24. Numerical indices that predict successful weaning from mechanical ventilation include:
    a. Respiratory rate <35/min
    b. Maximum inspiratory pressure >-25 cmH$_2$O
    c. $Pao_2/Fio_2 >200$ mmHg
    d. Minute ventilation >10 L/min
    e. $Pao_2/Pao_2 >0.35$

25. Following coronary artery bypass grafting 4 days previously, a patient suffers a cardiac arrest; appropriate management includes:
    a. Resternotomy performed only by a surgeon
    b. Resternotomy performed after three attempts at defibrillation for ventricular fibrillation (VF)
    c. Epicardial pacing wires set to DDD in context of asystole
    d. Prompt resternotomy in non-shockable rhythms
    e. Switch off pacemaker function in pulseless electrical activity (PEA)

26. Pericarditis:
    a. Is defined as chronic if present for more than 8 weeks
    b. When infectious is most commonly of fungal aetiology
    c. Causes a steep y descent on the jugular venous pressure (JVP) waveform
    d. Causes pathological Q-waves on ECG
    e. In acute presentation is negatively prognosticated by an elevated troponin I

27. Indications for vena cava filter insertions are:
    a. Severe coagulopathy
    b. Uncontrollable thromboembolic disease
    c. Limited life expectancy
    d. Patients with absolute contraindications to anticoagulation
    e. Patients undergoing pulmonary endarterectomy

28. Concerning respiratory gas analysis:
    a. Health and Safety Executive standards apply to monitoring during recovery
    b. The cathode in a fuel cell is sacrificial
    c. The glass in a Severinghaus electrode is H^+-selective
    d. Mass spectrometry involves ionizing molecules
    e. Molecules containing similar atoms absorb infrared radiation

29. Remifentanil:
    a. Is usually diluted to 50 mg/mL
    b. Continuous infusion dose range is $0.05-0.2$ $\mu g\,kg^{-1}\,min^{-1}$
    c. Is a non-selective opioid receptor
    d. Has a context-sensitive half-time of less than 4 minutes
    e. Exhibits altered pharmacokinetics in obesity

30. The following volatile agents cause a tachycardia:
    a. Isoflurane
    b. Desflurane
    c. Sevoflurane
    d. Halothane
    e. Enflurane

31. **The coeliac plexus:**
    a. Is the largest sympathetic plexus in the body
    b. Receives contributions from the glossopharyngeal and vagus nerves
    c. When blocked commonly results in hypertension
    d. Lies posterior to the abdominal aorta
    e. Can be blocked to diagnose sympathetically mediated pain

32. **Risk factors for postoperative nausea and vomiting (PONV) include:**
    a. Ketamine administration
    b. Opioid administration
    c. Old age
    d. Hip replacement surgery
    e. Anxiety

33. **Vasopressin:**
    a. Release is stimulated by noradrenaline
    b. Release is inhibited by noradrenaline
    c. Is available as DDAVP
    d. Shows reduced mortality in septic shock compared with noradrenaline
    e. Has been used successfully in place of adrenaline in cardiac arrests

34. **A 28-year-old intravenous drug user is admitted to hospital with suspected tetanus infection; the following management is appropriate:**
    a. If cardiovascularly stable, she does not require ICU admission
    b. Human tetanus immunoglobulin (HTIG) should be administered daily
    c. Metronidazole is the antibiotic of choice
    d. Episodes of hypertension should be treated with a β-blocker
    e. Recovery results in immunity

35. **When assessing patient need for liver transplantation, the Model for End-Stage Liver Disease (MELD) Score uses the following indices:**
    a. Alkaline phosphatase
    b. Serum creatinine
    c. International Normalized Ratio (INR)
    d. Bilirubin
    e. Haemoglobin

36. **Uraemia:**
    a. Is a cause of peripheral neuropathy
    b. Occurs when creatinine clearance falls to 60 mL/min
    c. Causes a prolonged bleeding time
    d. Leads to thrombocytopenia in approximately 50% of patients
    e. Toxicity is primarily due to accumulation of urea

37. **The following is correct of ventilators:**
    a. Pressure generators have a high internal impedance to flow
    b. The Manley MP3 ventilator is a Mapleson A during spontaneous ventilation
    c. The Manley MP3 ventilator is a time-cycled pressure generator
    d. Expiration is passive in high-frequency oscillatory ventilation (HFOV)
    e. Pressure generators compensate well for leaks

38. **The listed formulae for paediatric anaesthesia are correct:**
    a. Weight (kg) = [Age (years) + 4] × 2
    b. Endotracheal tube (ETT) external diameter (mm) = [Age (years)/4] + 4
    c. Oral ETT length (cm) = [Age (years)/2] + 15
    d. Dose of fluids for resuscitation = 20 mL/kg
    e. Resuscitation dose of atropine = 10 μg/kg

39. **When treating patients with chronic alcohol use:**
    a. Prolonged prothrombin time is a late manifestation of impaired synthetic liver function
    b. Regional techniques may be technically difficult
    c. Dose requirements for general anaesthetic agents decrease
    d. There is an increased incidence of postoperative bleeding
    e. Alcohol withdrawal syndrome (ANS) may be delayed for up to 5 days

40. **Concerning obesity:**
    a. Body mass index (BMI) >30 kg/m^2 with a comorbidity is considered morbid obesity
    b. Absolute blood volume increases
    c. Local anaesthetic doses for neuraxial blockade should be decreased
    d. Hormonal control of appetite includes adiponectin and inhibin
    e. Obesity and a collar size of more than 17 inches are a risk factor for obstructive sleep apnoea

41. **Risk factors identified for the development of phantom limb pain include:**
    a. Upper limb amputation
    b. Emergency amputation
    c. Pre-amputation pain
    d. Bilateral limb amputation
    e. Young age

42. **Thromboprophylaxis with low-molecular-weight heparin (LMWH) is not recommended for the following:**
    a. A previously warfarinized patient with an INR of 1.4
    b. A patient with suspected bacterial meningitis who has undergone a lumbar puncture 8 hours ago
    c. An elderly woman who suffered an episode of heparin-induced thrombocytopenia (HIT) 6 months ago
    d. An elderly man who suffered a thrombotic stroke 4 weeks ago
    e. A young man with haemophilia A admitted with sepsis

43. **The following changes would be expected of a brainstem-dead patient in intensive care:**
    a. Significant increase in cardiac output
    b. Ischaemic changes on ECG
    c. Hyperthermia
    d. Pulmonary oedema
    e. Rise in antidiuretic hormone (ADH)

44. **Sick sinus syndrome:**
    a. Is most commonly caused by drugs
    b. Is caused by hyperthyroidism
    c. Is often asymptomatic
    d. When symptomatic is an indication for a permanent pacemaker
    e. Mandates insertion of a pacing device prior to general anaesthesia

45. **With regards to cerebral aneurysms:**
    a. Hypertension is a risk factor
    b. The majority are small
    c. Risk of rupture is high if located around the basilar tip
    d. Following rupture, approximately one-third of patients die before reaching hospital
    e. 50% of ruptured aneurysms re-bleed within 6 weeks

46. **Hydrophobic bacterial and viral filters:**
    a. Are over 99.99% efficient
    b. Possess ports for 15 and 20 mm size tubings and connections
    c. Require a large surface area
    d. Provide humidification without a hygroscopic element
    e. Do not demonstrate inertial impaction

47. **The vagus nerve:**
    a. Lies between the internal jugular vein and internal carotid artery within the carotid sheath in the neck
    b. Supplies the cricothyroid muscle via the internal branch of the superior laryngeal nerve
    c. Internal branch of the superior laryngeal branch pierces the thyrohyoid membrane
    d. Recurrent laryngeal branch is closely related to the inferior thyroid artery
    e. Recurrent laryngeal branch originates anterior to the subclavian artery on the right

48. **Concerning the popliteal fossa:**
    a. It contains the posterior cutaneous nerve of the thigh
    b. Its medial border is formed by the biceps femoris
    c. The popliteal vein lies medial to the artery
    d. The tibial nerve is lateral and superficial to the popliteal artery
    e. Nerve stimulation during popliteal block should elicit foot inversion and/or plantar flexion

49. **Hyperbaric oxygen therapy (HBOT):**
    a. Is helpful in treating arterial air emboli as a function of Charles' law
    b. Increases the oxygen content of blood as a function of Henry's law
    c. Causes an increase in left ventricular afterload
    d. Is absolutely contraindicated in patients with a simple 'undrained' pneumothorax
    e. Is relatively contraindicated in patients with implantable pacemakers

50. **Following epidural anaesthesia for caesarean section, placental transfer of local anaesthetics:**
    a. Increases with the pK_a value
    b. Increases with maternal hyperventilation
    c. Is greater for lidocaine than procaine
    d. Decreases with fetal acidosis
    e. Increases when co-administered with bicarbonate

51. **'Liquid' ventilation:**
    a. Requires a specialized ventilator when 'partial'
    b. Uses fluorocarbons
    c. Exerts a mechanical effect
    d. Fills the lungs to closing capacity when 'partial'
    e. Increases the number of 'ventilator-free' days

52. **A 42-year-old motorcyclist presents to A&E with a crush injury following a road traffic incident; the following statements are correct:**
    a. Acidosis, hyperkalaemia and hypercalcaemia are expected
    b. Plasma creatine kinase (CK) concentration is proportional to muscle damage
    c. Intravenous fluid resuscitation should consist of 5% glucose
    d. Precipitation of the Tamm–Horsfall protein causes urinary casts
    e. Acute renal failure can be prevented by acidification of the urine

53. **Factors predictive of prolonged ventilation postoperatively in patients with myasthenia gravis are:**
    a. Forced vital capacity (FVC) <2.9 L
    b. Chronic respiratory disease
    c. SpO_2 <90% on air
    d. Long history (>6 years) of myasthenia gravis
    e. Requirement of >750 mg per day of pyridostigmine

54. **Diagnostic criteria for pre-eclampsia include:**
    a. Peripheral oedema
    b. Proteinuria >1 g/L
    c. Diastolic BP >100 mmHg on one occasion
    d. More than 20 weeks of pregnancy
    e. Uric acid >6 mg/dL

55. **Exponential processes:**
    a. Assume straight lines on semi-logarithmic paper
    b. Reduce to 37% of given value in one time constant
    c. Possess a rate constant that is the reciprocal of the time constant
    d. Include uptake of inhalational agents as an example of a positive process
    e. Are 95% complete in five time constants

56. **Association of Anaesthetists of Great Britain and Ireland Guidelines on Blood Transfusion (2005) state that:**
    a. Platelet transfusion for non-bleeding ICU patients should commence at $\leq 10\,000 \times 10^9/L$
    b. Thawed fresh frozen plasma (FFP) stored at 4°C can be used within 24 hours
    c. FFP stored at room temperature can be used within 12 hours
    d. Components should be used to facilitate regional anaesthesia where possible
    e. Vitamin K is recommended to reverse the effects of warfarin

57. **During cardiopulmonary bypass (CPB):**
    a. Activated clotting time (ACT) should be >150 s before CPB is commenced
    b. Minimal haemolysis occurs within the first 2 hours
    c. Type of surgery is a risk factor for development of a cerebrovascular event (CVE)
    d. 1 mg of protamine is administered for each international unit (IU) of heparin
    e. Hypothermia exerts a neuroprotective effect

58. **Concerning the right and left phrenic nerves:**
    a. Motor supply to the diaphragm is supplemented by the intercostal nerves
    b. Run posterior to the subclavian arteries
    c. Palsy results from stellate ganglion blockade on the side concerned
    d. Pierce the diaphragm via the caval orifice
    e. Give no branches in the thorax

59. **Examples of β-lactam antibacterial drugs are:**
    a. Flucloxacillin
    b. Ceftriaxone
    c. Meropenem
    d. Vancomycin
    e. Aztreonam

60. **The following have higher measured values in cerebrospinal fluid (CSF) than in plasma:**
    a. Magnesium
    b. Calcium
    c. Protein
    d. Chloride
    e. Osmolality

61. **Causes of hypovolaemic hyponatraemia include:**
    a. Cerebral salt-wasting syndrome (CSWS)
    b. Syndrome of inappropriate antidiuretic hormone secretion (SIADH)
    c. Diarrhoea
    d. Nephrogenic diabetes insipidus (DI)
    e. Acute renal failure

62. **The following is correct of infective endocarditis (IE):**
    a. It more commonly affects men
    b. It is diagnosed using the revised Jones criteria
    c. Erythema marginatum is a feature
    d. *Staphylococcus aureus* is the most common pathogen
    e. Antibiotic prophylaxis should be administered before dental surgery for patients previously affected

63. The following is correct of myotonic dystrophy:
    a. It exhibits autosomal dominant inheritance
    b. It improves with administration of dantrolene
    c. Nerve stimulator devices should be avoided
    d. There is increased sensitivity to propofol
    e. Neostigmine should be used to reverse residual neuromuscular blockade

64. Features of a modern scavenging system include:
    a. Pressure relief valves set at 1000 Pa in the collecting system
    b. 22 mm connectors between collecting and reservoir systems
    c. Dumping valves in a closed receiving system
    d. Active low-flow disposal
    e. Gas analysers

65. Regarding fluids:
    a. 0.9% saline is pH 5
    b. Gelofusine is pH 7.4
    c. Glucose 4%/saline 0.18% contains 30 mmol/L sodium
    d. Gelofusine contains 40 g gelatin per litre
    e. Haemaccel contains 2.65 mmol/L calcium

66. With regard to a 'Do Not Attempt Resuscitation' (DNAR) decision option:
    a. The senior clinician in charge of a patient's care can overrule an advance decision
    b. In England and Wales a patient who lacks capacity has access to independent advocacy
    c. For a patient who lacks capacity an Independent Mental Capacity Advocate has responsibility for decision making
    d. Survival rates following anaesthetic-related cardiac arrest are lower than for other in-hospital arrests
    e. It may be temporarily modified for the perioperative period

67. Following a road-traffic accident, a man is brought to A&E with multiple trauma. He has paradoxical chest wall movements, is mumbling incomprehensibly and is not eye-opening to pain; he is also extending his limbs in response to a painful stimulus. His vital signs are heart rate 120/min, blood pressure 84/56 mmHg, respiratory rate 42/min; the following applies:
    a. His GCS score is 5
    b. His GCS score is 6
    c. Rapid sequence induction is indicated immediately
    d. Head and chest CT scan is indicated without delay
    e. Trauma X-ray series of neck, thorax and abdomen is indicated

68. **Transcutaneous electrical nerve stimulation (TENS):**
    a. Requires a prescription
    b. Delivers monophasic pulsed currents
    c. Delivers pulse durations of 50–250 μs
    d. Delivers pulse frequencies of 1–200 Hz
    e. Can be applied over the anterior neck

69. **A 60-year-old patient undergoing an emergency laparotomy develops a thyrotoxic crisis intraoperatively; the following management options are appropriate:**
    a. Hyperpyrexia should be treated with tepid sponging, paracetamol or aspirin
    b. Ideal heart rate is less than 90/min
    c. Propranolol may precipitate further arrhythmias
    d. Dantrolene administration
    e. Steroids do not have a role

70. **A reduction in jugular venous saturation ($SjvO_2$) would be expected in:**
    a. Hyperoxia
    b. Hypocapnia
    c. Increased intracranial pressure
    d. Brain death
    e. Seizures

71. **Peripheral signs seen in severe aortic regurgitation include:**
    a. Quincke's sign
    b. Water hammer pulse
    c. Osler's nodes
    d. Janeway lesions
    e. Traube's sign

72. **Cataracts are features of:**
    a. Wilson's disease
    b. Congenital rubella syndrome
    c. Toxoplasmosis
    d. Amiodarone usage
    e. Hypercalcaemia

73. **The following is correct of spinal needles:**
    a. Sprotte is a non-cutting type
    b. Quincke is a non-cutting type
    c. Whitacre has an injection hole just proximal to the tip
    d. Postdural puncture headache is more common with Quincke than with Sprotte
    e. Greene is pencil-tipped

74. **During exercise:**
    a. $PaCO_2$ increases
    b. Ventilation increases in response to hypoxia
    c. The alveolar–pulmonary capillary PO_2 gradient increases
    d. A linear relationship exists between oxygen consumption and ventilation
    e. Pulmonary vascular resistance rises

75. **Approximate normal lung volumes for a 70 kg man are:**
    a. Inspiratory reserve volume: 1 L
    b. Residual volume: 0.5 L
    c. Total lung capacity: 6 L
    d. Vital capacity: 3 L
    e. Tidal volume: 2 L

76. **Acupuncture:**
    a. Needles are 27–29 G
    b. Is based on theories of energy flow across the body
    c. Involves 12 main and 8 secondary meridians
    d. Can involve passage of electrical currents at 100 Hz through the needle
    e. Is relatively contraindicated in burns

77. **The use of ultrasound for catheterization of the epidural space:**
    a. Has improved maternal satisfaction
    b. Resulted in longer times for the insertion procedure in children when done in 'realtime'
    c. Decreases the incidence of dural puncture in children
    d. Cannot assess the depth of the epidural space
    e. Reduces the number of attempts required for successful placement

78. **Following a percutaneous tracheostomy on ICU, an adult patient suddenly becomes hypoxic, hypotensive with increased airway pressure; immediate management should include:**
    a. Chest drain insertion
    b. Needle thoracocentesis
    c. Chest X-ray
    d. Rapid sequence induction with thiopentone and suxamethonium
    e. Administration of 100% oxygen and suction via the tracheostomy tube

79. **The following applies to the generic pacemaker code (NBG):**
    a. It consists of five letters
    b. Position I is chamber sensed
    c. Position II is chamber sensed
    d. Position III is programmability
    e. Position IV describes the antitachycardia function of the pacemaker

80. **Trigeminal neuralgia:**
    a. Most commonly affects the ophthalmic division of the trigeminal nerve
    b. Often occurs bilaterally
    c. Is more common in young females
    d. In 80% of cases is related to vascular compression of the gasserian ganglion
    e. Is best medically treated using carbamazepine

81. **Concerning abdominal wall defects:**
    a. Exomphalos is more common in males
    b. The majority of neonates with exomphalos have an associated congenital anomaly
    c. Surgical correction of gastroschisis should be performed as soon after birth as possible
    d. Neonates with gastroschisis should undergo an echocardiogram
    e. Nitrous oxide should be avoided in anaesthesia for surgical correction

82. **The properties below are correctly matched with their units of measurement:**
    a. Magnetic field strength: tesla
    b. Capacitance: coulomb
    c. Amount of substance: kilogram
    d. Charge: farad
    e. Power: watt

83. **For the provision of one-lung ventilation, the use of a Univent bronchial blocker has the following advantages when compared with a double-lumen tube:**
    a. Ease of ventilation
    b. Absence of a high-pressure cuff
    c. Use in small children
    d. No requirement for endotracheal tube (ETT) exchange for postoperative ventilation
    e. Selective lobar blockade

84. **Doxapram:**
    a. Is presented as 20 mg/mL
    b. Acts centrally and peripherally
    c. Should be given as a bolus of 1 mg/kg
    d. Displaces the CO_2 response curve to the right
    e. Can be used for postoperative shivering

85. Concerning major complications of central neuraxial blockade in the UK:
    a. It is the title of the 3rd National Audit Project of the Royal College of Anaesthetists
    b. Incidence of permanent injury is between 2 and 4.2 per 100 000
    c. Incidence of paraplegia or death was 0.7–1.8 per 100 000
    d. Only 20% of initially severe injuries resolved fully
    e. Most complications leading to harm occurred in obstetric practice

86. Regarding the nose:
    a. The floor consists of the palatine bone and the maxilla
    b. The paranasal sinuses and nasolacrimal duct open onto the medial wall
    c. Arterial supply comprises the maxillary and mandibular arteries
    d. Sensation to the septum is derived from the posterior ethmoidal nerve
    e. Topical anaesthesia is provided by Moffett's solution, which consists of 2 mL of 8% cocaine, 2 mL of 1% sodium bicarbonate and 1 mL of 1 : 1000 adrenaline

87. Concerning the Fontan circulation
    a. It is indicated for tricuspid and pulmonary atresia
    b. Conversion should be performed in the neonatal period
    c. Stage I consists of placing a systemic–pulmonary shunt
    d. Stage II consists of an anastomosis of superior vena cava to proximal left pulmonary artery
    e. After stage III the inferior vena cava is directed into the pulmonary circulation

88. Typical cerebrospinal fluid (CSF) findings for pyogenic meningitis are:
    a. Appearance: Turbid
    b. Predominant cell type: Polymorphs
    c. Cell count: $<500/mm^3$
    d. Protein: >1 g/dL
    e. CSF : blood glucose: $>60\%$

89. The following cylinder pressures are accurate at room temperature:
    a. N_2O: 137 bar
    b. CO_2: 50 bar
    c. Heliox: 40 bar
    d. Entonox: 137 bar
    e. O_2: 137 bar

90. Statins:
    a. All selectively inhibit HMG-CoA reductase
    b. Lead to increased hepatic LDL-receptor expression
    c. Lower LDL levels in a dose-dependent fashion
    d. Are associated with development of rhabdomyolysis
    e. Therapy should be monitored with regular plasma creatine kinase (CK) levels

4. Practice Paper 4: Answers

1a. False
1b. True
1c. True
1d. False
1e. True
Exclusion criteria for paediatric day surgery include:

- post-conceptual age <50 weeks
- inadequately controlled systemic disease
- uninvestigated cardiac murmur
- acute infection
- complex congenital heart disease
- sickle cell disease
- diabetes mellitus
- sleep apnoea
- *surgical criteria*: prolonged surgery, inexperienced surgeon, risk of excessive blood loss, body cavity surgery
- *social criteria*: lack of parental support, long journey time, no home telephone

Brennan LJ, Prabhu AJ. Paediatric day-case anaesthesia. *Contin Educ Anaesth Crit Care Pain* 2003; 3: 134–8.

2a. True
2b. False
2c. True
2d. True
2e. True
Ondansetron is a $5HT_3$ antagonist that is routinely used for antiemesis; *common reactions* include constipation, headache, flushing, injection-site reactions. *Less commonly*: hiccups, hypotension, bradycardia, chest pain, arrhythmias, movement disorders and seizures. *Rarely*: dizziness and transient visual disturbances. *Very rarely*: transient blindness.

British Medical Association, Royal Pharmaceutical Society of Great Britain. *British National Formulary 58*. Section 4.6: Drugs used in nausea and vertigo – Ondarsetron. London: Pharmaceutical Press, 2009.

3a. True
3b. False
3c. False
3d. True
3e. True
The following factors cause a leftward shift in the oxyhaemoglobin dissociation curve:

- *Hypothermia*
- *Increased blood pH* (the Bohr effect describes a reduction in pH leading to a rightward shift and better oxygen unloading)

- *Reduced 2,3-diphosphoglycerate (2,3-DPG) levels* (increased levels allow better oxygen unloading in states such as anaemia and pregnancy and at high altitude)
- *Fetal haemoglobin*
- *Carbon monoxide*
- *Methaemoglobinaemia*
- *Hypophosphataemia*: leads to reduced erythrocyte 2,3-DPG (compromising oxygen delivery to the tissues)

Ganong WF. *Review of Medical Physiology*, 22nd edn. Maidenhead: McGraw-Hill Medical, 2005.

4a. True
4b. True
4c. False
4d. True
4e. False
Hypothermia is defined as a core temperature below 36°C (NICE, 2008). Cutaneous vasoconstriction is mediated by increased sympathetic activity. Prolonged cooling results in a paradoxical vasodilatation by a direct cold-induced paralysis; blood vessels become less responsive to catecholamines. Hypothermia results in a decreased metabolic rate, cardiac output and heart rate, due to slowing of the rate of discharge of the sinoatrial node. In addition, O_2 utilization is decreased but solubility is increased; overall $\dot{D}O_2$ is decreased, with a leftward shift of the oxyhaemoglobin dissociation curve. Blood viscosity is increased. Below a core temperature of 28°C, cardiac arrhythmias are frequent, including refractory ventricular fibrillation that is typically unresponsive to drugs.

National Institute for Health and Clinical Excellence. *Perioperative Hypothermia (Inadvertent): Management of Inadvertent Perioperative Hypothermia in Adults*. London: NICE, 2008. Available at: guidance.nice.org.uk/CG65.
Power I, Kam P. *Principles of Physiology for the Anaesthetist*, 2nd edn. London: Arnold Publishers, 2007.

5a. True
5b. False
5c. True
5d. False
5e. True
Compliance is defined as volume change per unit change in pressure.

1/total thoracic compliance = 1/chest wall compliance + 1/lung compliance

Human lung compliance is approximately 1.5−2 L/kPa (150−200 mL/cmH$_2$O) and decreases while supine due to a decrease in functional residual capacity. Compliance increases with age and emphysema, and decreases with pulmonary fibrosis, vascular engorgement and pulmonary oedema. Increased pulmonary venous congestion decreases lung compliance.

Akhtar S. Pulmonary physiology. In: Wilson WC, Grande CM, Hoyt DB, eds. *Trauma: Critical Care*. New York: Informa Healthcare, 2007.

6a. True
6b. False
6c. False
6d. True
6e. False
HIV is an RNA retrovirus that is transcribed by reverse transcriptase into the host DNA and leads to AIDS. The Centers for Disease Control and Prevention classification divides patients into four groups:

- *Group I*: acute seroconversion illness that follows initial infection
- *Group II*: asymptomatic illness, which can persist for 10 years prior to development of AIDS
- *Group III*: persistent generalized lymphadenopathy
- *Group IV*: symptomatic HIV infection

Prout J, Agarwal B. Anaesthesia and critical care for patients with HIV infection. *Contin Educ Anaesth Crit Care Pain* 2005; 5: 153–6.

7a. False
7b. True
7c. False
7d. True
7e. False
Oesophageal varices develop most commonly owing to cirrhosis, occurring in 90% of cirrhotics within 10 years; bleeding represents a life-threatening complication with a 25–50% mortality. Varices develop when portal pressure rises above 10 mmHg, with rupture occurring above 12 mmHg. Portal hypertension occurs owing to increased intrahepatic vascular resistance and increased blood flow, leading to fibrosis and collagen deposition with subsequent liver dysfunction. As the portosystemic gradient increases, collaterals form at the gastroesophageal junction and the rectum. β-blockade is beneficial as primary prophylaxis, to reduce cardiac output and blood flow within the splanchnic circulation, thereby reducing portal pressure. It is not indicated as treatment in the acute setting of bleeding varices. Acute haemorrhage is treated with resuscitation with airway protection and volume replacement, transfusing blood products as necessary (avoiding over-transfusion, which may increase portal pressure). Medical treatment includes vasoconstrictors, sclerotherapy, band ligation and glue for gastric varices. Balloon tamponade stops the bleeding in about 90% of cases and is used as a bridging measure before more definitive management. Terlipressin has been shown to reduce the hepatic venous pressure gradient and mortality, band ligation is more effective in preventing recurrence of bleeding than sclerotherapy, which also has a higher complication rate. Finally, portosystemic shunting via a transjugular intrahepatic porto-systemic stented shunt (TIPSS) or surgical shunting diverts portal blood to the systemic circulation, reducing portal pressure but increasing the risk of hepatic encephalopathy.

McKay R, Webster NR. Variceal bleeding. *Contin Educ Anaesth Crit Care Pain* 2007; 7: 191–4.
Singer M, Webb AR. *Oxford Handbook of Critical Care*, 3rd edn. Oxford: OUP, 2009.

8a. False
8b. True
8c. False
8d. True
8e. True

The normal ICP waveform appears similar to an arterial blood pressure trace. It consists of three peaks (see Figure 4.1), named:

- *P1 (percussion wave)*: arterial pressure is transmitted from the choroid plexus to the ventricle
- *P2 (tidal wave)*: due to brain compliance; becomes larger than P1 as ICP increases and compliance decreases
- *P3 (dicrotic wave)*: due to closure of the aortic valve

Lundberg described the presence of fluctuations in ventricular patterns. These are:

- *A-waves (plateau waves)*: 50–100 mmHg, last 5–20 minutes; always pathological; represent vasodilatation in response to increased ICP and decreased cerebral perfusion pressure
- *B-waves*: 20–30 mmHg, 0.5–2/min; seen in normal individuals; their absence after a head injury is a poor sign
- *C-waves*: 4–8/min; little clinical significance

NICE guidance recommends that all patients with severe head injuries should be managed in specialized centres, even if they do not require immediate neurosurgery.

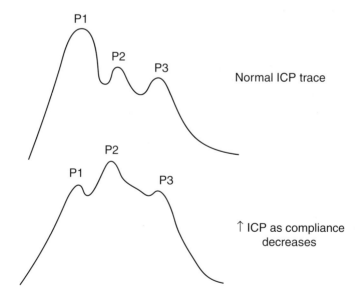

FIGURE 4.1   Intracranial pressure (ICP) waveforms.

Eynon A. Intracranial pressure monitoring. In: Waldmann N, Soni N, Rhodes A, eds. *Oxford Desk Reference: Critical Care*. Oxford: OUP, 2008.

National Institute for Health and Clinical Excellence. *Head Injury: Triage, Assessment, Investigation and Early Management of Head Injury in Infants, Children and Adults.* London: NICE, 2007. Available at: guidance.nice.org.uk/CG56.

9a. False
9b. False
9c. True
9d. False
9e. True

The hyperosmolar hyperglycaemic state (classically known as 'HONK', the hyperosmolar non-ketotic state) describes an extreme metabolic complication of type 2 diabetes mellitus, although it has been reported in type 1 diabetes (conversely, diabetic ketoacidosis is normally associated with type 1 diabetes, but may occur in type 2 diabetes). It can occur as a first presentation of diabetes (30–40%) or be precipitated by intercurrent illness and/or poor glycaemic control. It is characterized by the following as a result of insulin deficiency or resistance:

- serum osmolality: >320 mOsm/kg
- plasma glucose >33.3 mmol/L
- metabolic acidosis (pH ≤7.3)
- profound dehydration due to osmotic diuresis
- absence of ketoacidosis

The anion gap may be raised owing to profound dehydration and tissue hypoperfusion causing lactic acidosis, but if very high should prompt investigation of other causes: anion gap = $(Na^+ + K^+) - (Cl^- + HCO_3^-)$ mmol/L. Diuretic therapy will worsen the metabolic derangement and dehydration, which requires large amounts of fluid administration with an approximate overall deficit of 200 mL/kg. Hypernatraemia is almost universal, but over-rapid correction may result in cerebral oedema. Insulin therapy is required, with the aim of reducing glucose levels by 3 mmol L^{-1} h^{-1}; patients are often hypersensitive. Anticoagulation is warranted unless contraindicated, since this is a hypercoagulable state with 10–20% mortality.

Stoner GD. Hyperosmolar hyperglycemic state. *Am Fam Physician* 2005; **71**: 1723–30.

10a. True
10b. False
10c. True
10d. True
10e. True

MRI scanners can employ permanent magnets or electromagnets; permanent magnets are large and bulky with limited magnetic field strength and precision and cannot be turned off, which has implications for safety. Electromagnets are constructed with superconductors, which are certain metals and compounds whose electrical resistance falls to zero below a critical temperature. Superconducting magnets contains coils of wire that are maintained at near absolute zero using liquid helium (which boils at 4.2 K at atmospheric pressure) to maintain electrical current flow. Gadolinium is an MRI contrast agent, which as a compound does not pass the blood–brain barrier, however, as free ions it is highly toxic and can lead to nephrogenic systemic fibrosis.

Davis PD, Kenny GNC. *Basic Physics and Measurement in Anaesthesia*, 5th edn. Oxford: Butterworth-Heinemann, 2003.

11a. False
11b. False
11c. True
11d. False
11e. True
Liver lobules possess a central hepatic vein, connected by a network of sinusoids to portal tracts at the periphery, which consist of branches from the hepatic artery, *portal vein* and bile duct. The magnitude of its blood supply (20% of cardiac output) reflects the high level of metabolic activity. Flow increases after feeding and decreases during sleep or exercise. The liver receives blood from two sources: approximately one-third from the hepatic artery and two-thirds from the portal vein. The proportions of oxygen contributed by each may vary considerably under different conditions. Portal venous blood has a higher oxygen content than that of systemic venous blood and contributes 60% of total oxygen supply under normal circumstances.

Functions include:

- *Carbohydrate metabolism*: glycogen storage and breakdown
- *Protein metabolism*: synthesis of albumin, globulin, coagulation factors II, V, VII, IX–XIII (not all of these are vitamin K-dependent), complement and many others
- *Fat metabolism*: breakdown of triglycerides and fatty acids, production of lipoproteins
- *Metabolism*: bilirubin, hormones, drugs
- *Storage*: vitamins, blood reservoir
- *Haematological*: site of haematopoiesis in fetal and early neonatal life
- *Thermoregulation*
- *Immune*: Kupffer cells, reticuloendothelial system

Burt AD, Day CP. Pathophysiology of the liver. In: MacSween RNM, Burt AD, Portmann BC, et al., eds. *MacSween's Pathology of the Liver*, 5th edn. New York: Churchill-Livingstone, 2006.
Yentis S, Hirsch N, Smith G. *Anaesthesia and Intensive Care A to Z: An Encyclopaedia of Principles and Practice*, 4th edn. Oxford: Butterworth-Heinemann, 2009.

12a. False
12b. True
12c. True
12d. False
12e. False
Lidocaine is a tertiary amine (an amide derivative of diethylaminoacetic acid) that causes reversible neural blockade and Class Ib antiarrhythmic actions by

use-dependent sodium-channel blockade. All local anaesthetics consist of a lipophilic aromatic group, an intermediate chain and a hydrophilic tertiary or quaternary amine. Lidocaine is 64% protein-bound in plasma, predominantly to α-1 acid glycoprotein; V_D is 0.7–1.5 L/kg; pK_a is 7.7. Lidocaine is not removed by haemodialysis.

Sasada M, Smith S. *Drugs in Anaesthesia and Intensive Care*, 3rd edn. Oxford: OUP, 2003.

13a. True
13b. False
13c. False
13d. True
13e. True
Glucagon is a hormone secreted by the A (α)-cells of the pancreas. Its mechanism of action is hepatic adenylate cyclase stimulation, which causes glycogen breakdown and release of glucose; hepatic gluconeogenesis is increased. It stimulates release of growth hormone, insulin and somatostatin. It has positive chronotropic and inotropic effects and a half-life of less than 10 minutes. It may be administered for the treatment of hypoglycaemia or for β-blocker overdose; glucagon binds to its own receptor site, cAMP-signalling pathways are activated, resulting in L-type calcium channel activation, therefore bypassing cellular problems at the receptor level.

Mottram AR, Erickson TB. Toxicology in emergency cardiovascular care. In: Field JM, ed. *The Textbook of Emergency Cardiovascular Care and CPR*. Philadelphia: Lippincott Williams & Wilkins, 2009.

14a. True
14b. True
14c. False
14d. True
14e. True
Phaeochromocytomas are a catecholamine-secreting tumours derived from chromaffin tissue. They may secrete adrenaline, noradrenaline or dopamine and the most common presenting feature is sustained hypertension. Definitive treatment is surgical, but the patient's blood pressure should be controlled preoperatively using α-blockers; subsequent β-blockade can be used to control resulting tachycardia. Induction, endotracheal intubation and tumour manipulation can lead to increases in plasma catecholamine levels (up to 200 times) and can result in significant morbidity or death. Common postoperative complications include bleeding and hypotension, but surges in blood pressure can occur owing to incomplete tumour ligation or metastasis. Venous ligation results in a sudden drop in catecholamine levels, which can cause refractory hypotension.

Pace N, Buttigieg M. Phaeochromocytoma. *Contin Educ Anaesth Crit Care Pain* 2003; 3: 20–3.

15a. True
15b. True
15c. True
15d. False
15e. True
Delirium is an acute disturbance of attention, cognition and conscious level. Incidence is very high in the critical care setting (60–80%) owing to a combination of patient-related (age, psychological), illness-related (acidosis, sepsis, metabolic disturbances) and iatrogenic (drugs, sleep disturbance) factors. It can be hyperactive (positive), with symptoms of aggression and agitation, or hypoactive (negative), with signs of apathy and decreased awareness. Treatment is multifactorial and should first involve correction of any underlying causes (infection, medications, electrolyte disturbance), followed by psychological and pharmacological management of symptoms. The American Psychiatric Association recommends haloperidol as first-line treatment titrated to clinical effect up to a maximum dose. Side-effects are common and include extrapyramidal effects, QT prolongation and precipitation of torsades de pointes. Benzodiazepines are avoided since they may worsen symptoms and precipitate cardiorespiratory depression. ICU delirium is associated with a 3- to 11-fold increased risk of death at 6 months.

Ely EW, Shintani A, Truman B, et al. Delirium as a predictor of mortality in mechanically ventilated patients in the intensive care unit. *JAMA* 2004; **291**: 1753–62.
King J, Gratrix A. Delirium in intensive care. *Contin Educ Anaesth Crit Care Pain* 2009; **9**: 144–7.

16a. False
16b. True
16c. True
16d. False
16e. False
Ethylene glycol remains an important toxic alcohol, in addition to ethanol, methanol and isopropanol. It is a component of radiator fluid and antifreeze solutions and acts by altering the colligative properties of solutions (dependent on the number of particles present), thereby decreasing the freezing point and increasing the boiling point of the fluid to which it is added. Toxicity results from its metabolites, which are glycoaldehyde, glycolate and oxalate; oxalate is deposited as crystals in tissues including the renal cortex, leading to renal failure. Profound acidosis occurs and this is classically a Type B lactic acidosis (defined as occurring in the absence of poor tissue perfusion). A large anion gap and osmolar gap occur owing to unmeasured anionic compounds, along with hyperkalaemia and a consumptive hypocalcaemia. Blood levels above 500 mg/L are indicative of severe toxicity; treatment includes haemodialysis, ethanol therapy, thiamine and pyridoxine.

Yentis S, Hirsch N, Smith G. *Anaesthesia and Intensive Care A to Z: An Encyclopaedia of Principles and Practice*, 4th edn. Oxford: Butterworth-Heinemann, 2009.

17a. True
17b. False
17c. False
17d. True
17e. True
NICE recommends that treatment for rheumatoid arthritis start with non-steroidal anti-inflammatory drugs (NSAIDs) or cyclooxygnase 2 (COX-2) selective NSAIDs (prescribed with an appropriate proton pump inhibitor), while awaiting specialist review. Disease-modifying anti-rheumatic drugs (DMARDs) require 4–6 months to work, and early intervention is associated with a superior outcome. All DMARDs have potentially serious side-effects that limit their usefulness. Currently, methotrexate is used as an 'anchor' drug and other DMARDs added as necessary.

Side effects of DMARDs include:

- *Methotrexate*: blood dyscrasias, liver cirrhosis
- *Sulphasalazine*: bone marrow depression, hepatitis, oral ulcers
- *Cyclosporin*: tremor, gingival hypertrophy, hypertension
- *Gold*: bone marrow depression, proteinuria
- *Penicillamine*: blood dyscrasias, convulsions, renal and hepatic impairment, systematic lupus erythematosus-like syndrome
- *Hydroxychloroquine*: tinnitus, headache, permanent retinopathy

National Institute for Health and Clinical Excellence. *Rheumatoid Arthritis: The Management of Rheumatoid Arthritis in Adults*. London: NICE, 2009. Available at: guidance.nice.org.uk/CG79.

18a. False
18b. True
18c. False
18d. True
18e. False
Scoliosis is a lateral curvature and rotation of the thoracolumbar vertebrae with a resulting rib cage deformity. Most commonly it is idiopathic (70%); other aetiologies include neuromuscular (15%), congenital, traumatic, syndromes (Marfan's, osteogenesis imperfecta), neoplastic and infectious. The Cobb angle (see Figure 4.2) measures curvature using perpendicular lines from the *outer* surface of upper and lower, maximally tilted, vertebrae. A curvature is considered abnormal when $> 10°$. More severe curves result in a restrictive lung defect and exertional dyspnoea ($>65°$), respiratory failure, pulmonary hypertension and right heart failure ($>100°$). Surgery is indicated once the curvature has reached $>40°$.

Entwhistle MA, Patel DA. Scoliosis surgery in children. *Contin Educ Anaesth Crit Care Pain* 2006; 6: 13–16.

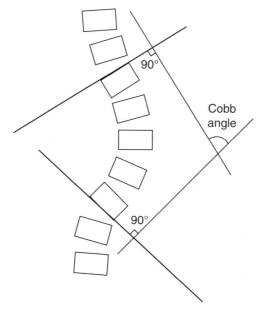

FIGURE 4.2   Cobb angle.

19a. True
19b. False
19c. False
19d. True
19e. True
Peripheral nerve stimulators are used to monitor neural transmission across the neuromuscular junction. This allows the user to establish depth, type and adequate reversal of neuromuscular blockade. A supramaximal stimulus is used to stimulate a peripheral nerve and ensures that all the motor fibres are recruited and depolarized. At the ulnar nerve, a current of 15–40 mA is used (higher in obese patients). Two electrodes are positioned on the nerve. The negative electrode is placed distally and the positive proximally. Ulnar nerve stimulation results in contraction of the *adductor* pollicis brevis muscle. Duration of the stimulus is less than 0.2 ms as a square wave to increase precision and avoid repetitive nerve firing.

Al-Shaikh B, Stacey S. *Essentials of Anaesthetic Equipment*, 3rd edn. London: Churchill Livingstone, 2007.

20a. False
20b. True
20c. False
20d. False
20e. True
The brachial plexus is derived from the anterior primary rami of the lower cervical and first thoracic spinal nerves (C5–T1). The four main mechanisms of nerve injury are compression, traction, ischaemia and metabolic derangements. Anaesthetized patients are more susceptible to brachial plexus injuries

when positioned with the arm supine and abducted. Optimal positioning consists of arm abduction below 90°, hand pronation and head turned towards the abducted arm. The roots C8 and T1 are prone to injury due to compression by the first rib, humerus and clavicle; since the ulnar nerve has the same roots, damage at this point could be mistaken for a distal ulnar injury. At the ulnar groove the nerve is exposed to direct compression and traction injuries.

Knight DJW, Mahajan RP. Patient positioning in anaesthesia. *Contin Educ Anaesth Crit Care Pain* 2004; 4: 160–3.

21a. True
21b. False
21c. False
21d. True
21e. False
The mediastinum is the central cavity of the chest; it lies between the pleurae and extends anteriorly from the sternum to the vertebral column posteriorly. It contains all the thoracic viscera and vessels, excluding the lungs. The anterior mediastinum lies only on the left, as the pleura diverges, and contains loose areolar tissue, part of the thymus gland that extends into the superior mediastinum, the internal mammary vessels and lymph nodes. The thyroid gland and aortic arch lie within the superior mediastinum.

Snell RS. *Clinical Anatomy: An Illustrated Review with Questions and Explanations.* Philadelphia: Lippincott Williams & Wilkins, 2003.

22a. True
22b. False
22c. True
22d. False
22e. True
Esmolol is a highly lipid soluble, cardioselective β-blocker with no intrinsic sympathomimetic activity. It is available only as an intravenous preparation and with a half-life of 10 minutes has extremely rapid onset and offset; its volume of distribution is 3.5 L/kg. It is metabolized by esterase hydrolysis in erythrocytes and has no active metabolites. In accordance with its class, it has negative inotropic and chronotropic effects.

Peck TE, Hill SA, Williams M. *Pharmacology for Anaesthesia and Intensive Care*, 3rd edn. Cambridge: CUP, 2008.

23a. True
23b. True
23c. False
23d. True
23e. False
IOP is between 15 and 20 mmHg and is influenced by external pressure and intraocular contents. Most intravenous anaesthetic agents reduce IOP, with the exception of ketamine; thus this agent is usually avoided. Volatile anaesthetic agents also reduce IOP; the true mechanism is unclear, although it is thought to also be due to reduced intraocular muscle tone; it is unaffected by

N_2O. All non-depolarizing muscle relaxants reduce IOP, while suxamethonium increases it; this increase lasts 6 minutes and still occurs after section of the eye muscles.

24a. True
24b. False
24c. True
24d. False
24e. True
Numerical indices that predict successful weaning from mechanical ventilation include:

Minute ventilation	< 10 L/min
Vital capacity/weight	> 10 mL/kg
Respiratory frequency	< 35/min
Tidal volume/weight	> 10 mL/kg
Maximum inspiratory pressure	< -25 cmH_2O
PaO_2/PAO_2	> 0.35
Respiratory rate/tidal volume	< 100/L
PaO_2/FiO_2	> 200 mmHg

Lermitte J, Garfield MJ. Weaning from mechanical ventilation. *Contin Educ Anaesth Crit Care Pain* 2005; 5: 113–17.

25a. False
25b. True
25c. True
25d. True
25e. True
For a shockable rhythm, defibrillation should ideally be performed three times before resternotomy and internal cardiac massage. For non-shockable rhythms, atropine administration and pacing (DDD at rate of 90 bpm on epicardial pacing wires for asystole and severe bradycardia) should be attempted. In the context of PEA, a functioning pacemaker should be briefly switched off to exclude underlying VF. Emergency resternotomy should form an integral part of cardiac arrest protocols up to the 10th postoperative day. If a surgeon is not readily available, other trained members of the arrest team may perform the procedure.

Dunning J, Fabbri A, Kolh PH, et al. on behalf of the EACTS Clinical Guidelines Committee. Guideline for resuscitation in cardiac arrest after cardiac surgery. *Eur J Cardiothorac Surg* 2009; 36: 3–28.

26a. False
26b. False
26c. False
26d. False
26e. False
Pericarditis is defined as chronic if present for ≥ 6 months and, although it can be idiopathic, causes include infection (most commonly viral: coxsackie B,

influenza), tuberculosis, uraemia, post-traumatic, post-myocardial infarction (10–15%), autoimmune disease or malignancy. The ECG in acute pericarditis classically shows saddle-shaped ST elevation in all leads, but does not cause pathological Q-waves. The steep y descent is characteristic of *constrictive* pericarditis and is due to fibrosis and calcification of the pericardial layers, causing rapid diastolic filling; there is also a rise in JVP with inspiration (Kussmaul's sign). Pericarditis itself will not cause these signs without conco-mitant pericardial effusion or tamponade. Troponin I can be elevated in acute pericarditis but has not been shown to be a negative prognostic marker.

Imazio M, Demichelis B, Cecchi E, et al. Cardiac troponin I in acute pericarditis. *J Am Coll Cardiol* 2003; **42**: 2144–8.

27a. False
27b. True
27c. True
27d. True
27e. True
Indications for insertion of vena cava filters vary widely between institutions. Essential indications are:

- uncontrollable thromboembolic disease
- pulmonary endarterectomy for chronic thromboembolic disease
- absolute contraindication for anticoagulation
- limited life expectancy

Retrievable filters may be used for interim prophylaxis. These devices stay in place for several months. A French study demonstrated that patients benefit only during the initial period. At 2-year follow-up it was found that post-thrombotic syndrome and recurrent venous thromboembolism occurred more frequently.

Decousus H, Leizorovicz A, Parent F, et al. A clinical trial of vena caval filters in the prevention of pulmonary embolism in patients with proximal deep-vein thrombosis. Prevention du Risque d'Embolie Pulmonaire par Interruption Cave Study Group. *N Engl J Med* 1998; **12**: 409–15.
van Beek EJR, Elliot CA, Kiely DG. Diagnosis and initial treatment of patients with suspected pulmonary thromboembolism. *Contin Educ Anaesth Crit Care Pain* 2009; **9**: 119–24.

28a. False
28b. False
28c. True
28d. True
28e. False
The Association of Anaesthetists of Great Britain and Ireland (AAGBI) produced guidelines titled *Recommendations for Standards of Monitoring during Anaesthesia and Recovery* (2007). The control of substances hazardous to health (COSHH) is the law produced by the Health and Safety Executive (HSE) that dictates standards for monitoring ambient anaesthetic agent concen-trations in hospitals.

The anode of a fuel cell is usually made of lead and is sacrificial, undergoing the following reaction:

$$Pb + 2OH^- \rightarrow PbO + H_2O + 2e^-$$

The cathode is gold and the following reaction occurs:

$$O_2 + 2H_2O + 4e^- \rightarrow 4OH^-$$

The Severinghaus electrode uses a glass pH electrode, is H^+-sensitive and measures the partial pressure of CO_2. Mass spectrometry involves removal of molecules, ionization and acceleration using a cathode. Magnets influence ions and allow separation on the basis of mass and charge. Photoreceptors detect signals, which are duly processed. Infrared radiation is absorbed by molecules containing dissimilar atoms. The molecules convert this energy into vibration, the frequency of which is dependent on mass and atomic bonding. Most molecules possess a specific wavelength at which they absorb ionizing radiation, which allows identification and the measurement of concentration.

Davis PD, Kenny GNC. *Basic Physics and Measurement in Anaesthesia*, 5th edn. Oxford: Butterworth-Heinemann, 2003.

29a. False
29b. True
29c. False
29d. True
29e. False
Remifentanil is a potent, highly-selective μ-opioid receptor agonist and is usually diluted to 50 μg/mL. Metabolism is via non-specific blood and tissue esterases. Pharmacokinetics are unaltered by obesity, hepatic or renal impairment.

	Fentanyl	Alfentanil	Morphine	Remifentanil
V_D (L/kg)	4	0.6	3.5	0.3
Clearance (mL min^{-1} kg^{-1})	13	6	16	40
Elimination half-life (min)	190	100	170	10
pK_a	8.4	6.5	8.0	7.1
Un-ionized at pH 7.4 (%)	9	89	23	68
Lipid solubility (from octanol–water coefficient)	600	90	1	20
Plasma protein-bound (%)	83	90	35	70

Egan TD. Remifentanil pharmacokinetics and pharmacodynamics. A preliminary appraisal. *Clin Pharmacokinet* 1995; **29**: 80–94.
Glass PSA. Remifentanil: a new opioid. *J Clin Anesth* 1995; **7**: 558–63.
Peck TE, Hill SA, Williams M. *Pharmacology for Anaesthesia and Intensive Care*, 3rd edn. Cambridge: CUP, 2008.

30a. True
30b. True
30c. False
30d. False
30e. True
Halothane causes a bradycardia secondary to vagal stimulation. It also
reduces myocardial contractility and can lead to atrioventricular block and
ventricular asystole; it also sensitizes the myocardium to catecholamines.
Sevoflurane has little effect on heart rate.

	Desflurane	Sevoflurane	Halothane	Enflurane	Isoflurane
Heart rate	↑	Nil	↓↓	↑	↑↑
Blood pressure	↓ ↓	↓	↓↓	↓↓	↓↓
Contractility	Minimal	↓	↓↓↓	↓↓	↓
Systemic vascular resistance	↓↓	↓	↓	↓	↓↓

Peck TE, Hill SA, Williams M. *Pharmacology for Anaesthesia and Intensive Care*,
3rd edn. Cambridge: CUP, 2008.

31a. True
31b. False
31c. False
31d. False
31e. True
The coeliac plexus receives contributions from the greater and lesser
splanchnics and the vagus nerve. It surrounds the root of the coeliac artery
at the level of L1. Superiorly are the crura of the diaphragm, posteriorly is the
aorta ('A2A', 'P2P': anterior to aorta, posterior to pancreas) and laterally lie
the adrenal glands. The coeliac plexus block is used to alleviate visceral
pain and chronic pain caused by pancreatitis and for postoperative analgesia. It
is also used to perform a diagnostic block for sympathetically mediated pain.
Complications include visceral damage, vascular injury, cardiovascular
instability, anterior spinal artery syndrome, paraplegia, and subarachnoid,
epidural or intravascular injection.

32a. True
32b. True
32c. False
32d. False
32e. True
Risk factors for PONV include:

- *Patient-related*: young age, female gender, motion sickness, previous PONV,
  anxiety and hypotension

- *Anaesthetic*: general $>$ regional anaesthesia, administration of nitrous oxide, opioids or ketamine
- *Surgical*: long duration, laparoscopy, strabismus and middle ear surgery

Janet M. Outpatient anesthesia. In: Miller RD, ed. *Miller's Anesthesia*, 7th edn. New York: Churchill Livingstone, 2009.

33a. True
33b. True
33c. False
33d. False
33e. True

Vasopressin (antidiuretic hormone, ADH) is a nonapeptide synthesized in the paraventricular and supraoptic nuclei of the posterior hypothalamus. It is released in response to increased plasma osmolality, decreased plasma volume, stress, hypoxaemia, hypercapnia, acidosis and various chemical mediators. At low concentrations, noradrenaline activates α_1 receptors, stimulating vasopressin release. At higher concentrations, actions at α_2 and β receptors inhibit vasopressin release. DDAVP is a trade name for desmopressin, a synthetic analogue of arginine vasopressin, and is used in the management of cranial diabetes insipidus and syndrome of inappropriate ADH secretion (SIADH). Desmopressin is a more potent antidiuretic and significantly less potent ($>1000\times$) vasoconstrictor. VASST (Vasopressin versus Noradrenaline Infusion in Patients with Septic Shock Trial) was a multicentre, randomized, double-blind trial that demonstrated that low-dose vasopressin did not reduce mortality rates compared with noradrenaline among patients with septic shock who were treated with catecholamine vasopressors. Vasopressin has been used successfully in cardiac arrests in various trials. Current European Resuscitation Council Guidelines suggest that there is insufficient evidence for the use of vasopressin in cardiac arrest. The Surviving Sepsis Guidelines (2008) recommend the use of vasopressin as an add-on therapy to first-line vasopressors.

European Resuscitation Council. Guidelines for resuscitation. *Resuscitation* 2005; **67**(Suppl. 1): 539–86.

Delinger RP, Leng MM, Cochet JM, et al. Surviving Sepsis Campaign: International guidelines for management of severe sepsis and septic shock. *Crit Care Med* 2008; **36**: 296–327.

Russell JA, Walley KR, Singer J, et al. Vasopressin versus norepinephrine infusion in patients with septic shock. *N Engl J Med* 2008; **358**: 877–87.

Sharman A, Low J. Vasopressin and its role in critical care. *Contin Educ Anaesth Crit Care Pain* 2008; **8**: 134–7.

34a. False
34b. False
34c. True
34d. False
34e. False

Tetanus is a disease mediated by the neurotoxins of *Clostridium tetani*, a Gram-positive anaerobe widespread in soil and dust. Infection occurs after abrasions or contamination of a wound. As a result of successful vaccination programmes, it is rare in the developed world, but is occasionally seen in high-risk groups such as intravenous drug users. Between 2003 and 2004 more than 20 cases were reported in the UK, all in drug users and thought to be a result of contaminated heroin. Tetanus toxin (tetanospasmin) binds to the neuromuscular junction and transport to the cell body occurs retrogradely, with subsequent trans-synaptic spread to adjacent motor and autonomic nerves. The primary targets are inhibitory pathways (glycine and GABAergic pathways), leading to increased muscle tone and rigidity. Disinhibited auto-nomic nervous system activity is seen, resulting in cardiovascular instability. Patients with suspected tetanus should be managed in a dark, quiet room, preferably in an ICU. Sudden laryngospasm, diaphragmatic paralysis and res-piratory insufficiency may occur; these patients need constant vigilance in an environment with immediate access to ventilatory support. HTIG neutralizes free-circulating neurotoxin but does not affect toxins already fixed to nerve terminals; it does not need to be repeated. Recovery from a tetanus infection does not confer immunity. Metronidazole and surgical debridement are effective at reducing the bacterial toxin load. Muscle spasms can be treated with benzodiazepine and opioids. If necessary, full sedation and even muscle relaxants may become necessary. Autonomic instability can result in cardio-vascular collapse. Typically there is prolonged sympathetic activity followed by parasympathetic activity (which can result in sinus arrest). Sedation, clonidine and magnesium have all been used with some success to control this instability. β-blocker use is associated with cardiovascular collapse, pulmonary oedema and death.

Taylor AM. Tetanus. *Contin Educ Anaesth Crit Care Pain* 2006; **6**: 101–4.
Thwaites L. Tetanus. In: Waldmann N, Soni N, Rhodes A, eds. *Oxford Desk Reference: Critical Care*. Oxford: OUP, 2008.

35a. False
35b. True
35c. True
35d. True
35e. False
The Model for End-Stage Liver Disease (MELD) Score indicates the severity of hepatic dysfunction and calculates the patient's risk of dying within 3 months from liver disease while waiting for a transplant. It is an unbiased assessment of patient need for liver transplantation. Calculation includes three blood indices:

- bilirubin
- prothrombin time
- creatinine

It is calculated as follows:

$$3.8 \log_e(\text{bilirubin, mg/dL}) + 11.2 \log_e(\text{INR}) + 9.6 \log_e(\text{creatinine, mg/dL})$$

The score ranges from 6 to 40, with 40 representing the sickest patient. It applies to patients over 12 years of age; a paediatric model (Paediatric End-Stage Liver Disease, PELD) also exists.

Fabbroni D, Bellamy M. Anaesthesia for hepatic transplantation. *Contin Educ Anaesth Crit Care Pain* 2006; **6**: 171–5.

36a. True
36b. False
36c. True
36d. True
36e. False

Uraemia describes the clinical syndrome of accumulation of waste products normally excreted via the kidneys; it is a non-specific term for a condition that accompanies deterioration in renal function. Cumulative retention of 'uraemic toxins' leads to the variable clinical picture of the uraemic syndrome; these include parathyroid hormone, β_2-microglobulin and advanced glycosylation end-products (AGEs); urea is not thought to be the primary cause of toxicity. Uraemia typically occurs when creatinine clearance falls to $10-20$ mL/min. It classically leads to reduced platelet function and reduced adhesiveness through changes in receptor expression, but up to 50% of uraemic patients are thrombocytopenic and bleeding time is prolonged. Uraemic encephalopathy and pericarditis can also occur.

Meyer TW, Hostetter TH. Uremia. *N Engl J Med* 2007; 357: 1316.
Michelson AD. *Platelets*. San Diego: Academic Press, 2006.

37a. False
37b. False
37c. True
37d. False
37e. True

There are many ways of classifying ventilators. They can be classified according to inspiratory characteristics (see Figure 4.3):

- *Pressure generators* deliver flow at a preset inspiratory pressure and have a low internal impedance to flow. Tidal volume will vary with lung compliance, but they compensate for leaks since they are set to always deliver the set pressure and this pressure will be reached less quickly with a leak
- *Flow generators* deliver preset flow rates despite differences in lung compliance and have an increased risk of barotrauma. They have a high internal impedance to flow

High-frequency ventilation can be positive, as in jet ventilation (HFJV), or negative, as in oscillatory ventilation (HFOV). With HFOV, inspiration and expiration are active via the cuirass, whereas with HFJV, expiration occurs passively. The Manley MP3 is a time-cycled, pressure generator (minute volume divider) and during spontaneous ventilation acts as a Mapleson D system.

Al-Shaikh B, Stacey S. *Essentials of Anaesthetic Equipment*, 3rd edn. London: Churchill Livingstone, 2007.

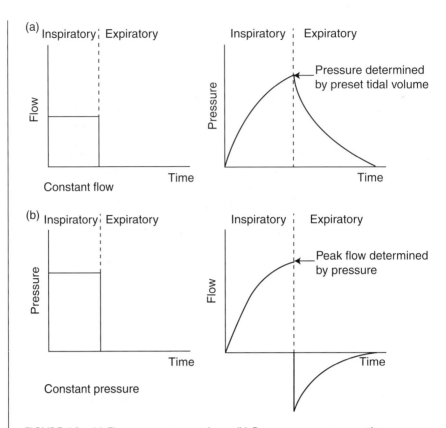

FIGURE 4.3   (a) Flow generator ventilator. (b) Pressure generator ventilator.

38a. True
38b. False
38c. False
38d. True
38e. False
Commonly used formulae are:

- Weight (kg) = [Age (years) + 4] × 2
- ETT internal diameter (mm) = [Age (years)/4] + 4
- Oral ETT length (cm) = [Age (years)/2] + 12
- Nasal ETT length (cm) = [Age (years)/2] + 15
- Resuscitation dose of atropine = 20 μg/kg
- Resuscitation dose of adrenaline = 10 μg/kg
- Dose of fluids for resuscitation = 20 mL/kg
- Systolic BP (mmHg) = 80 + [Age (years) × 2]

(b) is the correct formula for calculating ETT *internal* diameter. (c) is correct for calculating *nasal* ETT length.

Advanced Life Support Group. *Advanced Paediatric Life Support: The Practical Approach*, 4th edn. Oxford: Blackwell Publishing, 2004.

39a. False
39b. True
39c. False
39d. True
39e. True
30% of UK adults drink more than the recommended levels. Prolonged prothrombin time is an early manifestation of impaired synthetic liver function. Neuropathy, myopathy and Dupuytren's contractures can make regional techniques more difficult and dose requirements for general anaesthesia increase owing to enzyme induction. Impaired synthesis of coagulation factors and thrombocytopenia make postoperative bleeding more common; leukopaenia also results in increased postoperative infection rates. AWS is characterized by tremor, sweating, hypertension, hyperreflexia, anxiety and agitation leading to delirium, hallucinations and seizures. AWS is typically precipitated after 6–24 hours of abstinence but may be delayed up to 5 days; it can be fatal without treatment.

Chapman R, Plaat F. Alcohol and anaesthesia. *Contin Educ Anaesth Crit Care Pain* 2009; 9: 10–13.

40a. False
40b. True
40c. True
40d. False
40e. True
The WHO International Classification states the following BMI ranges (kg/m^2):

- normal: 18.5–24.9
- pre-obese: 25–29.9
- Class I obesity (overweight): 30–34.9
- Class II obesity (obese): 35–39.9
- Class III obesity (morbidly obese): >40
- morbidly obese has also been described as Class II with comorbidities

Absolute blood volume is increased, though corrected for body mass it is relatively reduced. Hormonal control includes adiponectin, leptin, ghrelin and insulin. Inhibin is secreted by the testes and ovaries to inhibit production of follicle-stimulating hormone. Local anaesthetic drugs for neuraxial blockade should be 75–80% of normal because engorged extradural veins and fat constrict these spaces. Obesity and a collar size of 17 inches in a man (16 inches in a woman) are risk factors for developing obstructive sleep apnoea.

Davies RJ, Stradling JR. The relationship between neck circumference, radiographic pharyngeal anatomy, and the obstructive sleep apnoea syndrome. *Eur Respir J* 1990; 3: 509–14.
French G, Low J, Thompson J. Endocrine and metabolic disease. In: Allman KG, Wilson IH, eds. *Oxford Handbook of Anaesthesia*, 2nd edn. Oxford: OUP, 2006.
Gastrointestinal surgery for severe obesity: National Institutes of Health Consensus Development Conference Statement. *Am J Clin Nutr* 1992; 55: 615–19.
World Health Organization. *WHO Expert Consultation on Obesity: Preventing and Managing the Global Epidemic.* Geneva: WHO, 3–5 June 1997.

41a. False
41b. False
41c. True
41d. True
41e. False
Following an amputation, surgical or traumatic, there is an estimated 4–78% incidence of pain in the region of the limb amputated. It normally starts within the first week after the amputation, although some studies have reported the development of pain months or years after the initial operation. Characteristically localized in distal areas of the amputated limb, phantom limb pain that persists beyond 6 months has a poor prognosis for spontaneous improvement. The pathophysiology is not completely understood, although various mechanisms have been proposed.

Peripheral mechanisms: alterations in the afferent nerve supply to the central nervous system

- ectopic discharge from nerves in the amputation site
- increased sensitivity of neuromas to mechanical/chemical stimuli
- ectopic discharge from cells in the dorsal root ganglia
- sympathetically maintained afferent input from the amputation site

Spinal cord mechanisms

- anatomical reorganization within the spinal cord: Aβ-fibres sprout connections to laminae 1 and 2, non-painful stimuli are experienced as pain
- central sensitization of dorsal horn cells in response to an increased barrage of painful stimuli from the amputation site

Supraspinal mechanism: cortical reorganization as a result of unmasking of occult synapses in the somatosensory cortex, rather than direct anatomical change.

There exist four identified risk factors for developing phantom pain:

- *pre-amputation pain*
- *lower limb amputation*
- *presence of persistent stump pain*
- *bilateral limb amputation*

Gender, age and site of amputation have not been identified as risk factors.

Jackson MA, Simpson KH. Pain after amputation. *Contin Educ Anaesth Crit Care Pain* 2004; 4: 20–3.

42a. False
42b. False
42c. True
42d. False
42e. True
The Intensive Care Society states that thromboprophylaxis with LMWH is indicated in all patients admitted to an ICU, unless there is a specific contraindication; this is a Grade A recommendation. The MEDENOX and PREVENT studies reported significant risk reduction in venous thromboembolism (VTE) in medical inpatients with enoxaparin and dalteparin,

respectively. In PREVENT the incidence of VTE was reduced from 4.96% in the placebo group to 2.77% in the treatment group; bleeding was not significantly higher in the treatment group. The recommendations for groups who should not have pharmacological thromboprophylaxis are empirical and have not been challenged in trials. They include:

- platelet count $<50 \times 10^9/L$
- coagulopathy: International Normalized Ration (INR) or activated partial thromboplastin time ratio (APTTR) >1.5
- active bleeding
- known bleeding disorder
- lumbar puncture/epidural/spinal within 4 hours
- haemophilia A or B
- severe von Willebrand's disease
- new ischaemic or haemorrhagic cerebrovascular accident (2 weeks after thrombotic stroke; 1 week after embolic stroke)

In addition, patients with a history of HIT in the last 6 months should not receive heparin in any form. Fondaparinux (a synthetic anti-Xa agent) may be used instead. Patients on LMWH should have full blood counts daily to check for the development of thrombocytopenia.

Intensive Care Society. *Guidelines for Venous Thromboprophylaxis in Critical Care*. London: ICS, 2008. Available at: www.ics.ac.uk.

43a. True
43b. True
43c. False
43d. True
43e. False
Critical ischaemia and subsequent infarction of the brainstem leads to intense autonomic activity and massive release of catecholamines. This is termed 'sympathetic storm' and leads to dramatic increases in heart rate, blood pressure, peripheral vascular resistance and cardiac output. ECG changes include ischaemia, arrhythmias and conduction abnormalities. Later, as infarction leads to death of the vasomotor centre, there is progressive vasodilatory hypovolaemia leading eventually to asystole. Neurogenic pulmonary oedema is also common. Endocrine failure ensues; owing to inhibition of the hypothalamo–pituitary axis, there is a decrease in ADH leading to diabetes insipidus. In addition, there is a fall in thyroid-stimulating hormone release causing decreased triiodothyronine concentrations. Hypothermia follows; coagulopathy often occurs.

Edgar P, Bullock R, Bonner S. Management of the potential heart-beating organ donor. *Contin Educ Anaesth Crit Care Pain* 2004; 4: 86–90.

44a. False
44b. True
44c. True
44d. True
44e. True
Sick sinus syndrome (tachy–brady syndrome) is characterized by sinus node dysfunction leading to severe bradycardia or sinus arrest and may also

exhibit alternating periods of tachyarrythmias. It is most commonly caused by idiopathic fibrosis of the sinoatrial (SA) node. Other causes can be intrinsic to the SA node, such as myocardial infarction, amyloidosis and cardiomyopathies, or extrinsic, including drugs such as digoxin, hyper- and hypothyroidism, hypothermia, potassium imbalance, sepsis and surgical damage. Patients are often asymptomatic or have non-specific complaints such as fatigue and dizziness, but can present with palpitations and chest pain or syncope. A pacing device should certainly be in place if the condition is diagnosed preoperatively, before general anaesthesia.

Adan V, Crown LA. Diagnosis and treatment of sick sinus syndrome. *Am Fam Physician* 2003; **67**: 1725–32.

45a. True
45b. True
45c. True
45d. True
45e. True

An aneurysm is an abnormal local dilatation in the wall of a blood vessel. It may be saccular, fusiform or dissecting. Saccular (or 'berry') aneurysms arise at the junction of vessels where there is a congenital deficiency in the muscle coat. These are particularly susceptible to degeneration, since elastic layers exist only in the internal lamina, unlike arteries elsewhere. Predisposing factors include hypertension, a family history of aneurysms, coarctation of the aorta, polycystic kidney disease and collagen diseases, including type II collagen deficiency. They are classified as small (<12 mm diameter), large (12–24 mm diameter) and giant (>24 mm), which make up 78%, 20% and 2% respectively. Aneurysms are commonly located at bifurcations of major arteries. Saccular aneurysms are mostly located on the circle of Willis or bifurcation of the middle cerebral artery (MCA). Common locations are:

Anterior circulation (85%)

- Anterior communicating artery
- Internal carotid artery
- MCA bifurcation
- Internal carotid artery (ICA) bifurcation
- Pericallosal/callosomarginal artery

Posterior circulation (15%)

- Basilar artery bifurcation
- Posterior inferior cerebellar artery

Following rupture, around one-third of patients will die before reaching hospital, one-third will have a poor outcome and one-third will survive with varying degrees of morbidity. Re-bleeding occurs in 50% within 6 weeks, and 25% in 2 weeks of the initial haemorrhage. Half of all patients who re-bleed will die as a result of the haemorrhage.

Kaye AH. *Essential Neurosurgery*. Oxford: WileyBlackwell, 2005.

46a. True
46b. False
46c. True
46d. True
46e. False

Bacterial and viral filters are designed to minimize the risk of cross-transmission between the patient and the anaesthetic breathing systems; they are electrostatic or hydrophobic. By addition of a humidification element, they can function as heat- and moisture-exchanging filters (HMEF); although hydrophobic filters provide some humidification, this can be improved with the addition of a hygroscopic element. Components of a filter include ports to accept (15 and 22 mm) tubings and connections, a sampling port and a filtration element. Mechanisms of action include:

- *Direct interception* (particles ≥ 1 μm): large particles are physically prevented from passing through pores
- *Inertial impaction* (0.5–1 μm): particles collide with the filter medium because of inertia and are held by van der Waals forces
- *Diffusional interception* (<0.5 μm): capture through Brownian motion; movement increases the apparent diameter of particles
- *Electrostatic attraction*: charged particles are attracted to fibres by coulombic attraction
- *Gravitational setting* (>5 μm): minimal effect in anaesthesia

Electrostatic filters exhibit 99.99% efficiency, although this decreases rapidly when they are wet, and they have a limited lifespan. Hydrophobic filters have a large surface area and low resistance and are 99.999% efficient; they have a longer lifespan.

Al-Shaikh B, Stacey S. *Essentials of Anaesthetic Equipment*, 3rd edn. London: Churchill Livingstone, 2007.

47a. True
47b. False
47c. True
47d. True
47e. True

The vagus nerve exits the skull base via the middle compartment of the jugular foramen to lie within the carotid sheath. Its superior laryngeal branch divides into the external branch, which is motor to the cricothyroid muscle, and the internal branch, which pierces the thryrohyoid membrane, supplying sensory innervation to the mucous membrane of the larynx down to the vocal cords. The right recurrent laryngeal nerve originates anterior to the subclavian artery and then loops posterior to it, to ascend in the tracheoesophageal groove, while the left originates inferolateral to the arch of the aorta, passing below the arch, posterior to the ligamentum arteriosum.

48a. True
48b. False
48c. False
48d. True
48e. True

The popliteal fossa is a diamond-shaped space containing popliteal vessels, the small saphenous vein, the common peroneal and tibial nerves and the posterior cutaneous nerve of the thigh, and the genicular branch of the obturator nerve, in addition to connective tissue and lymph nodes. The artery is deeply situated, lying medial to the vein. The tibial nerve passes in the fossa into the midline, lying markedly lateral to the artery and lateral to the vein.

Boundaries are as follows:

- *Above medial*: semimembranosus and semitendinosus
- *Above lateral*: biceps femoris
- *Below medial*: medial head of gastrocnemius
- *Below lateral*: lateral head of gastrocnemius and plantaris

Snell RS. *Clinical Anatomy for Medical Students*, 6th edn. Boston: Little, Brown and Company, 2000.

49a. False
49b. True
49c. True
49d. True
49e. True

The physics of HBOT for treatment of gas emboli lies in Boyle's law: PV is a constant; hence as pressure (P) increases, volume (V) decreases if temperature remains constant. HBOT relies upon the principles of Henry's law to increase the dissolved oxygen content of blood, as haemoglobin will be fully saturated. HBOT leads to vasoconstriction and thus an increase in afterload; it can also lead to a reduction in stroke volume and heart rate, leading to a fall in cardiac output. Untreated pneumothoraces constitute an absolute contraindication to HBOT, because of the risk of driving gas emboli into the vascular system, causing a tension pneumothorax or pneumomediastinum. Pacemakers are a relative contraindication and devices should have undergone pressure testing by manufacturers before exposure to HBOT.

Feldmeier J. *Hyperbaric Oxygen: Indications and Results – The Hyperbaric Oxygen Therapy Committee Report*. Kensington, MD: Undersea and Hyperbaric Medical Society, 2003.

50a. False
50b. True
50c. True
50d. True
50e. True

Factors affecting transfer of drugs across a cell membrane include membrane properties, which influence diffusion according to Fick's law, such as membrane thickness, surface area and concentration gradient; Graham's law states that passive diffusion is inversely proportional to the square root of the molecular size. Other factors include vascularity and blood flow, lipid solubility and protein binding. With increasing pK_a values, a greater proportion of the local anaesthetic agent is ionized and thus less lipid-soluble at physiological pH; thus lidocaine (pK_a 7.4) is less ionized at pH 7.35−7.45 than procaine (pK_a 8.9) with a similar molecular weight. In the presence of maternal hyperventilation and subsequent respiratory alkalosis, a greater fraction of drug will be un-ionized and thus more lipid-soluble, leading to increase in placental transfer; conversely fetal acidosis leads to the phenomenon of ion trapping as a greater fraction of ionized local anaesthetic is present.

51a. False
51b. True
51c. True
51d. False
51e. False
Liquid ventilation is a technique that has been used for patients in ICU suffering from acute lung injury/acute respiratory distress syndrome (ALI/ARDS). Based upon the principles of Henry's law, fluorocarbons bind large quantities of oxygen and carbon dioxide. In 'total' liquid ventilation the lungs are completely filled with perfluorocarbon and require a specialized ventilator; in 'partial' liquid ventilation they are filled up to functional residual capacity and a conventional gas ventilator can be used. The effect of the fluorocarbon is both mechanical (since it re-expands gravity-dependent alveoli, redirects blood to the non-dependent lung and eliminates surface tension) and physiological (gas exchange). It has also been shown to help with cleansing free radicals and inflammatory agents. Preliminary trials have shown no improvement in life expectancy or ventilator-free days for patients by using this method.

Mahajan RP. Acute lung injury. *Contin Educ Anaesth Crit Care Pain* 2005; 5: 52–5.

52a. False
52b. True
52c. False
52d. True
52e. False
Rhabdomyolysis describes the breakdown of striated muscle. Myocyte necrosis results in release of contents into the circulation, which can result in hyperkalaemia and acute renal failure (ARF). Hypocalcaemia, rather than hypercalcaemia, develops as a result of accumulation of calcium in damaged muscle. Plasma CK concentration represents the most sensitive test for the detection of rhabdomyolysis. CK is released as striated muscle is damaged, and CK concentration is proportional to the extent of muscle injury, with concentrations of >5000 u/L being associated with a 50% incidence of ARF. Potassium-containing solutions should be used with caution; 0.9% saline has been shown to reduce incidence of ARF. Urinary alkalization facilitates solubility of the Tamm−Horsfall protein−myoglobin complex (which causes tubular casts) and can help prevent ARF, although many patients will develop failure despite optimal management.

Hunter JD, Gregg K, Damani Z. Rhabdomyolysis. *Contin Educ Anaesth Crit Care Pain* 2006; **6**: 141–3.

53a. True
53b. True
53c. False
53d. True
53e. True
Myasthenia gravis is an autoimmune disease characterized by the presence of IgG autoantibodies directed against the post-synaptic acetylcholine receptors at the neuromuscular junction. Features include weakness and increased fatiguability of skeletal muscle. A study of 24 patients identified four risk factors:

- duration of myasthenia gravis (>6 years)
- chronic respiratory disease
- pyridostigmine dose (>750 mg/day)
- FVC <2.9 L

Leventhal SR, Orkin FK, Hirsh RA. Prediction of the need for postoperative mechanical ventilation in myasthenia gravis. *Anesthesiology* 1980; 53: 26–30.

54a. False
54b. True
54c. False
54d. True
54e. False
Pre-eclampsia is a major cause of poor outcome during pregnancy and an increased morbidity and mortality to mother and fetus. It is a multisystem disorder occurring after 20 weeks of pregnancy, affecting 2–3% of all mothers; the precise aetiology is unknown. The main features are pregnancy-induced hypertension (PIH) and proteinuria with or without oedema; virtually any organ system may be affected. Diagnostic criteria are:

- hypertension: diastolic ≥110 mmHg once, or ≥90 mmHg on two separate occasions (not in labour)
- proteinuria: >300 mg in 24 hours
- more than 20 weeks of pregnancy

Uric acid is raised in pre-eclampsia and is used as a marker of the disease. Eclampsia is the occurrence of one or more convulsions superimposed on pre-eclampsia. It is important to remember that women may present with eclampsia without any prodromal symptoms.

Hart E, Coley S. The diagnosis and management of pre-eclampsia. *Contin Educ Anaesth Crit Care Pain* 2003; 3: 38–42.
Royal College of Obstetricians and Gynaecologists. *Management of Severe Pre-Eclampsia and Eclampsia*. London: RCOG, 2006. Available at: www.rcog.org.uk/womens-health/clinical-guidance/management-severe-pre-eclampsiaeclampsia-green-top-10a.

55a. True
55b. True
55c. True
55d. False
55e. False
An exponential process describes one in which the rate of change of a variable at any one time is proportional to the value of the variable at that time. They are encountered often in medicine and anaesthesia, in particular:

- *exponential decay* (negative exponential): radioactive decay, washout curves
- *build-up* (wash-in): uptake of inhalational agents
- *positive exponential* (breakaway function): growth of bacteria

The half-time is the time taken for the variable to reach half of its original value. The time constant τ is the time taken for completion of the process at the initial rate of change; after 1 τ a process is 63% complete, after 3 τ it is 95% complete. The rate constant κ quantifies the speed of a reaction and is the reciprocal of τ.

Davis PD, Kenny GNC. *Basic Physics and Measurement in Anaesthesia*, 5th edn. Oxford: Butterworth-Heinemann, 2003.

56a. True
56b. True
56c. False
56d. False
56e. True
FFP stored at room temperature should be used within 4 hours. Components should not be used to facilitate regional anaesthesia where a general anaesthetic is possible. Vitamin K $\pm$ prothrombin complex concentrate (PCC) is recommended to reverse warfarin therapy. FFP can be given if bleeding is severe or PCC is unavailable. Platelet transfusion triggers recommended are:

- $<50 \times 10^9$/L if ongoing bleeding or urgent surgery is required
- $<10 \times 10^9$/L in a stable, non-bleeding ICU patient

Anaesthetic Association of Great Britain and Ireland Guidelines. *Blood Transfusion and the Anaesthetist*. London: AAGBI, 2005.

57a. False
57b. True
57c. True
57d. False
57e. True
A bolus dose of heparin 300 IU/kg is administered before commencing cardiopulmonary bypass. ACT must be greater than 400 s before cannulation of the aorta. Risk factors for the development of a CVE include:

- age
- aortic atheroma
- previous CVE
- diabetes

- type of surgery (aortic arch replacement > valve replacement > coronary graft)

Hypothermia confers cerebral protection, although many centres do not employ hypothermic techniques. Contact of the blood with the bypass circuits leads to inflammatory cascades, causing platelet dysfunction, fibrinolysis and complement activation. Haemolysis, platelet damage and consumption of coagulation factors are minimal in the initial 2 hours. Protamine is used to reverse the effects of heparin; 1 mg is given for each 100 IU heparin initially administered

Martin B, Sinclair M. Cardiac surgery. In: Allman KG, Wilson IH, eds. *Oxford Handbook of Anaesthesia*, 2nd edn. Oxford: OUP, 2006.

58a. False
58b. False
58c. False
58d. False
58e. False
The phrenic nerves are derived from the anterior primary rami of the C3, 4, 5 nerve roots and arise between the scalenus anterior and scalenus medius. They descend on the scalenus anterior from lateral to medial to enter the mediastinum behind the subclavian vein and thus can be damaged along their course by trauma, surgery, tumour infiltration or compression and are classically blocked by interscalene regional techniques. The right and left phrenic nerves then take different courses in the mediastinum:

Right:

- Passes over the lateral surface of the superior vena cava
- Lies within fibrous pericardium
- Pierces the diaphragm via the caval orifice (T8) (terminal branches)

Left:

- Descends with the internal thoracic artery
- Passes over the aortic arch anterior to the vagus
- Lies within fibrous pericardium to pierce the central tendon of the diaphragm

They give branches to the mediastinal pleura, fibrous and parietal pericardium and diaphragmatic pleura and are the sole motor supply to the diaphragm. The sensory fibres from the diaphragm explain the shoulder-tip referred pain caused by diaphragmatic irritation.

59a. True
59b. True
59c. True
59d. False
59e. True
β-lactam drugs are subdivided into

- penicillins
- cephalosporins
- carbapenems
- monobactams

These drugs contain a 4-atom β-lactam ring; which is hydrolysed by β-lactamase, rendering the drug ineffective against certain microorganisms. Vancomycin is a naturally occurring complex glycopeptide.

Peck TE, Hill SA, Williams M. *Pharmacology for Anaesthesia and Intensive Care*, 3rd edn. Cambridge: CUP, 2008.

60a. True
60b. False
60c. False
60d. True
60e. False
Concentrations/measurements are listed below. The shaded boxes show where values are higher in CSF than in plasma.

Substance	Unit	CSF	Plasma
pH		7.33	7.4
Protein	g/dL	0.2	60
Glucose	mmol/L	3.6	5.6
Na^+	mEq/kgH_2O	147	150
K^+	mEq/kgH_2O	2.9	4.6
Osmolality	mOsm/kg	289	289
Mg^{2+}	mEq/kgH_2O	2.2	1.6
Cl^-	mEq/kgH_2O	113	99
HCO_3^-	mEq/L	25.1	24.8
P_{CO_2}	kPa	6.6	5.3
Ca^{2+}	mEq/kgH_2O	2.3	4.7

Ganong WF. *Review of Medical Physiology*, 22nd edn. Maidenhead: McGraw-Hill Medical, 2005.

61a. True
61b. False
61c. True
61d. False
61e. False
Hyponatraemia is a serum sodium concentration of <135 mmol/L. Commonly associated with hypotonicity, hyponatraemia may occur in isotonic and hypertonic conditions. A major concern of hypotonic hyponatraemia is the creation of an osmotic gradient across the blood–brain barrier; water enters brain cells and cerebral oedema ensues. CSWS describes renal loss of sodium and water associated with intracranial pathology (head injury, subarachnoid haemorrhage) resulting in hypovolaemic hyponatraemia. SIADH is characterized by increased vasopressin levels and water retention, despite hypo-osmolality and *normo-* or *hypervolaemia*. DI, whether neurogenic or nephrogenic, is characterized by *hypernatraemia*. Causes of hyponatraemia are classified as follows:

Hypovolaemic hyponatraemia

- CSWS, diuretics, diarrhoea and vomiting, sweating, blood loss

Normovolaemic hyponatraemia

- SIADH (multiple causes, including traumatic brain injury, subarachnoid haemorrhage, drug-induced and pulmonary pathology), thiazide diuretics, adrenal insufficiency, hypothyroidism, iatrogenic

Hypervolaemic hyponatraemia

- SIADH, congestive heart failure, nephritic syndrome, cirrhosis, acute renal failure, iatrogenic

The following is an *aide-mémoire*:

Condition	Plasma sodium (mmol/L)	Urine sodium (mmol/L)	Plasma osmolality (mOsm/kg)	Urine osmolality (mOsm/kg)	Urine specific gravity
Normal	135–145	<10	285–295	600–1400	1.002 – 1.035
DI	↑	↑/normal	↑	↓	↓
SIADH	↓	↑/normal	↓	↑	↑
Cerebral salt wasting	↓	↑	↓	↑	↑

Bradshaw K, Smith M. Disorders of sodium balance after head injury. *Contin Educ Anaesth Crit Care Pain* 2008; 8: 129–33.

62a. True
62b. False
62c. False
62d. True
62e. False
IE results in formation of infective vegetations on the endocardial surface of the heart. Men are more commonly affected than women (2 : 1) and incidence increases with age. The primary pathogen is currently *S. aureus* and cases of prosthetic, nosocomial and intravenous drug-related IE have increased in recent years. Pathophysiology involves a primary bacteraemia followed by adherence of the organisms to the endocardial wall, made more likely by pre-existing thrombus or ulceration. Bacterial invasion of valvular leaflets ensues, leading to valvular insufficiency and cardiac failure, in addition to the wide array of systemic signs and symptoms. Up to 90% of patients present with fever; cardiac murmurs are found in 85%. Classical signs include Roth spots (retinal haemorrhages), Janeway lesions (haemorrhagic spots on palms and soles) and Osler's nodes (painful lesions on finger or toe pads). Erythema marginatum is a feature of rheumatic fever, diagnosed using the revised Jones criteria. Diagnosis of IE uses the modified *Dukes* criteria. The most recent NICE guidelines regarding antibiotic prophylaxis of IE state that routine dental prophylaxis is not warranted.

Beynon RP, Bahl VK, Prendergast BD. Infective endocarditis. *BMJ* 2006; **333**: 334–9.

National Institute for Health and Clinical Excellence. *Prophylaxis Against Infective Endocarditis*. London: NICE, 2008. Available at: guidance.nice. org.uk/CG64.

63a. True
63b. False
63c. True
63d. True
63e. False

Myotonic dystrophy is a complex multisystem genetic disorder. It is inherited in an autosomal dominant manner and exhibits variable penetrance and anticipation (increasing severity and earlier onset with successive generations). It is characterized by delayed muscle relaxation following contraction, with a prevalence of 4 per 100 000. Affected individuals have a characteristic facies with frontal balding, ptosis, cataracts, smooth forehead and proximal muscle wasting. The condition is associated with endocrine dysfunction, diabetes mellitus, gonadal atrophy, cardiac conduction defects and cardiomyopathy. Myotonia is provoked by cold, shivering, hyperkalaemia and exercise; drug triggers include suxamethonium and neostigmine, causing persistent muscle contraction. Similarly, nerve stimulators can also provoke generalized myotonic response, and thus should be avoided. Patients require reduced doses of intravenous induction agents and are at risk of tachyarrythmias and sudden death. Body temperature should be monitored and maintained and, although regional blockade avoids many anaesthetic drug triggers, the myotonic reflex is not blocked. Local anaesthetic infiltration directly to the muscle has been effective.

Russell SH, Hirsch NP. Anaesthesia and myotonia. *Br J Anaesth* 1994; **72**: 210–17.

64a. True
64b. False
64c. True
64d. False
64e. False

Modern scavenging consists of four main components:

Collecting system: gas-tight shroud enclosing the adjustable pressure limiting (APL) valve of the breathing circuit; 30 mm connectors are used. Some designs have an over-pressure relief valve (1 kPa, 1000 Pa)
Transfer system: wide-bore tubing between collecting and reservoir systems
Receiving system: contains reservoir, air brake, flow indicator and filter. A dumping valve is required to prevent excess negative pressure and a pressure relief valve to prevent excess positive pressure
Disposal system: in the UK these are active and *high-flow*. Sub-atmospheric pressure is generated by an exhauster unit

Sinclair CM, Thadsad MK, Barker I. Modern anaesthetic machines. *Contin Educ Anaesth Crit Care Pain* 2006; **6**: 75–8.

65a. True
65b. True
65c. True
65d. True
65e. False

Fluid	Sodium (mmol/L)	Potassium (mmol/L)	Chloride (mmol/L)	Calcium (mmol/L)	pH	Other
Hartmann's	131	5	111	2	6.5	Lactate 29
0.9% saline	154	–	154	–	5.0	–
Glucose 4%/ saline 0.18%	30	–	30	–	4–5	Glucose 40 g
Glucose 5%	–	–	–	–	4.0	Glucose 50 g
Bicarbonate 1.26%	150	–	–	–	7.0	HCO_3^- 150
Bicarbonate 8.4%	1000	–	–	–	8.0	HCO_3^- 1000
Gelofusine	154	<0.4	125	<0.4	7.4	Gelatin 40 g
Haemaccel	145	5.1	145	6.25	7.4	Gelatin 35 g

66a. False
66b. True
66c. False
66d. False
66e. True

The law provides a clear hierarchy in terms of legal standing in making DNAR decisions.

1. The competent patient's direct instructions
2. The patient's advance decision or proxy decision maker if competence is lacking
3. The senior clinician in charge of the patient's care, acting in the patient's best interests, if there is no legally valid advanced decision or proxy decision maker for a patient lacking competence

An independent mental capacity advocate (IMCA) is appointed by the local authority or health board; their role is to indicate to decision-makers the patient's wishes, feelings, beliefs and values. Survival rates following anaesthetic-related cardiac arrest can be as high as 92%; by comparison, survival rates for other in-hospital arrests are 15–20%.

Association of Anaesthetists of Great Britain and Ireland Guidelines. *Do Not Attempt Resuscitation (DNAR) Decisions in the Perioperative Period*. London: AAGBI, 2009. Available at: www.aagbi.org/publications/guidelines/docs/dnar_09.pdf.

Olsson GL, Hallen B. Cardiac arrest during anaesthesia. A computer-aided study in 250543 anaesthetics. *Acta Anaesthesiol Scand* 1988; **32**: 653–64.

Sandroni C, Nolan J, Cavallaro F, Antonelli M. In-hospital cardiac arrest: incidence, prognosis and possible measures to improve survival. *Intensive Care Med* 2007; **33**: 237–45.

4. Practice Paper 4: Answers

67a. True
67b. False
67c. False
67d. False
67e. False
The GCS of the patient is 5 (E1, V2, M2). In multiple trauma situations, an
'ABC' approach is adopted as per ATLS guidelines. While intubation is
definitely indicated with his GCS below 8, a rapid sequence induction may be
hazardous before exclusion or decompression of a tension pneumothorax,
which may be a cause of his hypotension and is made more likely in view of the
flail chest. NICE guidelines recommend head CT imaging in patients with a
GCS <13 following head injury, which should be analysed within the hour;
however, his cardiovascular instability dictates completion of the primary
survey and treatment of life-threatening emergencies prior to any in-hospital
transfer for imaging. Trauma X-ray series includes cervical spine, chest and
pelvis.

National Institute for Health and Clinical Excellence Guidelines. *Head Injury:
Triage, Assessment, Investigation and Early Management of Head Injury in
Infants, Children and Adults*. London: NICE, 2007. Available at:
guidance.nice.org.uk/CG56.

68a. False
68b. False
68c. True
68d. True
68e. False
In the UK, standard TENS devices can be purchased without prescription. A
standard TENS device delivers biphasic pulsed currents in a repetitive manner
using pulse durations of 50–250 μs and pulse frequencies of 1–200 Hz.
TENS should not be applied over the anterior neck, since this may produce
laryngospasm or hypotension.

Jones I, Johnson MI. Transcutaneous electrical nerve stimulation. *Contin Educ
Anaesth Crit Care Pain* 2009; **9**: 130–5.

69a. False
69b. True
69c. True
69d. True
69e. False
Thyrotoxic crisis ('thyroid storm') is a medical emergency that presents in
thyrotoxic patients and is precipitated by an intercurrent illness, emergency
surgery or trauma. It is rarely encountered owing to effective antithyroid
therapy. Presentation is with hyperpyrexia (>41°C), tachycardia, hypotension,
heart failure, jaundice, confusion, agitation and coma. Management involves
prompt recognition, supportive therapy and treatment of the precipitating
cause. Management consists of:

- ABC with 100% O_2
- Rehydration with crystalloid to compensate for large insensible losses

- Treating hyperpyrexia with tepid sponging and paracetamol; aspirin is not used, since it displaces thyroid hormone further from protein-binding sites
- β-blockade: propranolol is given in 1 mg increments up to 10 mg. The goal is a heart rate below 90/min
- Hydrocortisone 200 mg four times daily treats adrenal insufficiency and reduces thyroxine release and peripheral conversion to triiodothyronine
- Dantrolene can be used to prevent the action of calcium ions, which is initiated by the thyroid hormones in the sarcoplasmic reticulum
- Antithyroid medication: carbimazole or propylthiouracil may be used

Mortality, even with prompt diagnosis, is estimated to be 20–50%.

Blanshard H, Bennett D. Metabolic and endocrine. In: Allman KG, McIndoe AK, Wilson IH, eds. *Emergencies in Anaesthesia*, 2nd edn. Oxford: OUP, 2009.
Burch HB, Wartofsky L. Life-threatening thyrotoxicosis. Thyroid storm. *Endocrinol Metab Clin North Am* 1993; 22: 263–77.
Farling PA. Thyroid disease. *Br J Anaesth* 2000; 85: 15–28.

70a. False
70b. True
70c. True
70d. False
70e. True
$SjvO_2$ provides a measure of global cerebral oxygenation. It is measured by retrograde introduction of a catheter through the internal jugular vein to the jugular bulb. The position can be confirmed radiologically with a lateral skull X-ray showing the tip at the level of and medial to the mastoid process. Normal values are 55–75%.

Causes of ↑$SjvO_2$ (oxygen supply exceeds demand)

- ↓Metabolic demand (hypothermia, sedation)
- Increased blood supply
- Hypercapnia
- Arterial hyperoxia
- Brain death

Causes of ↓$SjvO_2$ (oxygen demand exceeds supply)

- ↑Metabolic demand (seizures, pyrexia)
- Hypotension
- Arterial hypoxia
- Hypocapnia
- Cerebral vasospasm

71a. True
71b. True
71c. False
71d. False
71e. True
Peripheral signs of aortic regurgitation due to a wide pulse pressure are:

- Watson's water hammer pulse (bounding peripheral pulses)
- collapsing pulse

- Corrigan's sign (dancing carotids)
- De Musset's sign (to-and-fro head nodding synchronous with cardiac pulse)
- Quincke's sign (capillary pulsations in nail beds)
- Traube's sign (systolic and diastolic sounds over femoral arteries with compression known as 'pistol-shot')
- Durozier's sign (double bruit over femoral artery with distal compression)
- Hill's sign (increase of femoral artery pressure over brachial pressure by > 10 mmHg above normal)

Osler's nodes are painful red lesions, while Janeway lesions are non-painful erythematous nodules on both the palms and soles, classically indicative of infective endocarditis.

72a. True
72b. True
72c. True
72d. True
72e. False
Causes of cataract formation include congenital syndromes such as Down's, genetic disorders such as myotonic dystrophy, trauma, radiation damage, UV light exposure and drugs such as amiodarone, phenytoin and steroids. Wilson's disease (hepatolenticular degeneration) is a rare recessively inherited disorder characterized by accumulation and deposition of copper within the liver and basal ganglia and other tissues. Infectious causes include rubella, which is a notifiable disease caused by an RNA virus; maternal infection can lead to the congenital rubella syndrome, typical features of which include congenital heart defects, eye lesions, deafness and microcephaly. Toxoplasmosis is a protozoal infection caused by *Toxoplasma gondii* and is a cause of cateract formation.

73a. True
73b. False
73c. True
73d. True
73e. False
Spinal needles can be classified as:

Cutting type

- *Quincke*: a short-bevelled cutting tip less often used because of its increased incidence of postdural puncture headache

Non-cutting type

- *Sprotte*: a smooth-sided pointed tip with a wide lateral hole proximal to the tip
- *Whitacre*: pencil-tip shaped with the hole just proximal to the tip
- *Greene*: oblique bevel with rounded edges

Yentis S, Hirsch N, Smith G. *Anaesthesia and Intensive Care A to Z: An Encyclopaedia of Principles and Practice*, 4th edn. Oxford: Butterworth-Heinemann, 2009.

74a. False
74b. False
74c. True
74d. True
74e. False

During exercise, O_2 supply and CO_2 excretion rely upon pulmonary ventilation, alveolar–capillary diffusion, transport and subsequent diffusion to active tissues and homeostatic regulation of these processes. O_2 consumption and CO_2 production increase during exercise and pulmonary capillary blood Po_2 falls, thus increasing the gradient and facilitating oxygen diffusion from the alveolus to capillary. Pulmonary ventilation increases proportionally to the oxygen consumption (Vo_{2max}) to a point and blood flow increases from 5 to up to 35 L/min; oxygen delivery thus increases up to a maximum beyond which an oxygen debt is incurred and lactic acid accumulates. Most lactic acid is transported to the liver and converted to pyruvate, but some remains, causing muscle cramp and fatigue. With increases in lactic acid production, the hyperventilation maintains alveolar and arterial Pco_2 at fairly constant levels owing to 'isocapnic buffering'; with further increases in lactic acid, there is a decline in alveolar and arterial Pco_2, as production is outstripped by the increase in ventilation. CO_2 production can rise from 200 to 8000 mL/min. Pulmonary vascular resistance falls during exercise owing to recruitment and dilatation of the pulmonary capillaries to allow for increased blood flow and increased oxygen delivery. The exact cause of increased ventilation during exercise is largely unknown.

Ganong WF. *Review of Medical Physiology*, 22nd edn. Maidenhead: McGraw-Hill Medical, 2005.
Tipton CM. *ACSM's Advanced Exercise Physiology*. Philadelphia: Lippincott Williams & Wilkins, 2005.

75a. False
75b. False
75c. True
75d. False
75e. False

A spirometer can measure the following values (normal values for a 70 kg male):

- *Tidal volume* (TV): volume of gas inspired or expired during normal breathing (500 mL)
- *Inspiratory reserve volume* (IRV): maximum volume of gas inspired from the normal end-inspiratory position (2500 mL)
- *Expiratory reserve volume* (ERV): maximum volume expired from the normal end-expiratory position (1500 mL)
- *Inspiratory capacity* (TV + IRV): 3000 mL
- *Vital capacity* (VC) (TV + IRV + ERV): 4500 mL

Lung volumes that cannot be measured via spirometry, but require plethysmography, N_2 washout or helium dilution, are:

- *Residual volume* (RV): volume of gas remaining in the lungs after maximal expiration (1200–1500 mL)
- *Total lung capacity* (VC + RV): volume of gas in the lung after maximal inspiration (6000 mL)

- *Functional residual capacity* (RV + ERV): volume of gas in the lungs at resting end-expiratory level (3000 mL standing to 2000 mL supine)

Atkinson RS, Rushman GB, Davies NJH. *Lee's Synopsis of Anaesthesia*, 11th edn. Oxford: Butterworth-Heinemann, 1993.

76a. False
76b. True
76c. True
76d. True
76e. False
Modern acupuncture is based on an ancient Chinese theory that there exists a delicate balance between two opposing forces in the body. The 'yin' is the cold or passive principle and the 'yang' is the hot or active principle. When there is an imbalance between these two, there is a blockage of vital energy flow or 'Qi' between 12 main and 8 secondary meridians in the body, which can be corrected by inserting needles in specific acupoints that connect them. The needles are 32–36 G. Techniques involve basic needling, electroacupuncture, which involves passage of current (1–3 mA, 1–100 Hz) either directly or through needles, moxibustion (application of heat to the needles), laser acupuncture or acupressure. Absolute contraindications include severe bleeding disorders, needle phobia, systemic sepsis, cellulitus, burns, ulceration and (for electroacupuncture) pacemakers.

Wilkinson J, Faleiro R. Acupuncture in pain management. *Contin Educ Anaesth Crit Care Pain* 2007; 7: 135–8.

77a. True
77b. False
77c. False
77d. False
77e. True
NICE has produced guidance on the use of ultrasound for epidural catheterization. Ultrasound can be used in a 'prepuncture' technique to locate the midline and middle of the interspinous spaces and assess the depth of the epidural space; once this is marked on the skin, placement continues in the traditional method. Alternatively, a 'realtime' technique can be employed to observe the passage of the needle into the epidural space. In a randomized control trial (RCT) of 300 women in labour, the number of attempts at successful epidural placement was 1.3 in the ultrasound group, compared with 2.2 in the control group. Maternal satisfaction was 1.3 in the ultrasound group, 1.8 in the control group (on a six-point verbal scale where 1 is very good and 6 is insufficient). One RCT involving 64 children reported that the mean time to successful placement was 162 s using a realtime technique, compared with 234 s using a prepuncture technique. In a further study of 180 children, there were no reports of dural puncture in either group. NICE specialist advice is that ultrasound guidance can be successful for patients in whom conventional techniques have failed and is associated with improved patient comfort during catheter insertion.

National Institute for Health and Clinical Excellence. *Ultrasound-Guided Catheterisation of the Epidural Space*. London: NICE, 2008. Available at: www.nice.org.uk/IPG249.

78a. False
78b. True
78c. False
78d. False
78e. True
Hypoxia and hypotension following tracheostomy should immediately raise suspicion of a tension pneumothorax and immediate management should include administration of 100% oxygen and establishment of a patent airway. Immediate suctioning via the tracheostomy may reveal a migrated tube, false passage or blockage with blood or secretions. Examination of the chest for movement, breath sounds and distended neck veins indicate a diagnosis of tension pneumothorax, for which a needle decompression should be performed without delay on the affected side. Chest X-ray and chest drain insertion can follow, but should not be performed before life-threatening airway and breathing problems have been addressed. A rapid sequence induction would be hazardous before tension pneumothorax has been excluded.

79a. True
79b. False
79c. True
79d. False
79e. False
Pacemakers have a generic code: NBG, which is derived from the NASPE (North American Society of Pacing and Electrophysiology), BPEG (British Pacing and Electrophysiology Group) and is generic. The code is as follows:

I   Chamber paced (O – none, A – atrium, V – ventricle, D – dual)
II Chamber sensed (O, A, V, D)
III Response to Sensing (O – none, T – trigger, I – inhibit, D – dual)
IV Programmability (O – none, P – simple, M – multi, C – communicating, R – rate modulation)
V   Antitachycardia function (O – none, P – pacing, S – shock, D – dual)

The first three letters describe anti-bradycardic functions, the fourth describes programmability (including rate modulation) and the fifth antitachycardia functions.

Diprose P, Pierce JMT. Anaesthesia for patients with pacemakers and similar devices. *Contin Educ Anaesth Crit Care Pain* 2001; **1**: 166–70.

80a. False
80b. False
80c. False
80d. True
80e. True
Trigeminal neuralgia (tic douloureux) is the prototype of neuropathic pain, with a prevalence of 3–5 per 100 000, more commonly in females over 50. It is almost always unilateral, most commonly affecting the mandibular division of

the trigeminal nerve. Diagnostic criteria by the International Headache Society are as follows:

- Paroxysmal attacks of facial/frontal pain, lasting a few seconds to less than 2 minutes
- Pain has at least four of the following:
  - ○ *distribution along one or more divisions of the trigeminal nerve*
  - ○ *sudden, intense, sharp, superficial, stabbing, or burning in quality*
  - ○ *severe pain intensity*
  - ○ *precipitation from trigger areas or by certain innocuous daily activities (e.g. eating, talking, washing)*
  - ○ *no symptoms between paroxysms*
  - ○ *no neurological deficit is present*
  - ○ *attacks are stereotyped in the individual patient*
  - ○ *other causes of facial pain are excluded*

Trigeminal neuralgia is either idiopathic or secondary; secondary causes include malignancy (acoustic neuroma), vascular (arteriovenous malformation) or inflammatory (multiple sclerosis, sarcoidosis) causing compression of the trigeminal sensory ganglion. Treatment can be medical or surgical but should include psychological support.

Farooq K, Williams P. Headache and chronic facial pain. *Contin Educ Anaesth Crit Care Pain* 2008; 8: 138–42.
The International Headache Society. *IHS Classification ICHD-II*. Available at: ihs-classification.org/en/.

81a. True
81b. True
81c. True
81d. False
81e. True
Exomphalos is a central abdominal wall defect caused by herniation of abdominal contents through the extraembryonic part of the umbilical cord, which covers it in a membrane. It occurs in 1 per 13 000 births in a 3 : 2 male-to-female ratio and the majority of affected neonates have associated defects (74.4% versus 16% for gastroschisis); thus an echocardiogram, renal ultrasound, chromosomal analysis and brain imaging are performed prior to surgical correction. Gastroschisis is a congenital defect of the abdominal wall, usually to the right of the umbilical cord; abdominal contents herniate through the defect into the amniotic cavity with no covering membrane. These neonates are operated on within hours of birth and are at great risk of heat and evaporative losses and of infection. Surgery may be staged or definitive; nitrous oxide should be avoided in both cases since it may result in further bowel distension with subsequent difficult closure.

Kilby MD, Lander A, Usher-Somers M. Exomphalos (omphalocele). *Prenat Diagn* 1998; 8: 1283–8.
Poddar R, Hartley L. Exomphalos and gastroschisis. *Contin Educ Anaesth Crit Care Pain* 2009; 9: 48–51.

82a. True
82b. False
82c. False
82d. False
82e. True
The correct units are:

- Magnetic field strength (tesla, T)
- Capacitance (farad, F)
- Amount of substance (mole, mol)
- Charge (coulomb, C)
- Power (watt, W)

The kilogram (kg) is the base SI unit for mass.

83a. False
83b. False
83c. True
83d. True
83e. True
Bronchial blockers are balloon-tipped luminal catheters that achieve one-lung isolation and are often placed fibre-optically through a single-lumen ETT. They allow oxygen insufflation and suctioning through the lumen. Double-lumen tubes are available from a smallest size of 26 FG, which allows paediatric usage in 8–12-year-olds.

Advantages of a bronchial blocker

- Ease of insertion in difficult airways
- Allows placement in various patient positions (i.e. lateral decubitus)
- No requirement for exchange to a single-lumen ETT
- Selective lobar blockade

Disadvantages of a bronchial blocker

- Slow inflation and deflation of isolated lung because of the narrow lumen
- Blockage by blood clots and secretions
- High-pressure cuff
- Risk of intraoperative leak due to displacement

Benumof JL. Anesthesia for thoracic surgery. In: Miller RD, ed. *Miller's Anesthesia*, 7th edn. New York: Churchill Livingstone, 2009.

84a. True
84b. True
84c. True
84d. False
84e. True
Doxapram is used primarily as a respiratory stimulant for the treatment of postoperative respiratory depression and acute-on-chronic respiratory failure. It can also be used in the treatment of laryngospasm, to facilitate blind nasal intubation and in the treatment of postoperative shivering. It acts primarily by stimulating the peripheral chemoreceptors and has a secondary

action on the respiratory centre. The CO_2 response curve is displaced to the left.

Sasada M, Smith S. *Drugs in Anaesthesia and Intensive Care*, 3rd edn. Oxford: OUP, 2003.

85a. True
85b. True
85c. True
85d. False
85e. False
The 3rd National Audit Project (NAP3) reported on major complications of central neuraxial blockade in the UK. The incidences of harm are as stated. Two-thirds of injuries initially reported as severe resolved fully and most complications leading to harm (such as haematoma or nerve damage) occurred in the perioperative setting. The incidence of complications in children, chronic pain and obstetrics was extremely low.

Cook TM, Counsell D, Wildsmith JAW. Major complications of central neuraxial block in the UK: report on the Third National Audit Project of the Royal College of Anaesthetists. *Br J Anaesth* 2009; **102**: 179–90.

86a. True
86b. False
86c. False
86d. False
86e. True
The nose is divided into external nose and cavities. It consists of:

- *Roof*: nasal and frontal bones, ethmoid and palatine
- *Floor*: palatine and maxillary bones
- *Medial wall*: nasal septum
- *Lateral wall*: ethmoidal labyrinth, maxilla and palatine bone consisting of superior, middle and inferior conchae. The paranasal sinuses (frontal, ethmoidal, maxillary and sphenoid) and nasolacrimal duct open onto the lateral wall
- *Arterial supply*: ophthalmic and maxillary (sphenopalatine) arteries, facial (superior labial) artery to anteroinferior septum
- *Venous supply*: facial vein and pterygoid venous plexus
- *Nerve supply*: olfactory zone by olfactory nerve, generalized sensation by ophthalmic and maxillary divisions of trigeminal nerve; nasal septum is supplied by the nasopalatine branch of the maxillary division (V_2). The posterior ethmoidal nerve (V_1) supplies the sphenoid and posterior ethmoidal sinuses.

87a. True
87b. False
87c. True
87d. False
87e. True

Conversion to a Fontan circulation is indicated for patients with tricuspid atresia, pulmonary atresia with intact ventricular septum, double-inlet left ventricle, hypoplastic left heart syndrome, double-outlet right ventricle and complete atrioventricular septal defects. Conversion occurs progressively, but must occur when pulmonary vasculature resistance is low, and hence is contraindicated in the neonate. Stage I consists of a systemic–pulmonary shunt, usually between the right subclavian artery and the right pulmonary artery; Stage II is a Glenn-type operation, or anastomosis between the *right* pulmonary artery and superior vena cava. Finally, Stage III is completion whereby inferior vena caval blood is directed into the pulmonary circulation.

Gewillig M. The Fontan circulation. *Heart* 2005; **91**: 839–46.
Nayak S, Booker PD. The Fontan circulation. *Contin Educ Anaesth Crit Care Pain* 2008; **8**: 26–30.

88a. True
88b. True
88c. False
88d. True
88e. False

Bacterial meningitis is primarily diagnosed by CSF examination. Typical CSF values are as follows:

	Viral	Pyogenic	Tuberculosis
Predominant cell type	Lymphocytes	Polymorphs	Lymphocytes
Cell count (/mm^3)	<500	>1000	50–1500
CSF : blood glucose	>60%	<60%	<60%
Protein (g/dL)	0.5–1	>1	1–5
Appearance	Clear	Turbid	Fibrin web

Singer M, Webb AR. *Oxford Handbook of Critical Care*, 3rd edn. Oxford: OUP, 2009.

89a. False
89b. True
89c. False
89d. True
89e. True
Absolute pressure = gauge pressure + atmospheric pressure; thus cylinder pressures are gauge pressures. A gas above its critical temperature cannot be liquefied no matter how much pressure is applied; this applies to heliox, Entonox (*pseudo*critical temperature $-6°C$, at which it separates into liquid N_2O and gaseous O_2) and O_2 (critical temperature $-118°C$). Boyle's law applies (PV = constant). Substances in a gaseous phase below their critical temperature are *vapours*; this applies to N_2O and CO_2 with critical temperatures of $36.5°C$ and $31.1°C$ respectively. The following cylinder pressures apply for various gases and vapours at room temperature:

- O_2, air, heliox, Entonox: 137 bar
- N_2O: 44 bar
- CO_2: 50 bar

Al-Shaikh B, Stacey S. *Essentials of Anaesthetic Equipment*, 3rd edn. London: Churchill Livingstone, 2007.

90a. True
90b. True
90c. True
90d. True
90e. False
Statins are a class of lipid-lowering agents that selectively inhibit HMG-CoA reductase, the rate-limiting enzyme in cholesterol biosynthesis. They lead to increased low-density lipoprotein (LDL)-receptor expression, which increases LDL clearance and reduces levels in a dose-dependent manner. Studies have shown that lipid reduction with statin therapy in high-risk patients is beneficial regardless of baseline LDL levels. Severe myopathy and rhabdomyolysis have been reported to be associated with statin therapy, particularly in combination treatment with drugs interfering with the cytochrome p450 3A4 metabolism of statins, but CK levels need not be monitored routinely.

Topol EJ, Califf RM. *Textbook of Cardiovascular Medicine*, Vol. 355. Philadelphia: Lippincott Williams & Wilkins, 2006.

5. Practice Paper 5: Questions

1. The following applies for antiretroviral drugs:
   a. The aim of therapy is to achieve an undetectable viral load
   b. Treatment should be initiated only when CD4 cell counts are <350 cells/mm^3
   c. Zidovudine is a nucleoside reverse transcriptase inhibitor
   d. Indinavir inhibits processing of viral proteins
   e. Triple therapy consists of two protease inhibitors combined with a nucleoside reverse transcriptase inhibitor

2. The following conditions are associated with the following vitamin disorders:
   a. Beriberi and vitamin B$_6$ deficiency
   b. Pellagra and vitamin B$_3$ deficiency
   c. Pernicious anaemia and vitamin B$_{12}$ deficiency
   d. Xerophthalmia and vitamin A deficiency
   e. Hepatosplenomegaly and hypervitaminosis D

3. Regarding innervation of the lower leg:
   a. The terminal branch of the femoral nerve supplies sensation to the majority of the skin of the forefoot
   b. The lateral cutaneous nerve of the thigh is a branch of the femoral nerve
   c. The deep peroneal nerve pierces the anterior intermuscular septum
   d. The deep peroneal nerve lies medial to the dorsalis pedis artery in the foot
   e. The sural nerve accompanies the long saphenous vein

4. Thiopentone:
   a. Is a stereoisomer of methohexitone
   b. Has a pK_a of 10.5
   c. Has active metabolites
   d. Is contraindicated in porphyria
   e. Is removed by dialysis

5. Concerning prone positioning under anaesthesia:
   a. The most common ocular injury is a pressure injury
   b. There is a decrease in cardiac index
   c. There is increased risk of abdominal compartment syndrome
   d. There is a decrease in functional residual capacity due to chest compression
   e. The upper limb can be safely abducted to $110°$

6. **The following statements on breathing systems are correct:**
   a. Coaxial Mapleson A is efficient for mechanical ventilation
   b. Mapleson D requires a fresh gas flow (FGF) of $70-100$ mL kg^{-1} min^{-1} for mechanical ventilation
   c. Magill requires an FGF of $70-100$ mL kg^{-1} min^{-1} for spontaneous ventilation
   d. Mapleson C is efficient for spontaneous ventilation
   e. Lack requires an FGF of $70-100$ mL kg^{-1} min^{-1} for spontaneous ventilation

7. **A subdural block:**
   a. Occurs when an epidural catheter is misplaced between the dura mater and ligamentum flavum
   b. Is definitively diagnosed by a positive aspiration test
   c. May cause Horner's syndrome
   d. Is characterized by a fast onset
   e. Is typically dense and widespread

8. **A 60-year-old man presents with bleeding varices; appropriate management includes:**
   a. Administration of vasopressin
   b. Application of a Sengstaken-type tube
   c. Insertion of a large-bore nasogastric tube
   d. Transjugular intrahepatic portosystemic stented shunting
   e. Administration of propanolol

9. **Concerning neonatal fluid and electrolyte management:**
   a. The Holiday and Segar regimen describes maintenance requirements
   b. Sodium should be administered at 3 mmol kg^{-1} day^{-1}
   c. Potassium should be administered at 3 mmol kg^{-1} day^{-1}
   d. Phototherapy warrants an additional 10 mL kg^{-1} day^{-1} of fluid
   e. Pyrexia makes no difference to maintenance fluid requirements

10. **Inguinal field block for hernia repair targets the following nerves:**
    a. Ilioinguinal
    b. Lateral femoral
    c. Iliohypogastric
    d. Genital branch of genitofemoral
    e. Medial branch of obturator

11. **Paget's disease:**
    a. Is characterized by disordered osteoblastic resorption
    b. Can affect any bone
    c. Shows raised calcium and phosphate on serum biochemistry
    d. Requires no treatment if asymptomatic
    e. Is asymptomatic in the majority of patients

12. A 2-year-old child presents to A&E with acute stridor; appropriate initial management includes:
    a. Humidified oxygen
    b. Measuring SpO_2
    c. Intramuscular adrenaline
    d. Intravenous access and cautious fluid administration
    e. Heliox

13. The baroreceptor reflex:
    a. Regulates long-term control of blood pressure
    b. Involves inhibitory signals to the medulla
    c. Involves excitatory signals to the medulla
    d. Results in lowering of heart rate
    e. Results in lowering of blood pressure

14. Oxygen:
    a. Is responsible for the Paul–Bert effect
    b. Cylinders are available in six sizes
    c. Supports combustion
    d. Can be explosive
    e. Has a critical pressure of 50.8 atm

15. Concerning laryngoscopes:
    a. Left-sided blades are not designed for left-handed anaesthetists
    b. The polio blade is at a 60° angle to the handle
    c. Magill's blade is straight
    d. Miller's blade is curved
    e. Robertshaw's blade is designed for paediatric use

16. A 48-year-old woman presents to A&E with diabetic ketoacidosis (DKA); the following statements are correct:
    a. She does not have type 2 diabetes
    b. Excess acetyl-CoA is converted to acetoacetate and γ-hydroxybutyric acid
    c. Plasma glucose may not be high
    d. Initial replacement of 0.9% saline must not exceed 10 mL kg^{-1} h^{-1}
    e. Total body potassium is reduced

17. With regard to fluid therapy:
    a. Crystalloid resuscitation should involve balanced salt solutions
    b. Haemodynamic status should be reviewed in patients whose urinary sodium is >20 mmol/L postoperatively
    c. High-molecular-weight (HMW) hydroxethylstarches should be used in patients with severe sepsis
    d. HMW hydroxethylstarches should be avoided in brain-dead kidney donors
    e. Carbohydrate-rich beverages 2–3 hours before induction of anaesthesia may facilitate recovery from surgery

18. Typical features of botulism include:
    a. Spastic paralysis
    b. Bulbar palsy
    c. Constipation
    d. Postural hypotension
    e. Respiratory failure

19. The following are correct of patients with Down's syndrome:
    a. Birth weight is increased
    b. Trisomy 21 abnormality is universal
    c. Hyperthyroidism is common
    d. Atrial septal defects are the most common cardiac anomaly
    e. It is the most common chromosomal disorder in the UK

20. The pin-index values listed are correct:
    a. Air: Positions 1 and 5
    b. O_2: Positions 2 and 6
    c. CO_2: Positions 1 and 6
    d. N_2O: Positions 2 and 5
    e. Entonox: Position 5

21. The sympathetic nervous system:
    a. Supplies postganglionic fibres to the coeliac plexus via the greater splanchnic nerve
    b. Provides outflow from the spinal cord from the lateral horns of T2–L1
    c. Supplies the cervical sympathetic ganglia with white rami originating from the thoracic levels only
    d. Causes vasoconstriction of the vertebral artery and its branches via the inferior cervical ganglion
    e. Is potentiated by digoxin in high doses

22. Base SI units include:
    a. Kelvin
    b. Ampere
    c. Watt
    d. Joule
    e. Kilogram

23. Physiological changes in pregnancy include:
    a. Reduction in plasma cholinesterase
    b. Reduction in minimum alveolar concentration (MAC) values at sea level
    c. Microcytic anaemia
    d. Reduction in antithrombin II levels
    e. Significant reduction in gastric emptying

24. Dalteparin:
    a. Is depolymerized heparin
    b. Is safe in renal failure
    c. Bioavailability is 90% following subcutaneous injection
    d. Is strongly basic
    e. Is active against factor Xa and factor IIa

25. Predictors for mortality without transplantation in a patient with hepatic encephalopathy are:
    a. Prothrombin time (PT) >100 s
    b. Serum bilirubin >225 μmol/L
    c. Age <40 years
    d. Hepatitis B
    e. Paracetamol toxicity associated with blood pH <7.3

26. A patient on ICU, admitted for respiratory failure, develops severe sepsis; contraindications to the administration of recombinant human activated protein C (rhAPC) include:
    a. Epidural catheter in situ
    b. Haemorrhagic stroke 6 months ago
    c. Platelet count <100 × 10^9/L
    d. Intracranial neoplasm
    e. Multi-organ failure

27. A patient is admitted with an Addisonian crisis; the following features are expected:
    a. Hypertension
    b. Hypokalaemia
    c. Hypernatraemia
    d. Hyperglycaemia
    e. Pyrexia

28. Beck's triad consists of:
    a. Tachycardia
    b. Hypotension
    c. Retrosternal pain
    d. Narrowed pulse pressure
    e. Muffled heart sounds

29. The following factors increase the risk of electrocution in the operating theatre:
    a. Current of high rather than low frequency
    b. Earthed patient contact
    c. Capacitative coupling
    d. Line isolation monitor
    e. High humidity

30. **Dobutamine:**
    a. Is a naturally occurring catecholamine
    b. Is an analogue of dopexamine
    c. Increases sinoatrial node automaticity
    d. Is contraindicated in aortic stenosis
    e. Is metabolized by monoamine oxidase (MAO)

31. **Concerning measurement of body fluid volumes:**
    a. Plasma volume can be measured with radiolabelled albumin
    b. Intracellular volume can be measured directly with deuterium oxide
    c. Extracellular fluid volume can be measured using mannitol
    d. Extracellular fluid volume is most accurately measured with inulin
    e. Intersititial fluid volume cannot be measured directly

32. **Concerning body weight:**
    a. Ideal body weight can be calculated using Broca's index
    b. Lean body weight is the weight of all the soft tissue organs, excluding bone and fat
    c. Suxamethonium should be dosed according to ideal body weight
    d. The Devine formula for ideal body weight takes age into account
    e. Body surface area can be calculated from the Mosteller formula

33. **A mountain climber ascends to an altitude of 3500 m in 12 hours; the following would be expected:**
    a. Lower percentage of inspired oxygen than at sea level
    b. Hypoxic pulmonary vasoconstriction
    c. High-altitude pulmonary oedema
    d. Alkaline urine
    e. Cheyne–Stokes breathing pattern during sleep

34. **The following is correct of renal replacement therapy (RRT):**
    a. Synthetic haemofilters are associated with superior outcomes
    b. For veno-venous catheters the 'arterial' port removes blood from holes on the side
    c. Patients with a platelet count $<80 \times 10^9$/L should receive prostacyclin
    d. Haemofiltration is based on the principle of diffusion
    e. Improvement in outcome has been demonstrated in septic shock

35. **Recognized risk factors for post-extubation stridor (PES) in ICU include:**
    a. Obesity
    b. Large endotracheal tubes
    c. Presence of a nasogastric tube
    d. Myasthenia gravis
    e. Intubation for more than 36 hours

36. **Risk factors for developing a postpartum haemorrhage (PPH) include:**
    a. Multiple pregnancy
    b. Prolonged labour
    c. Polyhydramnios
    d. Previous PPH
    e. Protein C deficiency

37. **A 65-year-old man presents for emergency surgery; on examination he has a slow-rising pulse and a loud ejection-systolic murmur; haemodynamic management for general anaesthesia includes:**
    a. Normal to high pulse rate
    b. Isoprenaline administration for persistent hypotension
    c. High to normal systemic vascular resistance (SVR)
    d. Low preload
    e. Atropine administration for heart rates <60/min

38. **The following statements regarding the measurement of lung volumes are correct:**
    a. A Vitalograph only measures expiratory volumes and flows
    b. Clinical measurements are performed at STP
    c. Functional residual capacity = residual volume + inspiratory reserve volume
    d. A Benedict–Roth is a 'wet'-type spirometer
    e. A Wright respirometer is inaccurate for continuous flow

39. **Doxapram:**
    a. Is contraindicated in thyrotoxicosis
    b. Causes an increase in cardiac output
    c. Can be given orally
    d. Is used as an adjunct for intubation
    e. Increases cerebral blood flow

40. **In evidence-based medicine:**
    a. Level Ib is based on at least one randomized controlled trial
    b. Level III is based on case reports
    c. Level IV is based on clinical experience of respected authorities
    d. Grade C recommendations are based on level III evidence
    e. Grade of recommendation does not reflect clinical importance of recommendation

41. **The following lead to an increase in pulmonary artery occlusion pressure (PAOP):**
    a. Mitral stenosis
    b. Acute respiratory distress syndrome (ARDS)
    c. Pulmonary fibrosis
    d. Left ventricular failure
    e. Use of positive end-expiratory pressure (PEEP)

42. Concerning the vertebrae:
    a. The gap between the odontoid peg and atlas is normally ≤5 mm in children
    b. Intervertebral joints are synovial
    c. The anterior longitudinal ligament connects C1 to the sacrum
    d. Ligamentum flavum connects the laminae of adjacent vertebrae
    e. The vertebral artery does not pass through the foramen transversarium of C7

43. A 74-year-old man is admitted to the ICU following return of spontaneous circulation (ROSC) after a prolonged in-hospital asystolic cardiac arrest. He is comatose and normothermic; reliable predictors of outcome include:
    a. Absent motor responses on day 1 post-arrest
    b. Burst suppression on electroencephalography
    c. His age
    d. Absent corneal reflexes on day 1 post-arrest
    e. The circumstances surrounding his cardiac arrest

44. National Institute of Health and Clinical Excellence (NICE) Guidelines recommend immediate CT scanning in head-injured adult patients with the following criteria:
    a. >1 episode of vomiting
    b. Amnesia for all events following impact
    c. GCS <13 on immediate examination
    d. Battle's sign
    e. GCS <14 on assessment in A&E 1 hour following injury

45. Duchenne's muscular dystrophy:
    a. Is a sex-linked recessive condition
    b. Typically presents at the age of 7 years
    c. Is associated with normal plasma creatine kinase (CK) levels
    d. Is associated with severe kyphoscoliosis
    e. Is commonly associated with autonomic dysfunction

46. Heart failure during pregnancy can be safely treated with:
    a. Digoxin
    b. Diuretics
    c. ACE inhibitors
    d. Nitrates
    e. Hydralazine

47. **Regarding oxygen measurement:**
    a. Beer's law states that the absorption of radiation by a given thickness of a solution of given concentration is the same as that of twice the thickness of solution of half the concentration
    b. Lambert's law states that each layer of equal thickness absorbs an equal fraction of radiation that passes through it
    c. The isobestic point depends on haemoglobin concentration and temperature
    d. Oxygen is a paramagnetic gas
    e. Clark's electrode consists of an Ag/AgCl anode and a gold mesh cathode

48. **With regard to a sub-Tenon's block:**
    a. Tenon's capsule fuses posteriorly with the dura of the optic nerve
    b. Warfarin therapy constitutes an absolute contraindication
    c. Globe perforation is not a risk
    d. Akinesia is volume-dependent of local anaesthetic
    e. It is ineffective anaesthesia for vitreoretinal surgery

49. **Injury of the ulnar nerve at the elbow results in:**
    a. A claw hand deformity worse than ulnar lesions at the wrist
    b. Paralysis of the medial half of the flexor digitorum profundus
    c. Inability to flex the wrist joint
    d. Inability to abduct the thumb
    e. Paralysis of the 3rd and 4th lumbricals causing hyperextension of the metacarpophalangeal joints

50. **Ketamine:**
    a. Is a pentazocine derivative
    b. Is contraindicated in porphyria
    c. Acts by competitive antagonism of NMDA receptors
    d. Does not affect postoperative nausea and vomiting
    e. Increases circulating catecholamine levels

51. **The following are boundaries of the femoral triangle:**
    a. Fascia iliaca forms the roof
    b. The inguinal ligament forms the superomedial border
    c. The lateral border is the medial border of sartorius
    d. The femoral vein lies outside the femoral sheath
    e. The psoas muscle forms part of the floor

52. **American College of Cardiology/American Heart Association guidelines (2003) state that the following are Category I indications for echocardiography in the critically ill patient:**
    a. Suspected myocardial contusion
    b. Haemodynamic instability
    c. Suspected aortic dissection
    d. Suspected pericardial tamponade
    e. Follow-up investigation in major trauma

53. **Regarding subarachnoid haemorrhage (SAH):**
    a. It occurs more frequently in women
    b. WFNS Grade 1–2 patients should be treated with surgical clipping
    c. Risk factors include smoking
    d. WFNS Grade 4–5 patients should be intubated and ventilated
    e. The highest risk of re-bleeding is at days 3–7 following haemorrhage

54. **Regarding a child with patent ductus arteriosus (PDA):**
    a. Treatment consists of indometacin
    b. True persistence is recognized after 1 month
    c. Accounts for 30% of congenital heart disease
    d. Thoracotomy, when performed, is usually right-sided
    e. Cyanosis is an early sign

55. **Necrotizing fasciitis:**
    a. Is polymicrobial in type I infections
    b. Is most commonly caused by group B streptococci
    c. Speed of spread is directly proportional to the thickness of the subcutaneous layer
    d. Is an absolute indication for surgery
    e. Leads to tissue destruction due to release of exotoxins

56. **The Wright respirometer:**
    a. Is used for measuring forced expiratory volumes
    b. Consists of a vane moved by gas flow
    c. Has a vane that rotates in both directions
    d. Measures continuous flow accurately
    e. Produces an electrical output for analysis

57. **Clonidine can be used for:**
    a. Intravenous regional anaesthesia (IVRA)
    b. Menopausal flushing
    c. Control of high intracranial pressure
    d. Seizure control
    e. Migraine

58. **Regarding heat loss during anaesthesia:**
    a. The linear phase precedes the redistribution phase
    b. Patients with autonomic neuropathy do not exhibit the plateau phase
    c. Both general and regional anaesthesia are causes
    d. Specific heat capacity of blood is 1.2 kJ kg^{-1} °C^{-1}
    e. Convection is the primary method under anaesthesia

59. The following is correct of the lumbar plexus:
    a. It is formed by T12–L4 roots
    b. The femoral and obturator nerves have the same origins
    c. The lateral cutaneous nerve of the thigh is formed from L3–4
    d. The genitofemoral nerve receives a contribution from T12
    e. The ilioinguinal and iliohypogastric nerves receive contributions from T12 and L1

60. Sodium:
    a. Is the principal extracellular anion
    b. Is mainly reabsorbed in the distal convoluted tubule
    c. Antidiuretic hormone (ADH) is released in response to serum osmolality of 280 mOsm/kg
    d. Correction can cause central pontine myelinolysis, which is diagnosed by CT
    e. Daily requirements are 0.1 mmol kg^{-1} day^{-1} in an adult

61. Fondaparinux:
    a. Is derived from heparin
    b. Has antithrombin activity
    c. Causes heparin-induced thrombocytopenia (HIT)
    d. Is safe in renal failure
    e. Is not reversed by protamine

62. A young man is brought to A&E following a motorcycle accident. He is very pale, hypotensive and tachycardic and complaining of difficulty breathing, with left-sided chest pain. The following is correct:
    a. Stony dullness is a likely finding on left chest examination
    b. Hyperresonance is a likely finding on left chest examination
    c. Definite absence of tracheal deviation excludes tension pneumothorax
    d. Spinal shock is likely
    e. A mediastinum >8 cm width at the aortic arch on chest X-ray is abnormal

63. Regarding Nissen's fundoplication:
    a. It is an effective treatment for a primary oesophageal carcinoma
    b. Mortality rate is less than 1%
    c. Dumping syndrome is a recognized postoperative risk
    d. Achalasia is effectively treated
    e. Patients who require fundoplication are at increased risk of bronchiectasis

64. Proximal muscle weakness is classically a feature of:
    a. Polymyositis
    b. Guillain–Barré syndrome
    c. Polymyalgia rheumatica
    d. Hypothyroidism
    e. Huntington's disease

65. The following is correct of intravenous cannulae:
    a. Flow rates are calculated through 110 cm tubing at a pressure of 10 kPa
    b. Flow rates are calculated using sterile 0.9% saline at 22°C
    c. 16 G cannulae have flow rates of 130–220 mL/min
    d. G is based on the wire-gauge system
    e. G is based on the French gauge system

66. In invasive arterial pressure monitoring:
    a. The fundamental frequency of the pressure waveform is equal to the heart rate
    b. The fundamental frequency is the frequency at which the monitoring system resonates
    c. Critical damping has a damping factor of 1
    d. The natural frequency should be within the range of the fundamental frequency
    e. Resonance is more likely with a highly non-compliant system

67. In the management of severe local anaesthetic toxicity:
    a. Seizures should be controlled with a phenytoin infusion
    b. Arrhythmias should be managed using standard protocols
    c. In the event of cardiac arrest an intravenous bolus of Intralipid 20% 5 mL/kg should be administered
    d. Propofol is a suitable substitute for Intralipid
    e. Cases from the UK must be reported to the National Patient Safety Agency

68. Prevention of catheter-related bloodstream infection (CRBSI) in central lines should include:
    a. Use of multiple-lumen catheters
    b. Preferable cannulation of the subclavian vein
    c. Cutaneous asepsis
    d. Routine tunnelling of lines
    e. Replacement of central lines every 5 days

69. Concerning laryngeal innervation:
    a. All innervation is derived from the vagus nerve
    b. The cricothyroid muscle is innervated by the recurrent laryngeal nerve
    c. The right recurrent laryngeal nerve runs below and posterior to the right subclavian artery
    d. Complete section of both external laryngeal nerves results in a cadaveric position of the vocal cords
    e. Partial section of the recurrent laryngeal nerve results in a hoarse voice

70. **The following are correct of sevoflurane:**
    a. It is a halogenated methyl ether
    b. MW = 200.1
    c. BP = 48.5°C
    d. SVP (20°C) = 32 kPa
    e. Oil : gas partition coefficient = 80

71. **Teicoplanin:**
    a. Is highly effective against Gram-positive bacteria
    b. Can be given to penicillin-allergic patients
    c. Is an aminoglycoside
    d. Is effective against MRSA
    e. Has predominantly bacteriocidal properties

72. **A man presents to A&E with stridor after being extracted from a house fire; he has burns to the face and torso. The following management is appropriate:**
    a. Rapid sequence induction using suxamethonium
    b. Asleep fibreoptic intubation
    c. Crystalloid fluid therapy of 4 mL/kg per % body surface area (BSA) burn given over the first 24 hours
    d. Immediate escharotomy to relieve stridor
    e. Prophylactic antibiotics

73. **The Q-wave on the ECG:**
    a. Represents septal repolarization
    b. In lead III is a normal finding
    c. Is pathological if ≥25% of the height of the succeeding R-wave
    d. Is normal if width is ≤0.03 seconds
    e. Is always associated with abnormal ST elevation in acute myocardial infarction

74. **In the management of heart failure (HF):**
    a. Digoxin should be considered as add-on therapy for symptomatic patients in sinus rhythm
    b. Cardiac resynchronization therapy is recommended
    c. Patients are often hyponatraemic
    d. Diuretics improve survival
    e. A left ventricular ejection fraction (LVEF) <35% is a predictor of perioperative mortality and morbidity

75. **Regarding the Clark electrode:**
    a. The anode is silver/silver chloride
    b. The cathode is platinum
    c. Electrons formed at the cathode move towards the anode to combine with oxygen
    d. There is a plastic membrane separating the anode from direct contact with blood
    e. False low readings may be seen in the presence of halothane

76. Appropriate management of a bleeding patient following 'on-pump' coronary artery bypass surgery includes:
    a. Return to theatre for resternotomy
    b. Administration of aprotinin
    c. Administration of protamine
    d. Platelet transfusion
    e. Clamping of surgical drains

77. The following agents cause epileptiform activity on EEG monitoring:
    a. Desflurane
    b. Propofol
    c. Enflurane
    d. Suxamethonium
    e. Methohexitone

78. Critical temperature:
    a. Is the temperature at which a gas cannot be liquefied no matter how much pressure is applied
    b. Is the temperature at which the latent heat of vaporization is zero
    c. A substance exists as a vapour above the boiling point but below the critical temperature
    d. Of CO_2 is $31°C$
    e. Of O_2 is $-180°C$

79. A patient with a haemoglobin (Hb) of 6 g/dL would be expected to have the following:
    a. Left shift in the oxyhaemoglobin dissociation curve
    b. Decreased mixed-venous oxygen saturation
    c. Decreased arterial oxygen saturation
    d. Increased mixed-venous oxygen content
    e. Increase in 2,3-DPG levels

80. Extracorporeal membrane oxygenation (ECMO):
    a. Can be discontinued in adults at flows of 5 L/min
    b. Shows most benefit for patients requiring $FiO_2 > 0.8$ for >7 days
    c. Has undergone cost–benefit analysis in the CESAR trial
    d. Carries embolization as its main risk
    e. Is not appropriate for patients with pulmonary fibrosis

81. Initial management of a bleeding patient following a warfarin overdose includes:
    a. Administration of 50 mL/kg fresh frozen plasma (FFP)
    b. Administration of recombinant factor VIIa
    c. Replacement of clotting factors II, VII, IX and X
    d. Administration of protamine
    e. Administration of tranexamic acid

82. Features of systemic lupus erythematosus (SLE) include:
    a. Autoantibodies to β_2-glycoprotein
    b. False-positive test for syphilis
    c. Discoid rash
    d. Association with human leukocyte antigen (HLA) B27
    e. Increased serum complement

83. A 58-year-old man presents with a 5-day history of a hot, swollen, tender knee with a restricted range of movement; he is afebrile. The following are appropriate:
    a. Empirical antibiotics should be given immediately
    b. Joint aspiration should not be performed if the patient is taking warfarin
    c. Measurement of serum urate concentration is not indicated
    d. MRI is the imaging modality of choice
    e. Intra-articular steroids should be administered

84. The following are consistent with a diagnosis of diabetes insipidus (DI):
    a. Plasma sodium of 155 mmol/L
    b. Urinary sodium of 170 mmol/L
    c. Urine specific gravity of <1.005
    d. Plasma osmolality of 325 mOsm/kg
    e. Urine osmolality of 450 mOsm/kg

85. A 12-year-old boy presents to A&E with a penetrating eye injury; the following statements are correct:
    a. The intraocular pressure (IOP) of the injured eye is atmospheric
    b. Isoflurane will reduce IOP
    c. Suxamethonium is contraindicated
    d. Ketamine is a useful agent for induction of anaesthesia
    e. The rise in IOP following suxamethonium is sustained for 6–8 hours

86. In the lateral position:
    a. There is increased compliance of the non-dependent lung in an awake patient
    b. The non-dependent lung is better ventilated under anaesthesia
    c. Perfusion is greater in the dependent lung under anaesthesia
    d. Functional residual capacity (FRC) is greater in the non-dependent lung in an awake patient
    e. Ventilation/perfusion $(\dot{V}/\dot{Q})$ mismatch is greater than in the supine position under anaesthesia

87. The following anaesthetic techniques are appropriate for a patient with a complete C7 spinal cord section presenting for elective cystoscopy and urethral stricture dilation:
    a. Spinal anaesthesia
    b. Epidural anaesthesia
    c. No anaesthesia is needed since the procedure is below the level of the lesion
    d. General anaesthesia
    e. Topical anaesthesia only

88. The cranial efferents of the parasympathetic nervous system consist of the:
    a. Optic nerve
    b. Vagus nerve
    c. Vestibulocochlear nerve
    d. Glossopharyngeal nerve
    e. Trigeminal nerve

89. The following are correct of amniotic fluid embolism (AFE):
    a. The majority present in labour
    b. Signs include hypertension
    c. Risk factors include primiparity
    d. Cases should be reported to the National Audit Project
    e. It is a cause of direct death only

90. A 55-year-old man presents for emergency surgery for a ruptured abdominal aortic aneurysm; he lost consciousness on arrival to A&E and investigations show sinus tachycardia (no ischaemia) on ECG, haemoglobin 10 g/dL, creatinine 200 μmol/L. The following applies:
    a. The Hardmann Index Score is 3
    b. He has a predicted mortality of 80%
    c. Cigarette smoking is the single most important risk factor for disease progression
    d. 10 units of packed red cells should be cross-matched
    e. Intraoperative hypothermia is indicated to reduce blood loss

5. Practice Paper 5: Answers

1a. True
1b. False
1c. True
1d. True
1e. False
Antiretroviral drugs fall into three categories according to the part of the retrovirus life-cycle that they inhibit:

- *NRTI* (nucleoside reverse transcriptase inhibitors): inhibit synthesis of DNA by reverse transcriptase by acting as a false nucleotide (e.g. zidovudine, didanosine); may cause gastrointestinal upset and less commonly neurological or hepatic impairment
- *NNRTI* (non-nucleoside reverse transcriptase inhibitors): bind to reverse transcriptase and inhibit enzyme activity (e.g. nevirapine)
- *PI* (protease inhibitors): prevent the processing of viral proteins into functional forms (e.g. indinavir, ritonavir); may have the same side-effects as NRTIs; may also cause inhibition of hepatic cytochrome p450 and thus cause interaction with other drugs

A typical therapeutic regimen comprises three agents: two NRTIs combined with one PI/NNRTI. It is also called highly active antiretroviral therapy (HAART) and the aim is to achieve an undetectable viral load and prolong duration and quality of life. HAART is recommended for individuals with WHO stage III or IV disease irrespective of CD4 counts, and should be considered in asymptomatic individuals with CD4 counts <350 cells/mm^3.

Cook GC, Zumla A. *Manson's Tropical Diseases*. London: Elsevier Health Sciences, 2008.
Prout J, Agarwal B. Anaesthesia and critical care for patients with HIV infection. *Contin Educ Anaesth Crit Care Pain* 2005; 5: 153–6.

2a. False
2b. True
2c. True
2d. True
2e. False
The following conditions are characteristically associated with the vitamin deficiencies:

Vitamin A:	Night blindness, xerophthalmia, dry skin
Vitamin B$_1$ (thiamin):	Beriberi, neuritis
Vitamin B$_2$ (riboflavin):	Glossitis, angular stomatitis
Vitamin B$_3$ (niacin):	Pellagra (diarrhoea, dermatitis, dementia)
Vitamin B$_6$ (pyridoxine):	Convulsions, hyper-irritability
Folates:	Sprue, anaemia, neural tube defects in pregnancy
Vitamin B$_{12}$ (cyanocobalamin):	Pernicious anaemia
Vitamin C:	Scurvy

Vitamin D:	Rickets
Vitamin E:	Muscular dystrophy
Vitamin K:	Bleeding diathesis

Hypervitaminosis A leads to hepatosplenomegaly due to excessive vitamin A intake (retinoids) overwhelming liver storage sites.

Ganong W. *Review of Medical Physiology*, 22nd edn. Maidenhead: McGraw-Hill Medical, 2005.

3a. False
3b. False
3c. True
3d. False
3e. False
The saphenous nerve is the terminal branch of the femoral nerve, supplying sensation to the skin of the medial knee, calf and shin, and medial forefoot; the superficial peroneal nerve supplies the majority of forefoot sensation. The lateral cutaneous nerve of the thigh is a branch of the lumbar plexus (L2, 3) supplying the lateral skin of the thigh. The deep peroneal nerve accompanies the anterior tibial vessels and lies lateral to the more medial dorsalis pedis artery in the foot. The sural nerve arises in the popliteal fossa as a branch of the tibial nerve and runs with the short saphenous vein to lie behind the lateral malleolus, supplying sensation to the lower lateral aspect of the calf and lateral foot.

4a. False
4b. False
4c. True
4d. True
4e. False
Thiopentone is a thiobarbiturate, while methohexitone is a methylated oxy-barbiturate. It is formulated as the sodium salt and prepared with 6% sodium carbonate; it is stored in nitrogen to reduce acidification and prevent formation of the undissociated acid. It has a pK_a of 7.6 and a pH of 10.5, and therefore is 60% un-ionized at physiological pH. It is metabolized by side-chain oxidation, to carbon fragments, pentobarbitone and urea, and induces liver enzymes.

5a. False
5b. True
5c. True
5d. False
5e. False
Optimal positioning for surgery is a compromise between best surgical access and patient safety. Prone positioning leads to a reduction in cardiac index, while mean arterial pressure is maintained through increased systemic vascular resistance. Abdominal compression presents a risk of abdominal compartment syndrome and vena cava compression leads to reduction in cardiac output and increased venous pressure with subsequent increased blood loss. Prone positioning has been used to improve $\dot{V}/\dot{Q}$ matching and

oxygenation in acute lung injury (ALI) and acute respiratory distress syndrome (ARDS) and consistently leads to an increase in functional residual capacity with reportedly unchanged compliance. Ocular injury is rare in anaesthesia; however, the most common complication is reported to be corneal abrasions in any position, with pressure injury and visual loss occurring with a reported incidence of 0.0008%, primarily owing to ischaemic neuropathy and central retinal artery occlusion. Careful positioning and adequate padding minimizes the risks associated with this position. The upper limbs should maintain slight anterior flexion and should be abducted and externally rotated to no more than 90°.

Edgcombe H, Carter K, Yarrow S. Anaesthesia in prone position. *Br J Anaesth* 2008; **100**: 165–83.

6a. False
6b. True
6c. True
6d. False
6e. True
Mapleson classified modern breathing systems into A, B, C, D and E (see Figure 5.1). Mapleson F was added after a revision to the classification. Mapleson A (Magill) is efficient for spontaneous ventilation (requiring an FGF

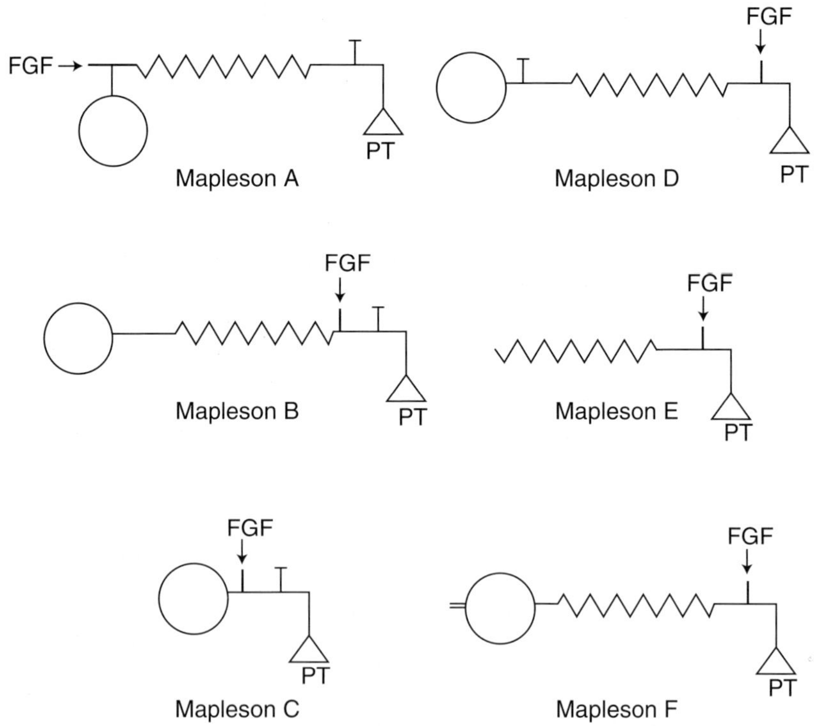

FIGURE 5.1   Mapleson's classification of breathing systems. FGF, fresh gas flow; PT, patient.

of 70–100 mL kg^{-1} min^{-1}) and inefficient for controlled ventilation (requiring an FGF three times minute alveolar ventilation). The coaxial version of Mapleson A is the Lack, which is also efficient for spontaneous ventilation. Mapleson D (Bain) is efficient for mechanical ventilation (FGF of 70–100 mL kg^{-1} min^{-1}), but requires FGF of 150–200 mL kg^{-1} min^{-1} for spontaneous ventilation. Mapleson B and C are used for remote locations or resuscitation and require 1.5–2 times minute volume for spontaneous ventilation.

Al-Shaikh B, Stacey S. *Essentials of Anaesthetic Equipment*, 3rd edn. London: Churchill Livingstone, 2007.

7a. False
7b. False
7c. True
7d. False
7e. False
A subdural block is an uncommon complication of epidural anaesthesia/analgesia and occurs when the catheter is placed between the dura and the arachnoid mater. Incidence is 1 : 1000 and it can be diagnosed definitively only by radiological methods (X-ray/CT contrast). The block has a classically slow onset, and can be widespread although patchy and asymmetrical with sparing of the motor fibres of the lower limb.

Eldridge J. Obstetric anaesthesia and analgesia. In: Allman KG, Wilson IH, eds. *Oxford Handbook of Anaesthesia*, 2nd edn. Oxford: OUP, 2006.

8a. True
8b. True
8c. True
8d. True
8e. False
Varices are portosystemic venous collaterals developed owing to elevated portal pressures ($>$12 mmHg). The vast majority of varices in the UK are a result of cirrhosis, but worldwide the main cause is schistosomiasis resulting in hepatic fibrosis. Management should follow an ABC approach initially. Following airway protection, an endotracheal tube facilitates placement of a Sengstaken–Blakemore tube; this tube possesses oesophageal and gastric balloons that are inflated to provide tamponade to bleeding varices. Balloon tamponade stops the bleeding in about 90% of cases and is used as a bridging measure before more definitive management. Pharmacological management consists of intravenous vasopressin or terlipressin to constrict mesenteric vessels; concurrent glyceryl trinitrate administration counters coronary vasoconstriction. A nasogastric tube can be placed with reasonable safety and reduces the risk of aspiration via gastric decompression. If bleeding continues after 2–3 days following attempts at control with balloon tamponade or endoscopic sclerotherapy, transjugular intrahepatic portosystemic stented shunt (TIPSS) may be performed. Surgical management includes portocaval anastamosis, which carries a greater risk of encephalopathy or oesophageal transection. β-blockade is beneficial as primary prophylaxis, to reduce cardiac output and blood flow within the splanchnic circulation, thereby reducing

portal pressure. It is not indicated as treatment in the acute setting of bleeding varices.

McKay R, Webster NR. Variceal bleeding. *Contin Educ Anaesth Crit Care Pain* 2007; 7: 191–4.
Singer M, Webb AR. *Oxford Handbook of Critical Care*, 3rd edn. Oxford: OUP, 2009.

9a. True
9b. True
9c. False
9d. False
9e. False
The Holiday and Segar paediatric fluid regimen uses the '4–2–1' calculation. Thus maintenance fluid is transfused at 4 mL kg^{-1} h^{-1} for the first 10 kg; 2 mL kg^{-1} h^{-1} for the next 10 kg and 1 mL kg^{-1} h^{-1} thereafter. Maintenance requirements make no allowance for sensible losses (diarrhoea, intestinal obstruction) or insensible losses (pyrexia). Added electrolytes include sodium at 3 mmol kg^{-1} day^{-1} and potassium at 2 mmol kg^{-1} day^{-1}. Up to 30 mmol kg^{-1} day^{-1} of fluid is added for infants receiving phototherapy. National Patient Safety Agency Alert 22 states that the maintenance fluids used for paediatric patients should not be hypotonic (glucose 4%, sodium 0.18%, glucose 5%, glucose 10%, sodium 0.45%, glucose 5%/sodium 0.45%), since their use can lead to severe hyponatraemia with potential mortality. Thus fluid used for maintenance or resuscitation should be 0.9% saline or Hartmann's solution.

National Patient Safety Agency. *Reducing the Risk of Hyponatraemia when Administering Intravenous Infusions to Children*, NPSA/2007/22. London: NPSA, 2007. Available at: www.nrls.npsa.nhs.uk/resources/ ?entryid45=59809.

10a. True
10b. False
10c. True
10d. True
10e. False
Inguinal field block targets:

- *Ilioinguinal nerve* (L1): found traversing the inguinal canal through the external ring
- *Iliohypogastric nerve* (L1): between the transversus abdominus and internal oblique
- *Genital branch of genitofemoral nerve* (L1/L2): entering the inguinal canal through the internal ring

Local anaesthetic infiltration should be performed at these points (in adults):

- 2 cm medial and inferior to the anterior superior iliac spine blocks ilioinguinal and iliohypogastric
- 1.5 cm above the midpoint of the inguinal ligament blocks genital branch of genitofemoral

- Subcutaneous infiltration at the symphysis pubis targets branches from the contralateral side
- Along incision site

Atkinson RS, Rushman GB, Davies NJH. *Lee's Synopsis of Anaesthesia*, 13th edn. Oxford: Butterworth-Heinemann, 2005.

11a. False
11b. True
11c. False
11d. True
11e. True
Paget's disease is characterized by marked increase in bone turnover in localized parts of the skeleton; excessive osteoclastic bone resorption is followed by disordered osteoblastic activity. This results in structurally abnormal and weak new bone formation leading to deformity and an increased risk of fracture and pain. The abnormal bone has increased metabolic activity and blood flow, which contributes to the pain. Serum biochemistry reveals raised alkaline phosphatase, with normal calcium and phosphate levels. In addition to biochemical changes, there are pressure effects (causing pain in other joints) and syndromes of nerve compression (including the skull, which can lead to deafness). Most patients are asymptomatic, with only 5% thought to be symptomatic.

Selby PL, Davie MWJ, Ralston SH, Stone MD. Guidelines on the management of Paget's disease of bone. *Bone* 2002; **31**: 10–19.

12a. True
12b. True
12c. False
12d. False
12e. True
Stridor is an airway emergency for which there are many causes. Priorities include avoidance of distress, since this can precipitate complete airway obstruction. A gentle examination including measurement of SpO_2 may be permitted. Intramuscular adrenaline is appropriate for the management of anaphylaxis; however, in a 2-year-old child the most likely causes are infection or inhaled foreign body. Heliox may be beneficial in providing better gas flow through a partial obstruction, due to its decreased density; however, it has an FiO_2 of 0.21, which limits its usefulness.

13a. False
13b. False
13c. True
13d. True
13e. True
Baroreceptors located within the carotid sinus and aortic arch are stretch receptors that mediate the baroreceptor reflex; this describes the lowering of heart rate and blood pressure in response to vessel distension caused by an increase in blood pressure. The glossopharyngeal and vagus nerves carry

afferent excitatory supply to the nucleus tractus solitarius within the medullary vasomotor centre. Inhibitory interneurons project from here to the C1 group of cells, which mediate increased sympathetic discharge to blood vessels and the heart. The net effect is a reduction in sympathetic outflow resulting in a temporary lowering of heart rate and blood pressure; the reflex is reset within approximately 30 minutes.

Ganong W. *Review of Medical Physiology*, 22nd edn. Maidenhead: McGraw-Hill Medical, 2005.

14a. True
14b. True
14c. True
14d. True
14e. True
O_2 is available as a compressed gas stored in cylinders, with a pressure of 137 bar at $15°C$. Cylinders are black with white shoulders and available in six sizes (C–J containing 170–8800 L). O_2 is explosive in the presence of grease. Its critical temperature is $-118.4°C$ and critical pressure 50.8 atm. The Paul–Bert effect describes acute oxygen neurotoxicity following administration of hyperbaric 100% O_2; symptoms include altered mood, vertigo, loss of consciousness and convulsions.

Sasada M, Smith S. *Drugs in Anaesthesia and Intensive Care*, 3rd edn. Oxford: OUP, 2003.

15a. True
15b. False
15c. True
15d. False
15e. True
Left-sided Macintosh blades are used for patients with right-sided facial deformities making the use of a standard right-sided blade difficult. The polio blade is mounted at an angle of 135° to the handle and was originally designed to intubate patients in a negative-pressure ventilator ('iron lung'). Magill and Miller are both straight blades, but Miller possesses a curved tip and a flatter flange and web. The Robertshaw blade has a straight tongue with a gentle curve near the tip and is designed to lift the epiglottis indirectly; it was designed for paediatric use.

Dorsch SA, Dorsch JE. *Understanding Anaesthesia Equipment*. Philadelphia: Lippincott Williams & Wilkins, 2008.

16a. False
16b. True
16c. True
16d. False
16e. True
The citric acid cycle (tricarboxylic acid cycle, Krebs cycle) is the final common pathway for oxidation of carbohydrate, fat and some amino acids to CO_2 and water. Acetyl-CoA enters the cycle to be metabolized, but may also form ketone bodies (acetone, acetoacetate and γ-hydroxybutyric acid) if present in excess or if a relative deficiency of oxaloacetate exists. Ketone bodies are normally utilized by the brain and heart, but levels increase when intracellular glucose is deficient or during starvation. DKA is a medical emergency and represents a life-threatening complication of diabetes mellitus. While normally associated with type 1 diabetes, it may occur in type 2 diabetes (although HONK – a hyperglycaemic, hyperosmolar non-ketotic state – is more likely). DKA occurs if insulin therapy is inappropriate for the physiological state or absent. Precipitants include infection, surgery or myocardial infarction. DKA manifests as severe uncontrolled diabetes and profound dehydration. Its management involves:

- Correction of dehydration with isotonic saline as a primary fluid not given too rapidly
- Intravenous insulin: critical for reducing ketosis; will decrease plasma glucose
- Early potassium replacement with frequent monitoring (total body potassium is likely to be low)
- When glucose levels are 10–15 mmol/L, add glucose-containing fluids (not more than 2 L in 24 hours) with higher rates of insulin infusions
- Treat the underlying illness

National Institute of Health and Clinical Excellence. *Diagnosis and Management of Type 1 Diabetes in Children, Young People and Adults.* London: NICE, 2004. Available at: guidance.nice.org.uk/CG15.

17a. True
17b. False
17c. False
17d. True
17e. True
Crystalloid resuscitation should involve balanced solutions such as Hartmann's to avoid hyperchloraemic acidosis, except in cases of hypochloraemia (Evidence level: **1b**). Patients in the perioperative period are at particular risk of developing conditions of sodium imbalance, and thus particular attention should be paid to the haemodynamic and fluid status, particularly when the urinary sodium concentration is <20 mmol/L (**1b**). In the absence of gastric-emptying disorders or diabetes, preoperative administration of carbohydrate-rich beverages 2–3 h before induction of anaesthesia may improve patient wellbeing and facilitate recovery from surgery. It should be considered in the routine preoperative preparation for elective surgery (**2a**). Based on current evidence, HMW hydroxyethylstarches (hetastarch and pentastarch, MW $\geq$200 kDa) should be avoided in patients with severe sepsis owing to an

increased risk of acute kidney injury (**1b**). These fluids should also be avoided in brain-dead kidney donors owing to reports of osmotic nephrosis-like lesions (**2b**).

Intensive Care Society. *British Consensus Guidelines on Intravenous Fluid Therapy for Adult Surgical Patients (GIFTASUP)*. London: ICS, 2009. Available at: www.ics.ac.uk.

18a. False
18b. True
18c. True
18d. True
18e. True

Botulism is a rare paralytic condition caused by the exotoxin of the Gram-positive anaerobe *Clostridium botulinum*; the toxin binds irreversibly to the pre-synaptic membrane of cholinergic neurons. Neurological signs begin with the cranial autonomics, causing diplopia, ptosis, dysphonia, facial weakness and bulbar palsy; in addition, nausea, vomiting and dry mouth are common. A descending flaccid paralysis ensues, leading to ventilatory failure with concomitant autonomic and motor nerve paralysis.

Wenham T, Cohen A. Botulism. *Contin Educ Anaesth Crit Care Pain* 2008; 8: 21–5.

19a. False
19b. False
19c. False
19d. False
19e. True

Described in 1866 by John Langdon Down, the syndrome is the most common chromosomal disorder, affecting 1 in 700 live births. There is an exponential increase in incidence with maternal age (1 in 1400 at 25 years; 1 in 46 by 45 years). Survival is approximately 90% at 1 year and 45% survive until the age of 60 years. 95% of individuals possess trisomy 21, 4% translocation and 1% mosaic trisomy 21. Down's syndrome is a multisystem condition. Features include:

General appearance

- Characteristic appearance: brachycephaly, flat nasal bridge, single palmar crease
- Low birth weight
- Obesity from childhood

Respiratory

- Dysfunctional central respiratory drive
- Subglottic or tracheal stenosis
- Recurrent lower respiratory tract infections
- Obstructive sleep apnoea secondary to craniofacial deformities

Cardiovascular

- Congenital heart disease (16–60%): commonly atrioventricular canal defects, atrial septal defects, ventricular septal defects (most commonly), patent ductus arteriosus and tetralogy of Fallot
- Pulmonary hypertension as a result of both shunts and obstructive sleep apnoea

Neurological

- Generalized hypotonia
- Laxity of joint ligaments
- Intellectual impairment (IQ 20–80)
- Epilepsy (10%)

Gastrointestinal

- Gastroesophageal reflux
- Anomalies (7%): obstruction, atresia, Hirschprung's

Others

- Immune system dysfunction making individuals prone to infections
- Polycythaemia (haematocrit values up to 70%)
- Hypothyroidism and type 1 diabetes are more common
- Atlantoaxial instability: excessive movement of spinal vertebrae can lead to compression of spinal cord in the spinal foramen

Allt JE, Howell CJ. Down's syndrome. *Contin Educ Anaesth Crit Care Pain* 2003; 3: 83–6.
Carvalho B. Miscellaneous problems. In: Allman KG, Wilson IH, eds. *Oxford Handbook of Anaesthesia*, 2nd edn. Oxford: OUP, 2006.

20a. True
20b. False
20c. True
20d. False
20e. False
The Pin Index System is an international system designed to prevent accidental connection of the wrong cylinder to yoke. The positions of holes on valve blocks are as follows:

Substance	Body colour	Shoulder colour	Pin index
Oxygen	Black	White	2 and 5
Helium	Brown	Brown	n/a
CO_2	Grey	Grey	1 and 6
Air	Grey	White/black check	1 and 5
N_2O	Blue	Blue	3 and 5
Entonox	Blue	White/blue check	7
Cyclopropane	Orange	Orange	3 and 6

Al-Shaikh B, Stacey S. *Essentials of Anaesthetic Equipment*, 3rd edn. London: Churchill Livingstone, 2007.

21a. False
21b. False
21c. True
21d. True
21e. True

The sympathetic outflow originates from the preganglionic cell bodies located within the lateral horns of the spinal cord from T1 to L2. These white rami communicantes enter the ganglia of the sympathetic chain; *preganglionic* fibres make up the greater splanchnic (T5–9), lesser splanchnic (T10–11) and least splanchnic nerves, which synapse in the coeliac, mesenteric and renal plexuses respectively; cardiac branches (T1–5) are postganglionic. Above the outflow level there are three cervical sympathetic ganglia: the superior, middle and inferior ganglia, which supply the head and neck with vasomotor, sudomotor, pilomotor and pupillary motor action. Preganglionic white rami communicantes connect the T1–L2 outflow with cervical ganglia above and lumbar ganglia below. Digoxin has dual autonomic effects, in addition to positive inotropy, it is also vagotonic and decreases conduction velocity through the atrioventricular (AV) node. Digoxin sensitizes the baroreceptors, thus reducing sympathetic activity for any given increase in arterial pressure; but potentiates sympathetic activity in higher doses, which may mediate aspects of digitalis toxicity.

Whitaker RH, Borley NR. *Instant Anatomy*, 3rd edn. Oxford: WileyBlackwell, 2005.

22a. True
22b. True
22c. False
22d. False
22e. True

The Système Internationale d'Unités (SI) is a system introduced in 1960 to standardize measurement. It is based on the metric system. The seven *base* SI units are: the metre, second, kilogram, ampere, kelvin, candela and mole. *Derived* units include the newton, pascal, joule, watt and hertz.

23a. True
23b. True
23c. False
23d. False
23e. False

The following physiological changes are seen in pregnancy:

Cardiovascular:	↑Cardiac output by 50% (↑35% stroke volume; ↑15% heart rate)
	↓Diastolic BP by mid-term, returning to pre-pregnant levels by term
	↓Systemic vascular resistance
	Significant aortocaval compression by the 20th week (or earlier)
Respiratory:	↑Minute ventilation by 50% at 2nd trimester (↑40% tidal volume; ↑15% respiratory rate)

	↓ Functional residual capacity (FRC) by 20%
	↓ Expiratory reserve volume, ↓ residual volume by mid-2nd trimester
	↓ $PaCO_2$
	↑ Oxygen consumption by 60%
Gastrointestinal:	Gastric emptying and acidity are little changed in pregnancy but significantly affected in labour
Renal:	↑ Renal blood flow by 75%
	↑ Glomerular filtration rate (GFR) by 50%
Central nervous system:	Greater susceptibility to local anaesthetics
	↓ MAC values
	↓ Plasma cholinesterase, but duration of succinyl choline little changed owing to ↑ volume of distribution
Haematological:	↑ Plasma volume by 50%
	↑ Red cell volume by 30%
	Physiological anaemia due to haemodilution
	Hypercoagulability due to ↑ factors I, VII, VIII, IX, X and XII
	↓ Antithrombin III levels

24a. True
24b. True
24c. True
24d. False
24e. True
Dalteparin (Fragmin) is a strongly acidic low-molecular-weight heparin (LMWH) with an average MW of 5000 Da. It works as an antithrombotic by potentiating the inhibition of factor Xa and factor IIa via antithrombin; it has a 4:1 activity against factor Xa compared with factor IIa. Onset of action is 1–2 hours and duration of action is >12 hours and is dose-related.

Douketis J, Cook D, Meade M, et al. Prophylaxis against deep vein thrombosis in critically ill patients with severe renal insufficiency with the low-molecular-weight heparin dalteparin. *Arch Intern Med* 2008; **168**: 1805–12.

25a. True
25b. True
25c. False
25d. False
25e. True
Patients unlikely to survive hepatic encephalopathy without transplantation can be identified by:

- PT >100 s

Or three of the following:

- age <10 or >40 years
- aetiology: hepatitis C, halothane, drug reaction
- duration of jaundice >2 days pre-encephalopathy
- PT >50 s
- serum bilirubin >225 μmol/L

When associated with paracetamol toxicity:

- pH <7.3 or PT >100 s and creatinine >200 μmol/L plus Grade 3 or 4 encephalopathy

Singer M, Webb AR. *Oxford Handbook of Critical Care*, 3rd edn. Oxford: OUP, 2009.

26a. True
26b. False
26c. False
26d. True
26e. False

In sepsis, the microcirculation undergoes unrestricted and/or inappropriate activation of coagulation and inflammatory pathways; the result is tissue hypoperfusion. Negative control of these pathways is through the protein C anticoagulation pathway (consisting of thrombin, thrombomodulin, endothelial protein C receptor, protein C and protein S). Activated protein C (APC) acts as a key regulator, restoring the microcirculation. rhAPC is a synthetic form of APC and is used in patients with severe sepsis with multi-organ failure. The PROWESS Trial (multicentre RCT, $n = 1690$) demonstrated an increased treatment effect as the number of dysfunctioning organs increased. There was, however, serious bleeding in both groups – mainly in those at a high risk of haemorrhage. Relative contraindications to administration of rhAPC include:

- current use of therapeutic anticoagulation
- active bleeding or coagulopathy
- platelet count <30 000
- recent major surgery
- recent (within 3 months) haemorrhagic stroke

- known hypersensitivity to rhAPC
- trauma with increased risk of bleeding
- epidural catheter
- intracranial mass or neoplasm
- recent (within 2 months) cranial procedure, spinal procedure or head trauma

The mortality benefit from PROWESS has not been replicated in all patient groups with severe sepsis. Coupled with the expense of rhAPC, this has led to the PROWESS Shock Trial, a second randomized double-blind placebo-controlled trial.

Bernard GR, Vincent JL, Laterre PF, et al. Efficacy and safety of recombinant human activated protein C for severe sepsis. *N Engl J Med* 2005; **344**: 699–709.
Shanker Hari M, Wyncoll D. Activated protein C. In: Waldmann N, Soni N, Rhodes A, eds. *Oxford Desk Reference: Critical Care*. Oxford: OUP, 2008.

27a. False
27b. False
27c. False
27d. False
27e. True
An Addisonian crisis is a potentially life-threatening condition caused by acute glucocorticoid (and to a lesser extent mineralocorticoid) deficiency. In chronic insufficiency states, a crisis can be precipitated by an acute stress or inter-current illness whereby the ability to secrete glucocorticoids is exceeded by demand. Most commonly the cause is abrupt cessation of steroid therapy coupled with hypothalamo–pituitary and adrenal suppression; other causes include adrenal destruction due to haemorrhage, infection (tuberculosis) or autoimmune disease. Features include the sequelae of gluco- and minera-locorticoid deficiency: *hypotension* unresponsive to catecholamines, *hyperka-laemia*, *hyponatraemia* (may be normal) and *hypoglycaemia*. Pyrexia is common and may be due to an underlying infection.

Chin R. Adrenal crisis. *Crit Care Clin* 1991; 7: 23–42.

28a. False
28b. True
28c. False
28d. False
28e. True
Cardiac tamponade is a result of fluid within the pericardium, which results in cardiac compression. Ventricular filling is restricted, with a decrease in stroke volume and cardiac output. Tamponade may present with Beck's triad:

* *hypotension*: impaired ventricular filling and reduced stroke volume
* *jugular venous distension*: impaired venous return to the heart
* *muffled heart sounds*: presence of pericardial fluid

Other signs include tachycardia, breathlessness, pulsus paradoxus (reduction in blood pressure of ≥ 10 mmHg on inspiration), narrowed pulse pressure and low-voltage QRS complexes on the ECG. Immediate management should consist of pericardiocentesis.

29a. False
29b. True
29c. True
29d. False
29e. False
Electrocution or macroshock can result from completion of an electrical circuit through bodily contact with two conducting parts at different voltage potentials. The effect of the current on the body depends on the *current density, duration of contact, current frequency* (higher frequencies present less hazard) and also on *location* of contact. An earthed patient represents a path for current completion; thus isolation transformers are used to isolate the operating theatre power supply from the patient. Two live unearthed lines exist for use with operating equipment; thus line isolation monitors are used to measure the potential for current flow from the isolated wire to earth.

An alarm is actuated if the current detected is high (2–5 mA); a circuit breaker interrupts flow in such circumstances, but these are not usually incorporated in operating theatre power supplies. Conductive flooring increases risk of electrical hazard; capacitive coupling occurs when electrosurgical equipment induces stray currents in nearby conductors. High levels of humidity (>50%) significantly reduce the risk of sparking .

Morgan GE, Mikhail MS, Murray MJ. *Clinical Anesthesiology*. New York: McGraw-Hill Medical, 2005.

30a. False
30b. False
30c. True
30d. True
30e. False
Dobutamine is a synthetic catecholamine derivative of isoprenaline; dopexamine is a synthetic analogue of dopamine. Cardiovascular effects include increases in cardiac contractility and sinoatrial node automaticity resulting in an increased heart rate via its actions on β_1-receptors. It also has action at β_2-receptors, causing a reduction in systemic vascular resistance and left ventricular diastolic pressure. It should not be used in patients with cardiac outflow obstruction and is metabolized rapidly by catechol O-methyl transferase (COMT), and thus is a safer option in patients taking MAO inhibitors.

Sasada M, Smith S. *Drugs in Anaesthesia and Intensive Care*, 3rd edn. Oxford: OUP, 2003.

31a. True
31b. False
31c. True
31d. True
31e. True
Total body water comprises 60% of body weight, which equates to 42 L in an average 70 kg man; this is divided into intracellular fluid (ICF: 40% body weight) and extracellular fluid (ECF: 20% body weight). ECF can be further subdivided into plasma (5%) and interstitial fluid (15%). Plasma volume can be measured using dyes bound to plasma proteins or using radiolabelled albumin. ECF can be measured using inulin, a polysaccharide with a molecular weight of 5200 Da, which is also used to accurately measure glomerular filtration rate since it is completely filtered at the glomerulus and not reabsorbed by the tubules; mannitol and sucrose can also be used to measure ECF. Interstitial and ICF volume cannot be measured directly and are calculated by subtraction. Deuterium oxide (heavy water) is used to measure total body water, from which ECF is subtracted to obtain a value for ICF volume.

Ganong W. *Review of Medical Physiology*, 22nd edn. Maidenhead: McGraw-Hill Medical, 2005.

32a. True
32b. False
32c. False
32d. False
32e. True

Broca's index:
Weight (kg) should equal Height (cm) − 100, ±15% for women or 10% for men

The Devine formula:
Men: Ideal body weight (IBW) (kg) = 50 + 2.3 kg per inch over 5 feet
Women: IBW (kg) = 45.5 + 2.3 kg per inch over 5 feet

The Mosteller formula:
Body surface area (BSA) (m^2) = [Height (cm) × Weight (kg)/3600]$^{1/2}$

Both Broca's index and Devine's formula are formulae for calculation of ideal body weight, but neither incorporates any method to allow for age. Lean body weight is the weight of all the organs, bone and muscles without fat.

Mosteller RD. Simplified calculation of body surface area. *N Engl J Med* 1987; 317: 1098.
Pai MP, Paloucek FP. The origin of the 'Ideal' body weight equations. *Ann Pharmacol* 2000; 34: 1066–9.

33a. False
33b. True
33c. False
33d. False
33e. True
At 3500 m (11 482 ft) the barometric pressure is 67 kPa and the inspired partial pressure of oxygen is reduced to 13.7 kPa but the percentage remains constant at 21%; thus hypoxic pulmonary vasoconstriction occurs owing to reduction in alveolar P_{O_2}. While high-altitude pulmonary oedema is possible, it is not likely, occurring in 1% of healthy individuals, particularly following rapid ascents. It is a potentially fatal, non-cardiogenic pulmonary oedema occurring usually 2–3 days following ascents above 2500 m in unacclimatized individuals. Respiratory alkalosis occurs with ascent to high altitude but renal excretion of bicarbonate increases over several days. Cheyne–Stokes breathing (periodic breathing) is common and non-pathological; typically 3–5 deep breaths will be followed by a period of shallow rapid breaths or apnoea.

West JB. *Respiratory Physiology: The Essentials*, 8th edn. Philadelphia: Lippincott Williams & Wilkins, 2008.

34a. False
34b. True
34c. True
34d. False
34e. True
RRT comprises peritoneal dialysis, intermittent haemodialysis and continuous RRT. In the modern ICU, continuous veno-venous haemofiltration (CVVH) and continuous veno-venous haemodiafiltration (CVVHDF) are the most common modalities used. A systematic review of RRT modality found no difference in mortality or dialysis dependence among survivors. There also exist no definitive randomized controlled trials demonstrating optimal starting times for RRT. Haemofiltration is based on the principle of convection, while haemodialysis is based on the principle of diffusion, and haemodiafiltration is a combination of the processes. RRT membranes are cellulose-based or synthetic. No evidence exists that either type is superior in terms of outcome.

In a venous catheter, the 'arterial' port removes blood from holes in the side of the catheter and blood is returned down the 'venous' lumen at the tip, minimizing recirculation of filtered blood. Anticoagulants are used to prolong filter life, usually heparin to target an activated partial thromboplastin time (APTT) of $1.5-2$ times control; when the platelet count is $<80 \times 10^9$/L prostacyclin should be used to avoid heparin-induced thrombocytopenia. High-volume haemofiltration (HVHF) has been used to produce reductions in plasma mediator concentrations, i.e. tumour necrosis factor (TNF), interleukins-1, -6 and -8 (IL-1, -6 and -8), platelet-activating factor (PAF) and complement. A prospective case review demonstrated a reduced 28-day mortality in patients with sepsis and two-organ failure using HVHF.

Davenport A, Will EJ, Davidson AM. Improved cardiovascular stability during continuous modes of renal replacement therapy in critically ill patients with acute hepatic and renal failure. *Crit Care Med* 1993; **21**: 328–38.

Hall NA, Fox AJ. Renal replacement therapies in critical care. *Contin Educ Anaesth Crit Care Pain* 2006; **6**: 197–202.

Tonelli M, Manns B, Feller-Kopman D. Acute renal failure in the intensive care unit: a systemic review of the impact of the dialytic modality on mortality and renal recovery. *Am J Kidney Dis* 2002; **40**: 875–85.

35a. False
35b. True
35c. True
35d. True
35e. True
PES occurs following $2-16$% of intubations. Recognized risk factors are:

Patient factors

• Female gender
• Muscle weakness
• Tracheal stenosis/ tracheomalacia

Surgical factors

• Nature of surgery (thyroid, airway surgery)
• Bleeding

ICU factors

- Intubation >36 hours
- Excessive cuff pressure
- Tracheal infection
- Large tube
- Aggressive suctioning causing oedema
- Mucus plugs
- Nasogastric tube

A Cochrane review found that in adults, multiple doses of corticosteroids begun 12–24 hours prior to extubation do appear beneficial for patients with a high likelihood of PES.

Karmarkar S, Varshney S. Tracheal extubation. *Contin Educ Anaesth Crit Care Pain* 2008; 8: 214–20.
Khemani RG, Randolph A, Markovitz B. Corticosteroids for the prevention and treatment of post-extubation stridor in neonates, children and adults. *Cochrane Database Syst Rev* 2009; (2): CD001000.

36a. True
36b. True
36c. True
36d. True
35e. False
World Health Organization definitions of PPH are:

- *Primary PPH*: >500 mL estimated blood loss from the genital tract within 24 hours of delivery
- *Secondary PPH*: abnormal bleeding from the genital tract, from 24 hours post-delivery to 6 weeks postpartum

Incidence is quoted at 5% and the most common cause is uterine atony in the UK; risk factors include macrosomia, multiple pregnancies, multiparity, polyhydramnios, prolonged labour and previous PPH. Pre-eclampsia, placenta praevia, retained products of conception, genital tract trauma or acute inversion can also lead to catastrophic haemorrhage. Protein C deficiency is a rare genetic condition that is associated with a hypercoagulable state.

Magann EF, Evans S, Hutchinson M, et al. Postpartum hemorrhage after vaginal birth: an analysis of risk factors. *South Med J* 2005; 98: 419–22.

37a. False
37b. False
37c. True
37d. False
37e. False
The cardiac pathology is aortic stenosis (AS), which generates a pressure gradient across the aortic valve that can be used to grade severity.

Haemodynamic management can be divided into the approach to preload, contractility and afterload:

- *Preload*: patients with AS have a *fixed cardiac output* (CO); it is thus essential to maintain preload, since they are less able to compensate by increasing stroke volume
- *Contractility*: tachycardia reduces diastolic coronary filling time and thus can lead to myocardial ischaemia even with normal coronary arteries. This is compounded by increased $\dot{V}O_2$ of the left ventricle, which undergoes hypertrophy as it ejects against a pressure gradient; low to normal heart rate is ideal and maintenance of sinus rhythm is paramount
- *Afterload*: since CO is relatively fixed, maintenance of systemic vascular resistance is vital for coronary perfusion. As systolic pressure falls, the gradient driving coronary flow also falls

Isoprenaline is arrhythmogenic and through β_1 effects may also lead to a tachycardia and should be avoided.

Martin B, Sinclair M. Cardiac surgery. In: Allman KG, Wilson IH, eds. *Oxford Handbook of Anaesthesia*, 2nd edn. Oxford: OUP, 2006.

38a. True
38b. False
38c. False
38d. True
38e. True
Clinical measurements are usually performed at ambient temperature and pressure; scientific measurements are made at standard temperature and pressure (STP = 273.15 K and 101.325 kPa). Functional residual capacity (FRC) is equal to the sum of residual volume (RV) and expiratory reserve volume (ERV); thus it is the volume in the lung at the end of a normal tidal expiration. It is increased by positive end-expiratory pressure (PEEP), asthma and exercise, and decreased by the supine position, obesity, pregnancy and anaesthesia. Tidal volumes can be measured using a Wright respirometer, which relies on the unidirectional rotation of a vane by gas flow; the movement of the vane produces a mechanical reading. Continuous flow causes inaccuracies in measurement and it does not produce an electrical output for analysis or recording. A wet spirometer (e.g. Benedict–Roth) consists of a lightweight cylinder suspended over a breathing chamber with a water seal. The Vitalograph (a dry spirometer) is used for bedside assessment, since it is more portable.

Davis PD, Kenny GNC. *Basic Physics and Measurement in Anaesthesia*, 5th edn. Oxford: Butterworth-Heinemann, 2003.

39a. True
39b. True
39c. False
39d. True
39e. True
Doxapram is a monohydrated pyrrolidinone derivative used in the treatment of respiratory depression, laryngospasm and postoperative shivering and as an

adjunct for blind nasal intubation. It is presented as a clear colourless solution for intravenous use as a bolus (1 mg/kg) or in an infusion. It acts primarily by stimulating the peripheral chemoreceptors and has direct actions on the respiratory centre; in low doses it increases minute volume and in higher doses rate of respiration. It increases stroke volume and metabolic rate is increased by up to 30%; increased oxygen consumption may therefore result in hypoxia. Cerebral blood flow is increased. Contraindications include thyrotoxicosis, epilepsy and asthma. Side-effects include restlessness, dizziness, hallucinations and perineal irritation.

Sasada M, Smith S. *Drugs in Anaesthesia and Intensive Care*, 3rd edn. Oxford: OUP, 2003.

40a. True
40b. True
40c. True
40d. True
40e. True
There exists more than one system for grading evidence. The National Institute for Health and Clinical Excellence (NICE) uses a hierarchical system for *levels of evidence* ranging from Ia to IV. Ia is the highest level, IV the lowest:

Ia: Evidence from meta-analysis of randomized controlled trials
Ib: Evidence from at least one randomized controlled trial
IIa: Evidence from at least one controlled study without randomization
IIb: Evidence from at least one other type of quasi-experimental study
III: Evidence from non-experimental descriptive studies, such as comparative studies, correlation studies and case–control studies
IV: Evidence from expert committee reports or opinions and/or clinical experience of respected authorities

Grading of recommendation does not reflect clinical importance of recommendation, but is the strength of the evidence. It is graded as follows:

A: Based on hierarchy I evidence
B: Based on hierarchy II evidence or extrapolated from hierarchy I evidence
C: Based on hierarchy III evidence or extrapolated from hierarchy I or II evidence
D: Directly based on hierarchy IV evidence or extrapolated from hierarchy I, II or III evidence

Marks DF. *Perspectives on Evidence Based Practice*. Health Development Agency; Public Health Evidence Steering Group, 2002.

41a. True
41b. False
41c. True
41d. True
41e. True
PAOP, or pulmonary artery wedge pressure (PAWP), is measured when the balloon at the tip of a pulmonary artery catheter is inflated in a branch of the pulmonary artery. It is normally 6–12 mmHg and is an indirect measure of left atrial pressure and left ventricular end-diastolic pressure (LVEDP). In mitral stenosis, the PAOP may exceed the LVEDP owing to the flow restriction before the left ventricle. In ARDS, criteria for diagnosis include PAOP ≤18 mmHg, as opposed to left ventricular failure, which can lead to cardiogenic pulmonary oedema and an increased PAOP. Pulmonary fibrosis leads toincreased venous resistance and increased PAOP. Use of PEEP can cause the PAOP to overestimate the LVEDP.

42a. True
42b. False
42c. False
42d. True
42e. True
There are 7 cervical vertebrae, 12 thoracic, 5 lumbar, 5 fused sacral and 3–5 vestigial coccygeal. The vertebral bodies are separated by fibrocartilaginous discs, which contain an inner nucleus pulposus and outer annulus pulposus, the former of which can extrude and cause nerve or even cord compression. The intervertebral joints are secondary cartilaginous joints while the superior and inferior articular processes are synovial, as are the costal facets between thoracic vertebrae and rib head and tubercles. The gap between the odontoid peg and atlas is normally ≤3 mm in adults and ≤5 mm in children on neck flexion. The vertebral arteries pass through the foramina transversaria of the cervical vertebrae except C7, through which only the vertebral veins pass. The ligaments are as follows:

• *Anterior longitudinal ligament*: C2 to sacrum over anterior vertebral bodies
• *Posterior longitudinal ligament*: attached to posterior vertebral bodies, C2 to sacrum
• *Ligamentum flavum*: between adjacent vertebral laminae and thicker in the lumbar region
• *Interspinous ligaments*: between adjacent vertebral spinous processes
• *Supraspinous ligaments*: from C7 to sacrum – attached to tips of spinous processes

Snell RS. *Clinical Anatomy for Medical Students*. Philadelphia: Lippincott Williams & Wilkins, 2000.
Yentis S, Hirsch N, Smith G. *Anaesthesia and Intensive Care A to Z: An Encyclopaedia of Principles and Practice*, 4th edn. Oxford: Butterworth-Heinemann, 2009.

43a. False
43b. True
43c. False
43d. True
43e. False
In the UK, approximately 50 000 patients are treated for cardiac arrest per annum. One in eight of these is admitted to an ICU, with one-third of these surviving to hospital discharge and 80% of those patients returning to their normal residence. Prognosis cannot be based on the circumstances of the cardiac arrest, and the decision to admit should be made on the basis of the patients' previous medical status. Reliable indicators for a poor prognosis in the comatose and normothermic patient are:

- absent pupil or corneal reflexes 1–3 days post-arrest
- absent or extensor motor responses 3 days post-arrest
- myoclonic status epilepticus within 1 day after primary cardiac arrest
- burst suppression or generalized epileptiform discharges on EEG
- a serum neuron-specific enolase (NSE) concentration >33 μg/L 1–3 days after cardiopulmonary resuscitation

Most studies do not show an association between age and survival after cardiac arrest. It has been shown that among comatose survivors there is an association between mortality and increasing age, but this is not an independent predictor of poor neurological outcome.

Intensive Care Society. *Standards for The Management of Patients after Cardiac Arrest*. London: ICS, 2008. Available at: www.ics.ac.uk.
Nolan J. Post-cardiac arrest management. In: Waldmann N, Soni N, Rhodes A, eds. *Oxford Desk Reference: Critical Care*. Oxford: OUP, 2008.
Rogove HJ, Safar P, Sutton-Tyrrell K, Abramson NS. Old age does not negate good cerebral outcome after cardiopulmonary resuscitation: analyses from the brain resuscitation clinical trials. The Brain Resuscitation Clinical Trial I and II Study Groups. *Crit Care Med* 1995; **23**: 18–25.

44a. True
44b. False
44c. True
44d. True
44e. False
NICE guidelines for management of head injury (2007) recommend immediate CT head scans for adults with any of the following:

- GCS <13 on immediate assessment in hospital
- GCS <15 in hospital, 2 hours following injury
- suspected open or depressed skull fracture
- any sign of basal skull fracture (Battle's sign, haemotympanum or cerebrospinal fluid leakage)
- >1 episode of vomiting
- post-traumatic seizure
- focal neurological deficit
- amnesia for events >30 minutes before impact

National Institute for Health and Clinical Excellence. *Head Injury: Triage, Assessment, Investigation and Early Management of Head Injury in Infants, Children and Adults*. London: NICE, 2008. Available at: guidance.nice.org.uk/CG65.

45a. True
45b. False
45c. False
45d. True
45e. False

Duchenne's muscular dystrophy (DMD) affects 1:3500 males and is a severe sex-linked recessive condition that leads to progressive muscle degeneration and death, usually occurring in the teens or early 20s due to cardiac failure or pneumonia. The *DMD* gene is located on the short arm of the X chromosome (Xp21) and it codes for the dystrophin protein, which is absent (or near-absent) in DMD. Presentation occurs in boys before the age of 6, with increasing clumsiness and proximal muscle weakness; muscle pseudohyper-trophy also occurs. Cardiac involvement leads to myocardial degeneration with heart failure and valve prolapse; skeletal deformities occur and CK levels are extremely high (40 times higher than normal). Autonomic dysfunction is not a typical feature.

Teasdale A. Neuromuscular disorders. In: Allman KG, Wilson IH, eds. *Oxford Handbook of Anaesthesia*, 2nd edn. Oxford: OUP, 2006.

46a. True
46b. True
46c. False
46d. True
46e. True

Cardiac disease was the most common cause of indirect maternal death in CEMACH 2003–05, and the most common cause of death overall. The physiological changes of pregnancy make significant demands on the cardio-vascular system. These include:

- Progesterone-induced drop in systemic vascular resistance
- Increased cardiac output (up 20% at 8 weeks, 40–50% by 20–28 weeks) due to increases in stroke volume and heart rate
- Expansion of plasma volume
- Cardiac output increases further during labour (50% in the second stage) due to pain, anxiety and an autotransfusion of uterine blood with each contraction
- Reduction in serum colloid oncotic pressure

Women with known cardiovascular disease should ideally undergo pre-conception counselling and obstetric care should be multidisciplinary, involving obstetricians, anaesthetists, intensivists, cardiologists and other relevant professionals. Regular follow-up throughout pregnancy is also required. The majority of women who die from heart disease have not been identified as being 'at risk' before labour. Management should comprise optimization of the cardiac condition, regular follow-up and monitoring for signs of deterioration. Excessive fluid loads should be avoided during delivery and the postpartum period.

Drugs considered safe for the treatment of heart failure are diuretics, digoxin and hydralazine. Nitrates can be used with hydralazine as vasodilators by off-loading the left ventricle. These drugs are not without side-effects and may necessitate fetal monitoring. Angiotensin-converting enzyme (ACE) inhibitors should be avoided because of the development of oligohydramnios and skull defects.

Burt CC, Durbridge J. Management of cardiac disease in pregnancy. *Contin Educ Anaesth Crit Care Pain* 2009; **9**: 44–7.

Lewis G, ed. The Confidential Enquiry into Maternal and Child Health (CEMACH). *Saving Mothers' Lives: Reviewing Maternal Deaths to make Motherhood Safer – 2003–2005*. The Seventh Report on Confidential Enquiries into Maternal Deaths in the UK. London: CEMACH, 2007. Available at: www.cmace.org.uk/getattachment/05f68346-816b-4560-b1b9-af24fb633170/Saving-Mothers'-Lives-2003-2005_ExecSumm.aspx.

Nelson-Piery C. Heart Disease. In: Nelson-Piercy C. *Handbook of Obstetric Medicine*, 3rd edn. Abingdon: Informa Healthcare, 2006.

47a. True
47b. True
47c. False
47d. True
47e. False
The laws are as stated. The isobestic points for oxy- and deoxyhaemoglobin are dependent only on haemoglobin concentration and occur at 590 and 805 nm. Oxygen is paramagnetic (it is attracted to a magnetic field, unlike most gases), this is the basis of the paramagnetic analyser. Clark's electrode consists of a silver (Ag/AgCl) anode and a platinum cathode. The fuel cell has a lead anode and a gold mesh cathode (and can be remembered as a 'poor cousin' of Clark in that lead and gold are cheaper than silver and platinum).

48a. True
48b. False
48c. False
48d. True
48e. False
Tenon's capsule is a layer of thin connective tissue surrounding the globe, fusing anteriorly with the conjunctiva at the limbus and extending posteriorly to fuse with the dura of the optic nerve. It is a safe and reliable alternative to retrobulbar and peribulbar techniques, but is not without risk and globe perforation has been reported during dissection with Westcott's spring scissors. Patients receiving anticoagulant medication can safely receive sub-Tenon's blocks, but the incidence of subconjunctival haemorrhage is higher in this group. Clotting profile should be available on the day of the procedure; an International Normalized Ratio (INR) of ≤ 3.5 is generally accepted in experienced hands.

Frieman BJ, Friedberg MA. Globe perforation associated with subtenon's anesthesia. *Am J Ophthalmol* 2001; **131**: 520–1.

Kumar N, Jivan S, Thomas P, McLure H. Sub-Tenon's anaesthesia with aspirin, warfarin and clopidogrel. *J Cataract Refract Surg* 2006; **32**: 1022–5.

49a. False
49b. True
49c. True
49d. False
49e. True

The ulnar nerve arises from the medial cord of the brachial plexus and enters the forearm, passing behind the medial epicondyle. Complete injuries at the elbow result in paralysis of the medial flexor digitorum profundus (FDP) and flexor carpi ulnaris, which leads to a claw deformity; injuries at the wrist are worse since the FDP is not affected and therefore causes marked flexion of the phalanges. In addition, the small muscles of the hand will be paralysed except for the thenar muscles and the 1st and 2nd lumbricals, supplied by the median nerve; inability to adduct the thumb will also result, but abduction and opposition are provided by the median nerve. On flexion of the wrist, a degree of abduction will result owing to flexor carpi radialis paralysis.

Snell RS. *Clinical Anatomy for Medical Students*, 6th edn. Boston: Little, Brown and Company, 2000.

50a. False
50b. False
50c. False
50d. False
50e. True

Ketamine is a phencyclidine derivative that is a non-competitive antagonist at the N-methyl-D-aspartate (NMDA) receptor calcium channel pores. It is used for intravenous anaesthesia, postoperative analgesia and sedation and in the treatment of chronic pain and severe asthma. It can be administered via intravenous, intramuscular, oral, nasal, rectal, epidural or intrathecal routes.

Actions:

Cardiovascular: ↑Heart rate, blood pressure, central venous pressure and cardiac output
Respiratory: ↑Respiratory rate and preservation of respiratory reflexes, bronchodilation
Central nervous system: Dissociative anaesthesia, ↑cerebral blood flow and cerebral metabolic rate
Gastrointestinal/genitourinary: Postoperative nausea and vomiting, ↑salivation, ↑uterine tone

Sasada M, Smith S. *Drugs in Anaesthesia and Intensive Care*, 3rd edn. Oxford: OUP, 2003.

51a. False
51b. True
51c. True
51d. False
51e. True
The femoral triangle is a compartment in the anterior upper thigh. It is anatomically relevant because of the structures it contains and its susceptibility to herniation. Its borders are:

- *Superomedial*: inguinal ligament
- *Medial*: medial border of the adductor longus
- *Lateral*: medial border of the sartorius
- *Roof*: fascia lata
- *Floor*: adductor longus, pectineus, psoas and iliacus

Its contents include the femoral artery, vein and canal within the sheath; the femoral nerve and lateral cutaneous nerve lie outside and lateral to the sheath.

52a. False
52b. True
52c. True
52d. True
52e. False
The ACC/AHA guidelines for performing an echocardiogram in critically ill patients were revised in 2003. Patient indications have been categorized as follows:

Category I: conditions for which evidence exists and/or general agreement that a given procedure is useful and effective:

- Haemodynamic instability
- Serious blunt or penetrating chest injury
- Suspected aortic dissection
- Suspected pre-existing valvular or myocardial disease with trauma
- Suspected aortic injury
- Suspected iatrogenic injury with guidewire, pacer electrode or pericardiocentesis needle

Category IIa: conflicting evidence or divergence of opinion but potentially in favour of the procedure:

- Follow-up of serious trauma
- Evaluation of multiple trauma with pulmonary artery catheter and haemodynamic stability but data findings not correlating clinically

Category III: evidence and/or general agreement that the procedure is not useful and may be harmful:

- Haemodynamic stability with no cardiac history
- Follow-up on haemodynamically stable patients
- Suspected myocardial contusion with normal ECG and clinical findings and haemodynamically stable

Cheitlin MD, Armstrong WF, Aurigemma GP, et al. *ACC/AHA/ASE 2003 Guideline Update for the Clinical Application of Echocardiography: A report of the American College of Cardiology/American Heart Association Task Force on Practice Guidelines*. American College of Cardiology Foundation and the American Heart Association, 2003. Available at: www.acc.org/qualityandscience/clinical/guidelines/echo/index_clear.pdf.

Roscoe A, Strang T. Echocardiography in intensive care. *Contin Educ Anaesth Crit Care Pain* 2008; 8: 46–9.

53a. True
53b. False
53c. True
53d. True
53e. False

SAH may be traumatic or spontaneous; classical presentation is sudden onset of a severe ('thunderclap') headache and is often associated with nausea and vomiting, reduced conscious level or seizures. Spontaneous SAH is more common in women and risk factors include smoking and hypertension; 85% of spontaneous SAH occur secondary to intracerebral aneurysms and 5% owing to arteriovenous malformations. The World Federation of Neurosurgical Societies (WFNS) Classification combines GCS and focal neurological deficit to grade severity as follows:

Grade	GCS	Focal neurological deficit
0	15	Unruptured
1	15	Absent
2	13–14	Absent
3	13–14	Present
4	7–12	Present or absent
5	3–6	Present or absent

The ISAT Trial compared endovascular coiling versus surgical clipping in patients with aneurysms < 10 mm of the anterior circulation and found that death or dependence was less likely in the group who had undergone endovascular coiling. Complications include re-bleeding (highest risk in the first 24 hours), vasospasm (highest risk from 3rd to 10th day following bleed), hydrocephalus and seizures.

de Rooij NK, Linn FH, van der Plas JA, Algra A, Rinkel GJ. Incidence of subarachnoid haemorrhage: a systematic review with emphasis on region, age, gender and time trends. *J Neurol Neurosurg Psychiatry* 2007; 78: 1365–72.

Molyneux AJ, Kerr RS, Yu LM, et al. International subarachnoid aneurysm trial (ISAT) of neurosurgical clipping versus endovascular coiling in 2143 patients with ruptured intracranial aneurysms: a randomized comparison of effects on survival, dependency, seizures, rebleeding, subgroups, and aneurysm occlusion. *Lancet* 2005; 366: 809–17.

54a. True
54b. True
54c. False
54d. False
54e. False
The ductus arteriosus (DA) normally constricts in response to increasing PaO_2 after the first breath, closure of the foramen ovale (FO) and decreasing prostaglandin E_1 (PGE_1) and PGE_2 concentrations; physiological closure occurs in 10–15 hours and permanent closure in 2–3 weeks. True persistence of a patent ductus arteriosus (PDA) is recognized after 3 months. It accounts for 10–15% of congenital heart disease (technically it is extracardiac). Shunt is initially left-to-right but with time pulmonary hypertension may develop, reversing the shunt and causing cyanosis. Management is medical or surgical. Intravenous indometacin has direct anti-prostaglandin action in addition to prostaglandin synthetase inhibition. A Cochrane review concluded that indometacin is the drug of choice for treatment of a PDA. PGE_1 has been used to prevent ductal closure for children awaiting surgery to prevent right-to-left shunting in patients with severe aortic coarctation or left-to-right shunting for pulmonary perfusion in severe Fallot's tetralogy. At ligation or clipping of the duct, *left* thoracotomy is performed. NICE has produced guidance stating that safety and efficacy of endovascular closure of PDA are adequate to support the use of this procedure.

National Institute for Health and Clinical Excellence. *Endovascular Closure of Patent Ductus Arteriosus*. London: NICE, 2004. Available at: guidance.nice.org.uk/IPG097.
Ohlsson A, Walia R, Shah S. Ibuprofen for the treatment of a PDA in preterm and/or low birth weight infants. *Cochrane Database Syst Rev* 2003; (2): CD003481.

55a. True
55b. False
55c. True
55d. True
55e. True
Necrotizing fasciitis is a rapidly progressive, inflammatory infection of the deep fascia with secondary skin and subcutaneous tissue necrosis; it occurs most commonly following trauma or surgery and most frequently affects the abdominal wall, extremities and perineum. Type I is a polymicrobial infection and type II is monomicrobial, most commonly caused by group A streptococci. There are many causative agents, including Gram-positive aerobes such as *Staphylococcus aureus* and MRSA, Gram-negative aerobes including *Pseudomonas* and *Escherichia coli*, and anaerobes such as *Bacteroides* and *Clostridia*. Soft tissue damage occurs with release of bacterial exotoxins and endogenous cytokines and the condition is almost universally fatal without surgical intervention and debridement.

Green R. Necrotising fasciitis. *Chest* 1996; **110**: 219–29.

56a. False
56b. True
56c. False
56d. False
56e. False
Tidal volumes can be measured using a Wright respirometer, which relies on unidirectional rotation of a vane by gas flow; the movement of the vane produces a mechanical reading. Continuous flow causes inaccuracies in measurement and it does not produce an electrical output for analysis or recording. At low tidal volumes the respirometer has a tendency to underestimate; at high volumes it overestimates owing to inertia.

Davis PD, Kenny GNC. *Basic Physics and Measurement in Anaesthesia*, 5th edn. Oxford: Butterworth-Heinemann, 2003.

57a. True
57b. True
57c. False
57d. False
57e. True
Clonidine is an aniline derivative; it stimulates presynaptic α_2-adrenoreceptors, thereby decreasing noradrenaline release from sympathetic nerve terminals. Sympathetic tone is reduced; it also increases vagal tone. Uses include:

- essential and secondary hypertension
- hypertensive crises
- migraine
- menopausal flushing
- chronic pain
- opiate and alcohol withdrawal
- IVRA for chronic regional pain syndrome

Sasada M, Smith S. *Drugs in Anaesthesia and Intensive Care*, 3rd edn. Oxford: OUP, 2003.

58a. False
58b. True
58c. True
58d. False
58e. False
Heat loss under anaesthesia is due to radiation (40%), convection (30%), conduction (5%), evaporation (15%) and respiration (10%). Both general and regional anaesthesia have been demonstrated to cause heat losses of 0.5–1°C in the first hour (redistribution) followed by approximately 0.3°C/h (linear). Metabolic production of heat is depressed under anaesthesia and the hypothalamus is 'reset' so that the compensatory mechanisms are activated at a much lower temperature. The three phases of heat loss are:

- *Redistribution*: movement of heat from core to periphery due to vasodilation
- *Linear phase*: heat loss exceeds heat production

- *Plateau phase*: temperature falls below the thermoregulatory threshold, peripheral vasoconstriction increases to limit the heat loss from the core compartment; patients with autonomic neuropathy or regional blockade do not exhibit this response.

The specific heat capacity of blood is **3.6 kJ kg^{-1} °C^{-1}**.

Sullivan G, Edmondson C. Heat and temperature. *Contin Educ Anaesth Crit Care Pain* 2008; 8: 104–7.

59a. True
59b. True
59c. False
59d. False
59e. True
Figure 5.2 illustrates the lumbar plexus.

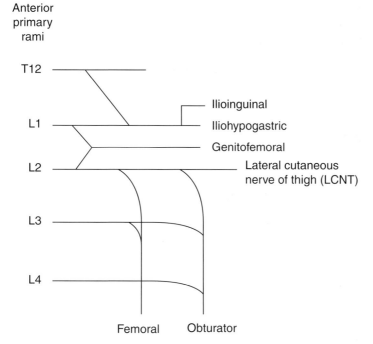

FIGURE 5.2   Lumbar plexus.

60a. False
60b. False
60c. True
60d. False
60e. False
Sodium is the principal extracellular cation and the major determinant of extracellular volume. It is freely filtered at the glomerulus and the majority is

reabsorbed in the proximal tubule. In the normal brain, ADH (vasopressin) is released in response to low serum osmolality (280 mOsm/kg) and low extra-cellular volume; thirst occurs when this reaches 295 mOsm/kg. The daily requirements for an adult of sodium (and potassium) are 1 mmol kg^{-1} day^{-1}. Central pontine myelinolysis is thought to occur with rapid correction of hyponatraemia, malnutrition, alcoholism and following liver transplants. 10% of the demyelination occurs outside the pons and it is diagnosed by magnetic resonance imaging.

61a. True
61b. False
61c. False
61d. False
61e. True
Fondaparinux is a synthetic pentasaccharide that consists of the antithrombin binding pentasaccharide sequence found in heparin. By binding with anti-thrombin, it induces a conformational change that enhances its activity against factor Xa; it has no antithrombin activity. It does not bind to platelet factor 4 and thus does not cause HIT. The Intensive Care Society suggests that fondaparinux can be used where contraindications to heparin exist, such as HIT within the last 6 months. It is administered subcutaneously and excreted renally; it is not recommended for patients with a creatinine clearance <30 mL/min. No specific reversal agent exists, although recombinant activated factor VII may reverse some of its anticoagulant effects.

Hunt B. Anticoagulants and heparin-induced thrombocytopenia. In: Waldmann N, Soni N, Rhodes A, eds. *Oxford Desk Reference: Critical Care*. Oxford: OUP, 2008.
Intensive Care Society. *Guidelines for Venous Thromboprophylaxis in Critical Care*. London: ICS, 2008. Available at: www.ics.ac.uk.

62a. True
62b. True
62c. False
62d. False
62e. True
Following major trauma, causes of profound hypotension with concurrent tachycardia include hypovolaemic shock (any source), tension pneumothorax and cardiac tamponade. Haemopneumothorax is likely; thus hyperresonance of non-dependent and stony dullness of dependent areas of the lung are both likely findings, in addition to decreased breath sounds and deteriorating gas exchange. Absence of tracheal deviation may indicate bilateral tension pneu-mothoraces, which can occur causing profound cardiovascular and respiratory compromise and which warrant urgent decompression. Spinal injury is highly possible following major trauma, but apart from a traumatic history, there are no other indicators of spinal shock (injuries >T6), which is characterized by severe autonomic dysfunction, with consequent hypotension, bradycardia, peripheral vasodilation and hypothermia with an associated spinal level. Aortic injury should be considered in unstable (or partially unstable) patients with

left-sided haemothorax. A widened mediastinum is reported as having a 53% sensitivity, 59% specificity and 83% negative predictive value for traumatic aortic injury.

Mirvis SE, Bidwell JK, Buddemeyer EU, et al. Value of chest radiography in excluding traumatic aortic rupture. *Radiology* 1987; **163**: 487–93.

63a. False
63b. True
63c. True
63d. False
63e. True
Nissen's fundoplication is first-line surgical treatment for gastroesophageal reflux (GOR) and hiatus hernia, performed when medical therapy has failed. It can be performed laparoscopically and involves wrapping the gastric fundus around the lower portion of the oesophagus, reinforcing the closing action of the lower oesophageal sphincter and preventing GOR. It is generally a safe procedure and complications include vomiting, dumping syndrome, bloating and dysphagia; dumping syndrome results from rapid emptying of osmotically active substances into the upper intestine. Achalasia is an oesophageal motility disorder treated surgically by Heller's myotomy; subsequent partial fundoplication can be performed in addition, to reduce the risk of GOR following myotomy. GOR is a risk factor for microaspiration and development of bronchiectasis.

Nissen R. Gastropexy and 'fundoplication' in surgical treatment of hiatal hernia. *Am J Dig Dis* 1961; **6**: 954–61.
Tsang KW, Lam WK, Kwok E, et al. *Helicobacter pylori* and upper gastrointestinal symptoms in bronchiectasis. *Eur Respir J* 1999; **14**: 1345–50.

64a. True
64b. False
64c. True
64d. True
64e. False
Classically these are all causes of proximal myopathy except Guillain–Barré syndrome, which presents with a distal ascending polyneuropathy causing sensory and motor deficits, and Huntington's disease, which is an autosomal dominant neurodegenerative condition, characterized by abnormal choreiform movements. Myopathies may be inherited or acquired; acquired causes can be further subdivided into metabolic, endocrine, drug-induced, inflammatory, infective and paraneoplastic aetiology. Polymyositis is a connective tissue disorder, presenting with proximal muscle weakness and often concomitant dermatomyositis; these conditions can be indicative of an underlying malignancy. Polymyalgia rheumatica classically presents in elderly females, with painful muscle weakness of the proximal pelvic and pectoral groups, and is strongly associated with temporal arteritis.

65a. True
65b. False
65c. True
65d. True
65e. False

Gauge is a measure of thickness/width; gauge of intravenous cannulae are based upon the wire-gauge system, while the French gauge system, originally used for sizing urinary catheters, equals external circumference in mm.

Flow rates for cannulae are calculated using distilled water at a temperature of $22°C$ under a pressure of 10 kPa through a 110 cm length of tubing with an internal diameter of 4 mm.

Al-Shaikh B, Stacey S. *Essentials of Anaesthetic Equipment*, 3rd edn. London: Churchill Livingstone, 2007.

66a. True
66b. False
66c. True
66d. False
66e. True

The arterial pressure waveform is composed of a series of waveforms that each have different frequencies and amplitudes; these can be broken down by Fourier analysis. The fundamental frequency is the 1st harmonic and is equal to the heart rate; a frequency range of 0.5–40 Hz is needed in any system used to measure and display the arterial waveform. The natural frequency of any system is the frequency at which the monitoring system itself resonates; thus this natural frequency should be outside the range of the fundamental frequency and should be at least 10 times the fundamental frequency. The natural frequency of the system increases further outside the range of the fundamental frequency with catheter diameter and decreases with increasing compliance of the system, increasing tubing length and increasing density of the fluid medium used. Hence a wide, short and stiff cannula is optimal. Damping is a progressive attenuation of the amplitude of oscillations within a system and is due to dissipation of the energy stored. It is inherent in any system, slowing the rate of change of signal between the patient and transducer. A damping factor (D) describes the degree of damping or resonance within a resonant system:

- *Optimally damped* ($D = 0.7$): system responds rapidly with small amount of overshoot
- *Critically damped* ($D = 1.0$): no overshooting, but may be too slow
- *Underdamped* ($D < 0.7$): resonance occurs, signal oscillates and overshoots
- *Overdamped* ($D > 1.0$): signal takes a long time to reach equilibrium, but will not overshoot

Al-Shaikh B, Stacey S. *Essentials of Anaesthetic Equipment*, 3rd edn. London: Churchill Livingstone, 2007.
Ward MA, Langton SA. Blood pressure measurement. *Contin Educ Anaesth Crit Care Pain* 2007; 7: 122–6.
Yentis S, Hirsch N, Smith G. *Anaesthesia and Intensive Care A to Z: An Encyclopaedia of Principles and Practice*, 4th edn. Oxford: Butterworth-Heinemann, 2009.

67a. False
67b. True
67c. False
67d. False
67e. True
Management of severe local anaesthetic toxicity should follow the Association of Anaesthetists of Great Britain and Ireland guidelines. Immediate management comprises stopping further injection of local anaesthetic, calling for help, securing the airway and ventilating with 100% oxygen. Seizures can be controlled with a benzodiazepine, thiopentone or propofol in small incremental doses. During cardiac arrest, management follows standard advanced life support (ALS) protocols, taking note that prolonged resuscitation may be required. Intralipid 20% is a new addition to the cardiac arrest algorithm and is administered:

- Initially as a dose of 1.5 mL/kg over 1 minute, followed by an infusion of 0.25 mL kg^{-1} min^{-1}
- Two further bolus injections may be administered at 5-minute intervals, then the rate of infusion is doubled to 0.5 mL kg^{-1}min^{-1}

Propofol is not a suitable alternative, despite some preparations being provided in Intralipid, since this will cause significant cardiovascular depression. In the UK cases should be reported to the National Patient Safety Agency (NPSA) and in Ireland to the Irish Medicines Board.

Association of Anaesthetists of Great Britain and Ireland. *Guidelines for the Management of Severe Local Anaesthetic Toxicity*. London: AAGBI, 2007. Available at: www.aagbi.org/publications/guidelines/docs/latoxicity07.pdf.
National Patient Safety Agency. *Epidural Injections and Infusions*. London: NPSA, 2007. Available at: www.nrls.npsa.nhs.uk/resources/type/alerts/?entryid45=59807&p=3.

68a. False
68b. True
68c. True
68d. False
68e. False
The prevention of infection of central lines can only be achieved with certainty by removal. The Hospital Infection Society guidelines include:

- single-lumen catheters if appropriate
- cannulation of the subclavian vein unless contraindicated
- aseptic technique during insertion
- disinfection of external surfaces of catheter hubs every time a catheter is accessed
- not to routinely replace tunnelled catheters as a method of CRBSI prevention

Pratt RJ, Pellowe C, Loveday HP, et al. Guidelines for the prevention of infection associated with the insertion and maintenance of central venous catheters. *J Hosp Infect* 2001; 47: S47–67.

69a. True
69b. False
69c. True
69d. False
69e. True
All divisions of the laryngeal nerves are derived from the vagus nerve.
The superior laryngeal nerve is divided into internal (sensory to mucous
membranes down to the vocal cords) and external (motor to the cricothyroid
muscle). The recurrent laryngeal nerve is sensory below the vocal cords and
motor to all intrinsic muscles of the larnyx *except* the cricothyroid. The left
recurrent laryngeal passes below and posterior to the aorta; the right
recurrent laryngeal passes below and posterior to the right subclavian artery.
Damage to the superior laryngeal nerve results in a slack vocal cord and a
weak voice. Partial damage to the recurrent laryngeal nerve causes the
cord to move into the midline, resulting in a hoarse voice. Complete damage
results in adoption of the cadaveric (intermediate) position and voice loss.

70a. False
70b. True
70c. False
70d. False
70e. True
Sevoflurane is a halogenated ether. Isoflurane (and enflurane) are halogenated
methyl ethers.

	Sevoflurane	Desflurane	Halothane	Enflurane	Isoflurane	N_2O
BP (°C)	58.5	23.5	50.2	56.5	48.5	−88
MAC (%)	1.8	6.6	0.75	1.68	1.17	105
SVP (20°C; kPa)	22.7	89.2	32.3	23.3	33.2	5200
B:G PC	0.7	0.45	2.4	1.8	1.4	0.47
O:G PC	80	29	224	98	98	1.4
MW	200.1	168	197	184.5	184.5	44

BP, boiling point; MAC, minimum alveolar concentration; SVP, saturated vapour pressure; B:G PC, blood : gas partition coefficient; O:G PC, oil : gas partition coefficient; MW, molecular weight.

Peck TE, Hill SA, Williams M. *Pharmacology for Anaesthesia and Intensive Care*, 3rd edn. Cambridge: CUP, 2008.
Sasada M, Smith S. *Drugs in Anaesthesia and Intensive Care*, 3rd edn. Oxford: OUP, 2003.

71a. True
71b. True
71c. False
71d. True
71e. True
Teicoplanin is a glycopepetide antibiotic it has a similar spectrum of activity to vancomycin, but with less toxicity. It is highly effective against Gram-positive bacteria, including MRSA and *Clostridium difficile*, but has limited action against Gram-negative species. The glycopeptides are bacteriocidal and act by inhibiting peptidoglycans formation and thus cell wall synthesis. Its side-effect profile is favourable and there is very rarely cross-reactivity with vancomycin. It has been safely used in patients who developed the 'red-man syndrome' associated with vancomycin administration; side-effects include rashes, fever, ototoxicity and thrombocytopenia. It is poorly absorbed orally; cerebrospinal fluid penetration is better than that with vancomycin. It can be given intramuscularly or intravenously with good bone penetration. Gentamicin is an aminoglycoside.

Peck TE, Hill SA, Williams M. *Pharmacology for Anaesthesia and Intensive Care*, 3rd edn. Cambridge: CUP, 2008.

72a. True
72b. False
72c. True
72d. False
72e. False
Burns can be classified on the basis of the extent or depth of the injury. The extent is expressed as a percentage of the total body surface area (BSA). Depth is classified as partial- or full-thickness. Criteria for a major burn include:

- full-thickness burn: >10% BSA (5% in children)
- partial-thickness burn: >25% BSA in adults (>20% at extremes of age)
- burns to the face, hands, feet, perineum or over a major joint

House fires should alert one to the possibility of smoke inhalation and consequent carbon monoxide or cyanide poisoning; stridor signals impending airway obstruction secondary to oedema. Stridor necessitates immediate airway intervention and although awake fibreoptic intubation has been advocated, complete obstruction of the narrowed airway can occur on instrumentation of the fibrescope. Suxamethonium is safe to use in burns within the first 24 hours. The Parkland formula is 4 mL/kg per %BSA burn in the first 24 hours, with half given over the first 8 hours, but fluid resuscitation should be titrated to clinical need. Finally, prophylactic antibiotics are not recommended but regular cultures should be taken.

Craft TM, Nolan J, Parr MJA. *Key Topics in Critical Care*. London: Informa Healthcare, 2004.

73a. False
73b. True
73c. True
73d. True
73e. True
'Septal' Q-waves on the ECG represent septal depolarization from left to right and can be a normal finding in lead III if no abnormal Q-waves are present in leads II and aVF. Pathological Q-waves have the following features:

- $\geq 25\%$ height of the succeeding R-wave
- ≥ 0.04 s in width

Pathological Q-waves indicate full-thickness myocardial infarction and occur 2–24 hours following infarction; they signal depolarization moving away from the infarcted tissue in opposing healthy myocardium. Pathological Q-waves in leads I, aVL, V5 and V6 indicate anterolateral myocardial infarction.

Khan MG. *Rapid ECG Interpretation*. Totowa, NJ: Humana Press, 2007.

74a. True
74b. True
74c. True
74d. False
74e. True
Pharmacological therapy for HF currently includes:

- Angiotensin-converting enzyme (ACE) inhibitors for all grades of HF
- β-blockers for HF due to left ventricular systolic dysfunction (LVSD) for all grades of severity
- Angiotensin II-receptor antagonists and aldosterone antagonists for moderate to severe HF due to LVSD (or patients who have suffered a myocardial infarction (MI) and have LVEF <40% and either diabetes or clinical signs of HF)

Cardiac resynchronization therapy with a pacing device (CRT-P) is recommended as a treatment option for people with HF who fulfil the following criteria:

- NYHA class III–IV symptoms
- Sinus rhythm with a QRS >150 ms or 120–149 ms and mechanical dyssynchrony on echocardiography
- LVEF of 35% or less
- Receiving optimal pharmacological therapy

There is no strong evidence that diuretics improve survival. A decrease in LVEF is associated with increased mortality and morbidity, with the highest-risk group being those with an LVEF <35%.

American College of Cardiology/American Heart Association 2007 Guidelines on Perioperative Cardiovascular Evaluation and Care for Noncardiac Surgery. *J Am Coll Cardiol* 2007; **50**: 159–202 and *Circulation* 2007; **116**: 1971–96. Available at: content.onlinejacc.org/cgi/content/full/j.jacc.2007.09.003 and at: circ.ahajournals.org/cgi/reprint/CIRCULATIONAHA.107.185699.

European Society of Cardiology. Guidelines for the diagnosis and treatment of chronic failure: executive summary. *Eur Heart J* 2005; **26**: 1115–40.

National Institute for Health and Clinical Excellence. *Cardiac Resynchronisation Therapy for the Treatment of Heart Failure*. London: NICE, 2007. Available at: www.nice.org.uk/TA120.

75a. True
75b. True
75c. False
75d. False
75e. False
The Clark electrode is used to measure oxygen concentration in blood gas analysers; it consists of a platinum cathode and a silver/silver chloride anode immersed in a solution of potassium chloride. A voltage of 0.6 V is applied between the electrodes; this generates electrons by the reaction of silver with potassium chloride solution. Electrons combine with oxygen and water at the cathode to form hydroxyl ions as follows:

$$O_2 + 4e^- + 2H_2O \rightarrow 4OH^-$$

A plastic protective cover is required at the cathode to prevent protein deposits due to direct blood contact. Halothane causes falsely high readings due to polarization.

Davis PD, Kenny GNC. *Basic Physics and Measurement in Anaesthesia*, 5th edn. Oxford: Butterworth-Heinemann, 2003.

76a. True
76b. False
76c. True
76d. True
76e. False
Postoperative bleeding is a major complication following cardiac surgery on cardiopulmonary bypass. Inadequate haemostasis can necessitate resternotomy, but a surgical cause is found in only 50% of re-explorations. Pharmacological causes include inadequate reversal of heparin, which can be checked using near-patient coagulation tests such as thromboelastography (TEG) or activated clotting time (ACT); this can be treated with protamine administration. Contact of the blood with the bypass circuits leads to inflammatory cascades, causing platelet dysfunction, fibrinolysis and complement activation. Clotting factors may be diluted, causing further bleeding, and administration of blood products should be tailored to the patient's need, by appropriate investigation and diagnosis of the problem. Use of aprotinin has been controversial, with some studies suggesting an increased mortality following cardiac surgery. Finally, clamping drains should never be undertaken, because of the risk of cardiac tamponade.

Henry DA, Carless PA, Fergusson D, Laupacis A. The safety of aprotinin and lysine-derived antifibrinolytic drugs in cardiac surgery: a meta-analysis. *CMAJ* 2009; **180**: 183–93.
Paparella D, Brister SJ, Buchanan MR. Coagulation disorders of cardiopulmonary bypass: a review. *Intensive Care Med* 2004; **30**: 1873–81.

77a. False
77b. False
77c. True
77d. False
77e. True

Desflurane causes cerebrovascular dilatation with subsequent increased blood flow, but decreases cerebral oxygen consumption; it does not cause epileptiform activity, unlike enflurane, which does, particularly in the context of hypocapnia; enflurane is thus avoided in patients with epilepsy. Propofol has potent anticonvulsant properties and, while associated with involuntary motor activity, there is no corresponding epileptiform activity on EEG studies. As a depolarizing muscle relaxant, suxamethonium causes fasciculations and also causes a rise in intracranial and intraocular pressure; however, it does not cross the blood–brain barrier and is not epileptogenic. Methohexitone is a methylbarbiturate and elicits excitatory activity on induction; it reduces both cerebral blood flow and oxygen consumption, but can lead to spike-and-wave patterns on EEG monitoring.

Sasada M, Smith S. *Drugs in Anaesthesia and Intensive Care*, 3rd edn. Oxford: OUP, 2003.

78a. False
78b. True
78c. True
78d. True
78e. False

The critical temperature is the temperature *above* which a substance cannot be liquefied, no matter how much pressure is applied.

	Critical temperature (°C)	Boiling point at 1 atm (°C)
Oxygen	-119	-180
CO_2	31	-78.5
N_2O	36.5	-88

Latent heat of vaporization is the heat required to convert a substance from liquid to vapour at a given temperature (in joules). The temperature where the latent heat is zero corresponds to the critical temperature, since this is the temperature where a substance spontaneously vaporizes with no additional energy required.

79a. False
79b. True
79c. False
79d. False
79e. True

Oxygen content is the total amount of oxygen expressed as mL/100 mL blood:

$$CaO_2 = \text{oxygen bound to Hb} + \text{oxygen dissolved in plasma}$$
$$CaO_2 = [Hb(g/dL) \times 1.34\,mL\ O_2/g\ Hb \times SaO_2/100]$$
$$+ [PaO_2(mmHg) \times 0.003\,mL\ O_2\ mmHg/dL]$$

Oxygen flux describes the amount of O_2 delivered to the tissues per unit time, this is derived by multiplying CaO_2 by cardiac output. The iron–porphyrin groups of the Hb molecule represent the binding sites for molecular oxygen and each molecule of Hb possesses four oxygen-binding sites. The percentages of available binding sites that are actually bound to oxygen represent the oxygen saturation. Thus arterial oxygen saturation is unchanged in anaemia since all available binding sites are occupied; however, the oxygen *content* of arterial and venous blood will be decreased. The mixed-venous saturation represents the balance between oxygen delivery and oxygen uptake at tissue level; extraction will increase in anaemia due to a reduced supply of oxygen and SvO_2 will decrease. 2,3-Diphosphoglycerate (2,3-DPG) is a product of glycolysis and is a highly charged anion that causes a right shift of the oxy-haemoglobin dissociation curve, causing more oxygen to be liberated. Levels increase in chronic anaemia, chronic hypoxia, following exercise, during ascent to high altitudes, by the action of thyroid hormones and in pregnancy.

Ganong W. *Review of Medical Physiology*, 22nd edn. Maidenhead: McGraw-Hill Medical, 2005.

80a. False
80b. False
80c. True
80d. False
80e. True

ECMO comprises an arteriovenous extracorporeal circuit designed to provide oxygenation and remove CO_2 from patients who are extremely hypoxaemic. The ECMO flow rate is reduced as the patient improves. At flow rates of 1 L/min they are considered ready to discontinue ECMO. Patients with high ventilatory pressures (peak inspiratory pressures >30 cmH$_2$O) and high FiO_2 (>0.8) for more than 7 days and those with advanced chronic lung disease or irreversible lung conditions are excluded since they are unlikely to recover. Bleeding is the main complication.

The CESAR (Conventional Ventilation or ECMO for Severe Adult Respiratory Failure) trial was a multicentre randomized controlled trial conducted in the UK to evaluate survival without disability at 6 months and the cost–benefit of ECMO versus conventional ventilation. Early reports suggest that mortality and disability were lower in the ECMO group (65% survived to 6 months without disability) compared with the control group (47%).

Charles B, Peek G. ECMO for adults in respiratory failure. In: Waldmann N, Soni N, Rhodes A, eds. *Oxford Desk Reference: Critical Care*. Oxford: OUP, 2008.
Peek GJ, Mugford M, Tiruvoipati R, et al. The CESAR Trial Collaboration. Efficacy and economic assessment of conventional ventilatory support versus extracorporeal membrane oxygenation for severe adult respiratory failure (CESAR): a multicentre randomised controlled trial. *Lancet* 2009; 374: 1351–63.

81a. False
81b. False
81c. True
81d. False
81e. False
Warfarin is a coumarin derivative that inhibits synthesis of the vitamin K-dependent clotting factors (factors II, VII, IX and X) in the liver; this is by preventing the reduction of oxidized vitamin K required for carboxylation of clotting factor precursors. The management of warfarin overdose, following initial resuscitation and stabilization, includes administration of prothrombin complex concentrate (PCC), which contains the necessary factors but is expensive; thus 15 mL/kg of FFP is often administered, but presents a risk of anaphylaxis and transmission of blood-borne pathogens and is the most common cause of transfusion-related acute lung injury (TRALI). Recombinant factor VIIa (rFVIIa) is increasingly being used in uncontrollable haemorrhage. The Israeli Multidisciplinary Task Force have recommended its use where the platelet count is $>50 \times 10^9$/L, pH >7.2 and fibrinogen >0.5; it has been shown to work in oral anticoagulant overdose. Protamine is used to neutralize the effects of heparin through a physicochemical pH-dependent interaction, but in high doses has anticoagulant and myocardial depressant action. Finally, antifibrinolytics, such as tranexamic acid, competitively inhibit activation of plasminogen to plasmin and are thus not helpful in this context. Vitamin K should also be given but will make reintroduction of warfarin difficult in the short term.

Martinowitz U, Michaelsons M. on behalf of the Israeli Multidisciplinary RVIIA Task Force. Guidelines for the use of recombinant activated factor VII (rFVIIa) in uncontrolled bleeding: a report by the Israeli Multidisciplinary rFVIIa Task Force. *J Thromb Haemost* 2005; 3: 640–8.
Ridley S, Taylor B, Gunning K. Medical management of bleeding in the critically ill patient. *Contin Educ Anaesth Crit Care Pain* 2007; 7: 116–21.

82a. False
82b. True
82c. True
82d. False
82e. False
SLE is the most common of the connective tissue disorders and is characterized by the presence of antinuclear antibodies (ANA). Autoantibodies to

β_2-glycoprotein are associated with *anti-phospholipid syndrome*. The term 'systemic' emphasizes the multisystem involvement. It affects $\sim$0.1% of the population, mainly women (9 : 1 female-to-male ratio) in their 20s and 30s, and is most common in the African-Caribbean population. Certain HLA types occur more commonly in SLE patients, -B8 and -DR3 in particular. HLA-B27 is associated with *ankylosing spondylitis*. Serum complement levels are reduced in active disease. The American College of Rheumatology Classification System suggests that the presence of four or more of the features below is consistent with a diagnosis of SLE:

- malar rash
- discoid lupus
- photosensitivity
- oral or nasal ulcers
- arthritis
- renal involvement with blood or protein in urine
- seizures or mental illness
- haematological disorders
- immunological disorders
- positive LE test
- serositis
- anti-Smith antibody
- false-positive test for syphilis
- positive antinuclear antibody
- anti-DNA antibody

American College of Rheumatology. *Guidelines for Referral and Management of Adults with Systemic Lupus Erythematosus.* Atlanta, GA: ACR, 1999.

83a. False
83b. False
83c. True
83d. True
83e. False

Septic arthritis describes an infection producing inflammation of a native or prosthetic joint. It is a serious condition with a case fatality rate of 11% and delay in treatment results in joint damage. Classic presentation is with a single hot, swollen and tender joint with a restricted range of movement with a history of less than 2 weeks; it may occur in the absence of fever. It is imperative to treat such patients as having septic arthritis. The most common affected joints are knee (50%), hip (20%), shoulder (8%), ankle (7%) and wrist (7%). Organisms are most commonly Gram-positive and include:

- *Staphylococcus aureus*
- *Streptococcus* spp.
- *Haemophilus influenzae* type b
- *Mycobacterium tuberculosis*
- *Neisseria gonorrhoeae*

Synovial fluid must be aspirated and sent for Gram-staining and culture prior to administration of antibiotics. Warfarin does not contraindicate joint aspiration. The serum urate concentration is of no value in sepsis, bloods should consist of blood culture, white cell count, erythrocyte sedimentation rate (ESR), C-reactive protein (CRP) and electrolytes. MRI is the diagnostic imaging modality of choice since it is sensitive at detecting osteomyelitis. Intra-articular steroids must not be injected into a joint with suspected sepsis.

Coakley G, Mathews C, Field M, et al. BSR & BHPR, BOA, RCGP and BSAC guidelines for management of the hot swollen joint in adults. *Rheumatology* 2006; 45: 1039–40.

84a. True
84b. False
84c. True
84d. True
84e. False
Central DI is characterized by reduced secretion of antidiuretic hormone (ADH, vasopressin) from the hypothalamo–pituitary axis, leading to an inability to concentrate urine with polyuria and polydipsia. It is associated with traumatic brain injury, subarachnoid haemorrhage, hypoxic encephalo-pathy and pituitary surgery; it also occurs with primary intracranial tumours and with endocrine failure in brainstem death. Nephrogenic DI occurs when there is a resistance to effects of ADH within the collecting tubules of the kidney and occurs in chronic renal insufficiency, lithium toxicity and as a rare X-linked mutation of the V2 receptor gene. The diagnosis is made with clinical and laboratory investigations, which are classically:

- production of large volume of dilute urine (3–18 L in 24 hours)
- high serum sodium (>145 mmol/L)
- high serum osmolality (>305 mOsm/kg) and
- inappropriately low urine osmolality (specific gravity of <1.005)

ADH assays can distinguish between central and nephrogenic DI.

Condition	Plasma sodium (mmol/L)	Urine sodium (mmol/L)	Plasma osmolality (mOsm/kg)	Urine osmolality (mOsm/kg)	Urine specific gravity
Normal	135–145	<10	285–295	600–1400	1.002 – 1.035
DI	↑	↑/normal	↑	↓	↓
SIADH[a]	↓	↑/normal	↓	↑	↑
Cerebral salt wasting	↓	↑	↓	↑	↑

[a]Syndrome of inappropriate ADH secretion.

85a. True
85b. True
85c. False
85d. False
85e. False
Penetrating eye injuries require immediate referral because of the risk of endophthalmitis or permanent visual loss. Risk-versus-benefit analysis is required concerning general anaesthesia, between airway protection from a full stomach and rises in IOP which may lead to extrusion of the globe con-tents. IOP is between 15–20 mmHg and is influenced by external pressure and intraocular contents. Most intravenous anaesthetic agents reduce IOP, with

the exception of ketamine; thus this agent is usually avoided. Volatile anaesthetic agents also reduce IOP and although thought to also be due to reduced intraocular muscle tone, the true mechanism is unclear. All non-depolarizing muscle relaxants reduce IOP slightly, while suxamethonium increases it; this increase lasts 6 minutes and still occurs after section of the eye muscles. Most surgeons prefer suxamethonium not to be used and in certain cases, particularly where visual loss is deemed irrevocable, full fasting guidelines are employed; thus liaison between surgical and anaesthetic teams is, as always, necessary.

Wilson A, Soar J. Anaesthesia for emergency eye surgery. *Update in Anaesthesia* 2000; Issue 11, Article 10.

86a. False
86b. True
86c. True
86d. True
86e. False
An awake patient in the lateral position has increased FRC of the non-dependent lung since the mediastinal contents are pushed to the dependent side by gravity. The upper lung has a lower compliance, lying on the steeper part of the compliance curve, and ventilation is greater in the dependent lung. Both ventilation and perfusion increase down the upright lung, according to gravity, but perfusion increases more than ventilation; perfusion is always greater in the dependent lung. Under anaesthesia, with reduced FRC, the dependent lung lies on the flatter part of the compliance curve and ventilation is greater in the non-dependent lung, which is also free from diaphragmatic compression owing to underlying abdominal viscera. Under anaesthesia, $\dot{V}/\dot{Q}$ mismatch will be greater in the lateral position, since the upper lung is better ventilated, but the dependent lung is better perfused. Compliance curves for dependent and non-dependent lungs in the lateral position are illustrated in Figure 5.3.

West J. *Respiratory Physiology: The Essentials*, 8th edn. Philadelphia: Lippincott Williams & Wilkins, 2008.

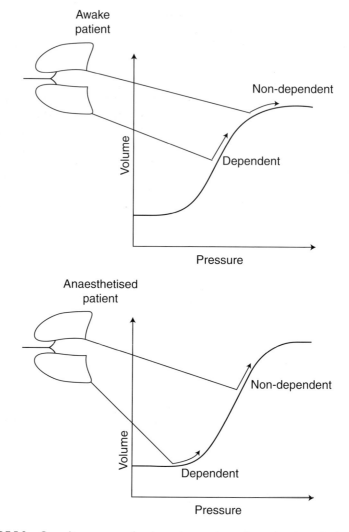

FIGURE 5.3   Compliance curves for dependent and non-dependent lungs in the lateral position.

87a. True
87b. True
87c. False
87d. True
87e. False
Following spinal cord injury, there are three phases:

- *Initial phase*: immediately following injury, with intense neuronal firing that can lead to hypertension, arrhythmias, myocardial infarction, left ventricular failure and pulmonary oedema
- *Spinal shock phase*: from 3 days to 8 weeks. Bradycardia and hypotension occur owing to disrupted sympathetics and unopposed vagal tone;

occurring with high cord lesions, most often above T7. Elective surgery is contraindicated during this phase
- *Reflex phase*: long-term synaptic changes lead to increased tone and hyperreflexia

Perioperative risks include autonomic dysreflexia, which is a syndrome of massive disordered autonomic discharge, due to stimulation below the level of the lesion. This is a medical emergency and is a risk if no anaesthesia is administered. The response is characterized by hypertension and bradycardia and can lead to sinus arrest. Other features include sweating, headache, nausea and priapism. Afferent impulses from urological, uterine and bowel distension or instrumentation are transmitted through pudendal nerves and hypogastric plexuses to elicit massive disordered sympathetic discharge. Topical anaesthesia has been described for urological procedures; however, it will not abolish the response due to bladder distension; epidural and spinal anaesthesia have both been used successfully and are often advocated.

Hambly PR, Martin B. Anaesthesia for chronic spinal cord lesions. *Anaesthesia* 1998; **53**: 273–89.
Teasdale A. Neuromuscular diseases. In: Allman KG, Wilson IH, eds. *Oxford Handbook of Anaesthesia*, 2nd edn. Oxford: OUP, 2006.

88a. False
88b. True
88c. False
88d. True
88e. False
The autonomic nervous system uses reflex pathways to regulate non-voluntary bodily functions. It is divided into parasympathetic and sympathetic nervous systems.

Parasympathetic nervous system 'craniosacral'

- Myelinated preganglionic efferents emerge with:
  - cranial nerves III, VII, IX and X
  - sacral nerves S2–4
- Acetylcholine is the neurotransmitter at all synapses
- Nicotinic at ganglia; muscarinic at postganglionic synapses

Sympathetic nervous system 'thoracolumbar'

- Myelinated preganglionic efferents emerge from T1–L2
- Pass into the sympathetic trunk
- Acetylcholine is the neurotransmitter at ganglia and adrenal medulla (and postganglionic at sweat glands)
- Noradrenaline is the neurotransmitter at postganglionic nerve endings

89a. True
89b. True
89c. False
89d. False
89e. False
AFE is a rare but devastating complication of pregnancy. It occurs as a result of amniotic fluid, fetal cells, hair or debris entering the maternal circulation. The incidence is thought to be between 1 per 8000 and 1 per 18 000 pregnancies. It is thought to occur as a reaction in part to biochemical markers; it occurs in two phases:

- *Phase 1*: as cells enter the maternal circulation, inflammatory mediators are released. This results in pulmonary artery vasospasm leading to pulmonary hypertension, increased right ventricular pressure and dysfunction. Hypoxaemia and hypotension ensue resulting in myocardial and capillary damage
- *Phase 2*: left ventricular failure and pulmonary oedema develop. The inflammatory mediators result in disseminated intravascular coagulation (DIC) and uterine atony

Mothers may complain of dyspnoea, cough, headache and chest pain. They may present with hypotension (or transient hypertension), fetal distress, pulmonary oedema, cyanosis, coagulopathy, seizures or cardiovascular collapse. 70% present in labour, 19% during caesarean section and 11% following vaginal delivery. In the last triennial CEMACH report (2003–05) there were 19 reported deaths from AFE, two of which were *late* since the mothers died some weeks later in a persistent vegetative state. There exist no proven risk factors, but certain factors are believed to have an association (increased maternal age, *multiparity*, meconium-stained liquor, intrauterine fetal death, polyhydramnios). Cases should be reported to the UK Obstetric Surveillance System (UKOSS).

Dedhia JD, Mushambi MC. Amniotic fluid embolism. *Contin Educ Anaesth Crit Care Pain* 2007; 7: 152–6.
Lewis G, ed. The Confidential Enquiry into Maternal and Child Health (CEMACH). *Saving Mothers' Lives: Reviewing Maternal Deaths to make Motherhood Safer – 2003–2005*. The Seventh Report on Confidential Enquiries into Maternal Deaths in the UK. London: CEMACH, 2007. Available at: www.cmace.org.uk/getattachment/05f68346-816b-4560-b1b9-af24fb633170/Saving-Mothers'-Lives-20003-2005_ExecSumm.aspx.

90a. False
90b. True
90c. True
90d. True
90e. False
The Hardmann Index for ruptured abdominal aortic aneurysms was published in 1996 and scores range from 0–5; studies have shown that a Hardmann

Index Score of ≥ 2 predict a mortality of 80%. He has a Hardmann Index Score of 2 as follows:

Hardmann index

Parameters	Score
Age >76 years	1
Serum creatinine >190 μmol/L	1
Haemoglobin <9 g/dL	1
Myocardial ischaemia on ECG	1
Loss of consciousness after arrival to hospital	1

Steps to maintain intraoperative patient temperature should be in place, since hypothermia will reduce myocardial contractility and exacerbate acidosis and coagulopathy.

Leo E, Biancari F, Nesi F, et al. Risk-scoring methods in predicting the immediate outcome after emergency open repair of ruptured abdominal aortic aneurysm. *Am J Surg* 2006; **192**: 19–23.

Loonard A, Thompson J. Anaesthesia for ruptured abdominal aortic aneurysm. *Contin Educ Anaesth Crit Care Pain* 2008; **8**: 11–15.

Relevant studies for the Final FRCA: Trials

Included below are landmark trials from recent years that are of relevance to the Final FRCA examination. A brief summary of findings is also included, and although critical appraisal of the papers is beyond the scope of this book, we have included full references for those wishing to further their reading.

Perioperative β-blockade

DECREASE-IV (Dutch Echocardiographic Cardiac Risk Evaluation Applying Stress Echocardiography)

Aim: Evaluated the effectiveness and safety of β-blockade and statins for the prevention of perioperative cardiovascular events; intermediate-risk patients undergoing non-cardiovascular surgery were selected

Method: Randomized open-label trial assigned 1066 patients to bisoprolol, fluvastatin, combination treatment, or control therapy for 34 days before surgery; primary outcome was the composite of 30-day cardiac death and myocardial infarction

Result: Bisoprolol use demonstrated a significant reduction of 30-day cardiac death and non-fatal myocardial infarction; fluvastatin demonstrated a trend for improved outcome

Reference: Dunkelgrun M, Boersma E, Schouten O, et al. Bisoprolol and fluvastatin for the reduction of perioperative cardiac mortality and myocardial infarction in intermediate-risk patients undergoing noncardiovascular surgery: a randomized controlled trial (DECREASE IV). *Ann Surg* 2009; **249**: 921–6

POISE (Perioperative Ischaemic Evaluation Study)

Aim: Investigated the effects of perioperative β-blockers in non-cardiac surgery; previous trials had given conflicting results

Method: Multicentre, randomized controlled trial comprising 8351 patients with, or at risk of, atherosclerotic disease assigned to metoprolol or placebo groups; treatment started 2–4 hours preoperatively and continued for 30 days; primary outcomes were cardiovascular death, non-fatal myocardial infarction and non-fatal cardiac arrest

Result: Fewer myocardial infarctions, but more deaths and strokes in the metoprolol group

Reference: Deveraux PJ, Yang H, Yusuf S, et al. POISE Study Group. Effects of extended-release metoprolol succinate in patients undergoing non-cardiac surgery (POISE Trial): a randomised controlled trial. *Lancet* 2008; **371**: 1839–47

General versus local anaesthesia

GALA (GA versus LA for carotid surgery)

Aim: Studied whether type of anaesthesia for carotid endarterectomy influences perioperative morbidity and mortality, quality of life and longer-term outcome in terms of stroke-free survival

Method: Multicentre randomized controlled trial of 3526 patients; primary outcome was proportion of patients alive, stroke-free and without myocardial infarction 30 days postoperatively

Result: No significant difference between groups for quality of life, length of hospital stay or the primary outcome

Reference: Gough MJ, Bodenham A, Horrocks M, et al. GALA: an international multicentre randomised trial comparing GA versus LA for carotid surgery. *Lancet* 2008; **372**: 2132–42

Operative delay

Operative Delay in Hip Fractures

Aim: Assessed whether operative delay increases mortality in elderly patients with hip fractures; surgical repair within 24 hours is recommended by the Royal College of Physicians' guidelines

Method: Over 250 000 patients from 16 observational studies were selected; primary outcomes were all-cause mortality at 30 days and 1 year

Result: Operative delay beyond 48 hours post-admission may increase mortality (30 days: 41%; 1 year: 32%)

Reference: Shiga T, Wajima Z, Ohe Y. Is operative delay associated with increased mortality of hip fracture patients? Systematic review, meta-analysis, and meta-regression. *Can J Anaesth* 2008; **55**: 146–54

Oesophageal Doppler Monitoring

Oesophageal Doppler Monitor in Major Surgery

Aim: Compared intraoperative intravenous fluid treatment guided by monitoring ventricular filling versus conventional parameters

Method: Data from 5 studies involving 420 patients undergoing major abdominal surgery were reviewed

Result: Use of oesophageal Doppler monitoring demonstrated a reduced hospital stay, fewer complications, fewer ICU admissions, less requirements for inotropes and faster return of normal gastrointestinal function

Reference: Abbas SM, Hill AG. Systematic review of the literature for the use of oesophageal Doppler monitor for fluid replacement in major abdominal surgery. *Anaesthesia* 2008; **63**: 44–51

Nitrous oxide

ENIGMA (Evaluation of Nitrous Oxide in the Gas Mixture for Anaesthesia)

Aim: Evaluated the effectiveness and safety of nitrous oxide in anaesthesia

Method: 2050 patients having major surgery expected to last at least 2 hours were randomly assigned to nitrous oxide-free (80% O_2, 20% N_2) or nitrous oxide-based (70% N_2O, 30% O_2) anaesthesia; primary outcome was length of hospital stay

Result: Median duration of hospital stay did not differ between the groups; patients in the nitrous oxide-free group had lower rates of major complications (pneumonia, pneumothorax, pulmonary embolism, wound infection, myocardial infarction, venous thromboembolism, stroke, awareness and death) and severe nausea and vomiting

Reference: Myles PS, Leslie K, Chan MT, et al. Avoidance of nitrous oxide for patients undergoing major surgery: a randomized controlled trial. *Anesthesiology* 2007; **107**: 221–31

ENIGMA–II (Evaluation of Nitrous oxide in the Gas Mixture for Anaesthesia) – *in progress*

Aim: To test the hypothesis that the avoidance of nitrous oxide in patients undergoing anaesthesia for major non-cardiac surgery will reduce the incidence of death and major cardiovascular events

Method: International randomized trial to involve 7000 patients at risk of coronary artery disease; primary outcomes are death and major non-fatal events (myocardial infarction, cardiac arrest, pulmonary embolism and stroke)

Bispectral index

B-Unaware

Aim: Assessed whether incidence of awareness is decreased with a BIS-based protocol versus measurement of end-tidal anaesthetic gas (ETAG)

Method: Randomized trial incorporating 2000 patients; assessed for awareness at 0–24 hours, 24–72 hours and 30 days post-extubation

Method: 2000 patients were enrolled in a randomized clinical trial; primary outcome was awareness at any time

Result: Did not reproduce results of B-Aware; awareness occurred equally in both groups, even when BIS values and ETAG concentrations were in target ranges

Reference: Avidan MS, Zhang L, Burnside BA, et al. Anesthesia awareness and the bispectral index. *N Engl J Med* 2008; **358**: 1097–108

B-Aware

Aim: Assessed whether bispectral index (BIS) monitoring reduced the incidence of awareness in adults undergoing general anaesthesia

Method: Prospective, multicentre, randomized, double-blind trial involving 2463 patients; assessed by a blinded observer at 2–6 hours, 24–36 hours and 30 days postoperatively; primary outcome was confirmed awareness at any time

Result: BIS-guided anaesthesia reduces the risk of awareness by 82%

Reference: Myles PS, Leslie K, McNeil J, et al. Bispectral index monitoring to prevent awareness during anaesthesia: the B-Aware randomised controlled trial. *Lancet* 2004; 363: 1757–63

Prevention of eclampsia

MAGPIE (Magnesium Sulphate for the Prevention of Eclampsia)

Aim: Evaluated effects of magnesium sulphate given to patients with pre-eclampsia to prevent convulsions

Method: 10 141 women in 33 countries were randomized to magnesium sulphate or placebo groups; primary outcomes were eclampsia and death of the baby

Result: Women given magnesium sulphate had a 58% lower risk of eclampsia, maternal mortality was also lower; no difference in risk of baby dying

Reference: Duley L, Carroli G, Farrell B, et al. Do women with pre-eclampsia, and their babies, benefit from magnesium sulphate? The MAGPIE Trial: A randomised placebo-controlled trial. *Lancet* 2002; 359: 1877–90

Epidural anaesthesia

MASTER (Multicentre Australian Study of Epidural Anaesthesia)

Aim: Compared adverse outcomes for high-risk patients undergoing major abdominal surgery with epidural block or alternative analgesic strategies with general anesthesia

Method: 915 high-risk patients assigned to intraoperative and 72 hours postoperative epidural analgesia with general anaesthesia, or control; primary outcome was death at 30 days or major postoperative morbidity

Result: Mortality was low in both groups; among eight categories of other morbid endpoints, only respiratory failure occurred with less frequency in patients managed with epidural techniques.

Reference: Rigg JRA, Jamrozik K, Myles PS, et al. Epidural anaesthesia and analgesia and outcome of major surgery: a randomised controlled trial. *Lancet* 2002; 359: 1276–82

Tracheostomy

TRACman (Tracheostomy Management in Critical Care) – *in progress*

Aim: To determine whether 'early' or 'late' tracheostomy placement for patients requiring ventilatory support influences hospital mortality

Method: Multicentre, prospective, open randomized controlled trial; patients assigned to 'early' (days 1–4 post-admission to ICU) or 'late' (not before day 10 post-admission to ICU) tracheostomy; primary outcome is 30-day mortality after randomization

Result: To be published

ECMO

CESAR (Conventional Ventilatory Support Versus Extracorporeal Membrane Oxygenation (ECMO) for Severe Adult Respiratory failure)

Aim: Assessed whether ECMO increased the rate of survival without severe disability and cost-effectiveness for patients with severe, but reversible, respiratory failure

Method: Multicentre, randomized trial comprising 180 patients recruited from various hospitals in UK; assigned to ECMO or conventional treatment; primary outcomes were death and severe disability at 6 months post-randomization or before hospital discharge

Results: Mortality and disability were lower in the ECMO group (63% survived to 6 months without disability, compared with 47% in conventional management group); strategy likely to be cost-effective

Reference: Peek GJ, Mugford M, Tiruvoipati R, et al. The CESAR Trial Collaboration. Efficacy and economic assessment of conventional ventilatory support versus extracorporeal membrane oxygenation for severe adult respiratory failure (CESAR); a multicentre randomised controlled trial. *Lancet* 2009; 374: 1351–63

Vasopressin and septic shock

VASST (Vasopressin and Septic Shock Trial)

Aim: Evaluated whether low-dose vasopressin as compared to noradrenaline would decrease mortality in patients with septic shock

Method: Multicentre, randomized, double-blind trial comprising 778 patients on 5 μg/min of noradrenaline; assigned to low-dose vasopressin (0.01–0.03 U/min) or noradrenaline (5–15 μg/min); primary outcome was 28-day mortality

Result: No significant difference between groups in 28- or 90-day mortality or overall rates of serious adverse events; in those with less severe septic shock, mortality was lower in the vasopressin group

Reference: Russell JA, Walley KR, Singer J, et al. VASST Investigators. Vasopressin versus norepinepherine infusion in patients with septic shock. *N Engl J Med* 2008; 358: 877–87

Steroids

CORTICUS (Corticosteroid Therapy of Septic Shock)

Aim: Studied value of hydrocortisone in patients with septic shock

Method: A multicentre, randomized, double-blind, placebo-controlled trial of 499 patients; assigned to 50 mg of intravenous hydrocortisone or placebo 6-hourly for 5 days; primary outcome was death amongst those not having a response to corticotropin at 28 days

Result: No significant difference in mortality between groups (both corticotropin responders and non-responders); in the hydrocortisone group, shock was reversed more quickly, but there were more episodes of new sepsis and septic shock

Reference: Sprung CL, Annane D, Keh D, et al. Hydrocortisone therapy for patients with septic shock. *N Engl J Med* 2008; **358**: 111–24

CRASH (Corticosteroid Randomization After Significant Head Injury)

Aim: Studied the effects of corticosteroids on death and disability after head injury

Method: A randomized placebo-controlled trial recruiting 10 008 adults within 8 hours of head injury and a GCS of 14 or less; treated with a 48 hour infusion of methylprednisolone or placebo; data collected at 6 months

Result: The risk of death and death or severe disability was higher in the corticosteroid group

Reference: Edwards P, Arango M, Balica L, et al. Final results of MRC CRASH, a randomised placebo-controlled trial of intravenous corticosteroid in adults with head injury-outcomes at 6 months. *Lancet* 2005; **365**: 1957–9

Acute respiratory distress syndrome (ARDS)

Nitric Oxide

Aim: Summarized effects of nitric oxide (NO) versus non-NO care for adults and children with acute lung injury (ALI) or ARDS

Method: Meta-analysis comprising 12 trials and 1237 patients; outcomes were mortality, duration of ventilation, oxygenation, pulmonary arterial pressure and adverse events

Result: No significant differences between groups in mortality, duration of ventilation, or ventilator-free days; NO group had increased Pao_2/Fio_2 on day 1, but increased risk of renal dysfunction

Reference: Adhikari NK, Burns KE, Friedrich JO, et al. Effect of nitric oxide on oxygenation and mortality in acute lung injury: systematic review and meta-analysis. *BMJ* 2007; **334**: 757–8

LaSRS (Late Steroid Rescue Study)

Aim: Assessed whether corticosteroids improve mortality rates in patients with ARDS

Method: Double-blinded, randomized controlled trial comprising 180 patients with ARDS of at least 7 days' duration; assigned to methylprednisolone or placebo groups; primary outcome was 60-day mortality

Result: No significant difference in mortality rates at 60 and 180 days between groups; methylprednisolone associated with higher 60- and

180-day mortality rates in patients enrolled at least 14 days after onset of ARDS; methylprednisolone group had increased ventilator- and shock-free days (in first 28 days) but higher rate of neuromuscular weakness

Reference: Steinberg KP, Hudson LD, Goodman RB, et al. National Heart, Lung and Blood Institute ARDS Clinical Trials Network. Efficacy and safety of corticosteroids for persistent acute respiratory distress syndrome. *N Engl J Med* 2006; **354:** 1671–84

ALVEOLI (Assessment of Low Tidal Volume and Elevated End-Expiratory Pressure to Obviate Lung Injury)

Aim: Conducted to compare effects of higher and lower positive end-expiratory pressure (PEEP) on clinical outcomes

Method: 549 patients with ALI and ARDS assigned to higher (13.2 $\pm$ 3.5 cmH$_2$O) or lower (8.3 $\pm$ 3.2 cmH$_2$O) PEEP

Result: Patients receiving a tidal-volume goal of 6 mL/kg of predicted body weight and an end-inspiratory plateau-pressure limit of 30 cmH$_2$O show similar clinical outcomes irrespective of lower or higher PEEP levels used.

Reference: Brower RG, Lanken PN, MacIntyre N, et al. National Heart, Lung and Blood Institute ARDS Clinical Trials Network. Higher versus lower positive end-expiratory pressures in patients with the acute respiratory distress syndrome. *N Engl J Med* 2004; **351:** 327–36

Proning

Aim: Studied the effect on survival of placing patients with ALI or ARDS in the prone position

Method: Multicentre, randomized controlled trial comprising 304 patients; assigned to either prone position for 6 hours or more per day for 10 days, or conventional (supine) groups

Result: Patients in the prone position had improved oxygenation; there was no significant difference in mortality during the 10-day study period or at 6 months between the groups

Reference: Gattinoni L, Tognoni G, Pesenti A, et al. Effect of prone positioning on the survival of patients with acute respiratory failure. *N Engl J Med* 2001; **345:** 568–73

ARMA

Aim: Evaluated if ventilation of ARDS patients with lower tidal volumes improved mortality

Method: Prospective, multicentre, randomized trial ventilating 861 patients; assigned to groups with higher tidal volumes (12 mL/kg predicted body weight and plateau pressure of 50 cmH$_2$O) or lower tidal volumes (6 mL/kg predicted body weight and plateau pressure of 30 cmH$_2$O); primary outcomes were death before discharge home, breathing without assistance and ventilator-free days (from days 1 to 28)

Result: Trial stopped early owing to reduced mortality and increased ventilator-free days in the lower-tidal-volume group

Reference: The Acute Respiratory Distress Syndrome Network. Ventilation with lower tidal volumes as compared with traditional tidal volumes for acute lung injury and the acute respiratory distress syndrome. N Engl J Med 2000; 342: 1301–8

Infections

Catheter-Related Bloodstream Infections (CRBSI)

Aim: Measured incidence of CRBSI before, during, and up to 18 months after implementation of evidence-based intervention

Method: Collaborative cohort study of 108 ICUs; rate of infections per 1000 catheter-days measured at 3-month intervals

Result: Up to 66% reduction in CRBSI sustained through 18 months

Reference: Pronovost P, Needham D, Berenholtz S, et al. An intervention to decrease catheter-related bloodstream infections in the ICU. N Engl J Med 2007; 355: 2725–32

Insulin

Intensive Insulin Therapy

Aim: Evaluated role of intensive insulin therapy in medical ICUs

Method: Prospective, randomized, controlled study of 1200 adult medical ICU patients expected to stay for 3 days; assigned to normalization (4.4–6.1 mmol/L) or correction of glucose ≥ 12 mmol/L

Result: Intensive insulin therapy reduced blood glucose levels but did not significantly reduce in-hospital mortality; the intensive insulin therapy group demonstrated less acute kidney injury, accelerated weaning from mechanical ventilation and faster discharge from ICU and hospital; for those in the intensive insulin therapy group and staying in ICU for under 3 days, mortality was increased; for those staying over 3 days, mortality and morbidity were decreased

Reference: Van den Berghe G, Wilmer A, Hermans G, et al. Intensive Insulin Therapy in the Medical ICU. N Engl J Med 2006; 354: 449–61

Pulmonary artery catheters

PAC-Man (Pulmonary Artery Catheters in Management of Patients in Intensive Care)

Aim: Studied whether mortality in critically ill patients is reduced when managed with a PAC

Method: Prospective, randomized controlled trial of 1041 subjects enrolled in 65 British ICUs

Result: No difference in hospital mortality; complications in 46 of 486 patients associated with PAC insertion, non of which were fatal; no clear evidence of benefit or harm by managing critically ill patients with a PAC

Reference: Harvey S, Harrison DA, Singer M, et al. Assessment of the clinical effectiveness of pulmonary artery catheters in management of patients in intensive care (PAC-Man): a randomised controlled trial. *Lancet* 2005; **366:** 472–7

Nutrition and fluids

Nutrition

Aim: Investigated effect of trial quality on conclusions when comparing standard enteral with standard parenteral nutrition in critically ill patients

Method: Meta-analysis of 465 publications, of which 11 were included

Result: Aggregation revealed a mortality benefit in favour of parenteral nutrition; parenteral nutrition was associated with increased infectious complications

Reference: Simpson F, Doig GS. Parenteral versus enteral nutrition in the critically ill patient: a meta-analysis of trials using the intention to treat principle. *Intensive Care Med* 2005; **31:** 12–23

SAFE (Saline versus Albumin Fluid Evaluation)

Aim: Studied the effects on mortality of fluid resuscitation with saline or albumin

Method: Multicentre, randomized, double-blinded trial comprising 6997 heterogenous ICU patients; received normal saline or 4% albumin during next 28 days; primary outcome was death from any cause during the 28-day period

Result: No significant difference between the two groups in deaths, new single- or multi-organ failure, mean number of days on ICU, in the hospital, on mechanical ventilation or renal replacement therapy

Reference: Finfer S, Bellomo R, Boyce N, et al. SAFE Study Investigators. A comparison of albumin and saline for fluid resuscitation in the intensive care unit. *N Engl J Med* 2004; **350:** 2247–56

Hypothermia

Out-of-Hospital Cardiac Arrest (OOHCA) with Induced Hypothermia

Aim: Studied whether moderate hypothermia in unconscious patients after OOHCA improved neurological outcome

Method: Randomized, controlled trial of 77 patients; assigned to hypothermia (33°C within 2 hours, maintained for 12 hours) or normothermia groups; primary outcome was survival to hospital discharge with sufficient neurological function (to allow discharge to home or rehabilitation facility)

Result: Hypothermia was associated with a better outcome than normothermia (odds ratio 5.25); groups showed no difference in frequency of adverse events

Reference: Bernard SA, Gray TW, Buist MD, et al. Treatment of comatose survivors of out-of-hospital cardiac arrest with induced hypothermia. *N Engl J Med* 2002; **346**: 557–63

Acute renal failure

Diuretics in Acute Renal Failure – PICARD (Project to Improve Care in Acute Renal Disease)

Aim: Studied whether use of diuretics is associated with adverse or favourable outcomes in critically ill patients with acute renal failure

Method: Cohort study comprising 552 patients; outcome measures were all-cause hospital mortality, non-recovery of renal function, and a combined outcome of death or non-recovery

Result: Diuretic use associated with significant increase in the risk of death or non-recovery of renal function; increased risk largely in those unresponsive to diuretics

Reference: Mehta RL, Pascual MT, Soroko S, Chertow GM. PICARD Study Group. Diuretics, mortality, and nonrecovery of renal function in acute renal failure. *JAMA* 2002; **288**: 2547–53

Dopamine in Acute Renal Failure Prevention

Aim: Studied whether low-dose dopamine reduces severity of acute renal failure, requirement for dialysis or mortality in critically ill patients

Method: Meta-analysis of 17 randomized controlled trials comprising 854 patients

Result: Onset of acute renal failure, requirement for dialysis or mortality were not prevented by administration of dopamine

Reference: Kellum JA, M Decker J. Use of dopamine in acute renal failure: a meta-analysis. *Crit Care Med* 2001; **29**: 1526–31

Sepsis

PROWESS (Recombinant Human Protein C Worldwide Evaluation in Severe Sepsis)

Aim: Assessed whether recombinant human activated protein C (rhAPC) reduced rate of death among patients with severe sepsis

Method: Multicentre, randomized, double-blind, placebo-controlled trial; 1690 patients with severe sepsis assigned to groups with infusions of rhAPC ($24\ \mu g\ kg^{-1}\ h^{-1}$) or placebo for 96 hours; primary outcome was 28-day mortality

Result: rhAPC demonstrated a reduced relative risk of death of 19.4%, with an increased incidence of bleeding

Reference: Bernard GR, Vincent JL, Laterre PF, et al. PROWESS Study Group. Efficacy and safety of recombinant human activated protein C for severe sepsis. N Engl J Med 2001; 344: 699–709

Early Goal-Directed Therapy (EGDT)

Aim: Evaluated efficacy of EGDT in septic or severe septic patients before ICU admission

Method: 263 patients randomized; assigned to 6 hours of EGDT or standard therapy before ICU admission; primary outcome was in-hospital mortality

Result: EGDT group demonstrated lower in-hospital mortality, higher mean central venous oxygen saturations, lower lactate concentration, lower base deficit, and higher pH; EGDT group had lower mean APACHE II scores

Reference: Rivers E, Nguyen B, Havstad S, et al. Early Goal-Directed Therapy Collaborative Group. Early goal-directed therapy in the treatment of severe sepsis and septic shock. N Engl J Med 2001; 345: 1368–77

Rofecoxib

VIGOR (Vioxx Gastrointestinal Outcomes Research)

Aim: Studied whether rofecoxib (Vioxx) is associated with a lower incidence of upper gastrointestinal events than with naproxen among patients with rheumatoid arthritis

Method: Randomly assigned 8076 patients to 50 mg of rofecoxib daily or naproxen 500 mg twice daily; primary outcome was upper gastrointestinal events (gastroduodenal perforation or obstruction, upper gastrointestinal bleeding and symptomatic gastroduodenal ulcers)

Result: Drugs had similar efficacy against rheumatoid arthritis; over 9 months the rofecoxib group had fewer gastrointestinal events, but a higher rate of myocardial infarction; rate of death from cardiovascular events was similar in the two groups

Reference: Bombardier C, Laine L, Reicin A, et al. Comparison of upper gastrointestinal toxicity of rofecoxib and naproxen in patients with rheumatoid arthritis. VIGOR Study Group. N Engl J Med 2000; 343: 1520–8

Transfusion

Transfusion Requirements

Aim: Studied effects of restrictive versus liberal red-cell transfusion strategies in critically ill patients

Method: A multicentre, randomized, controlled clinical trial comprising 838 euvolaemic patients with haemoglobin concentrations below 9.0 g/dL within 72 hours admission to ICU; the restrictive group were transfused at concentrations below 7.0 g/dL, the liberal group below 10.0 g/dL; primary outcomes were death at 30 days and severity of organ dysfunction

Result: 30-day mortality was similar between groups; rates were significantly lower in the restrictive group in those less acutely ill, or below 55 years of age, but not with cardiac disease; mortality during hospitalization in restrictive group was lower

Reference: Hébert PC, Wells G, Blajchman MA, et al. A multicenter, randomized, controlled clinical trial of transfusion requirements in critical care. *N Engl J Med* 1999; **340**: 409–17